Confidential Enquiry into Maternal and Child Health
Improving care for mothers, babies and children

Why Mothers Die 2000–2002

The Sixth Report
of the Confidential Enquiries into Maternal
Deaths in the United Kingdom

Director and Editor
Gwyneth Lewis MSc MRCGP FFPH FRCOG

Clinical Director
James Drife MD FRCOG FRCPEd FRCSEd

Central Assessors and Authors

Thomas Clutton-Brock MRCP FRCA
Griselda Cooper FRCA FRCOG
Marion Hall MD FRCOG
Ann Harper MD FRCPI FRCOG
Mary Hepburn MRCGP FRCOG
James Neilson MD FRCOG
Catherine Nelson-Piercy FRCP
John McClure FRCA
Margaret Oates DPM FRCPsych
Gillian Penney MD FRCOG MFFP
Kate Sallah RN RM ADM MPH
Michael de Swiet MD FRCP
Harry Millward-Sadler FRCPath MHSH
Robin Vlies FRCSEd FRCOG

Other authors and contributors

Victoria Brace MRCOG
Nirupa Dattani BSc MPhil
Alison Macfarlane BA Dip Stat Cstat FFPH
Nigel Physick
Carine Ronsmans MD DrPH
Lisa Hunt MD PhD
Jessica Chamberlain BA (Hons) MSc
Tania Corbin BSc (Hons) MSc

CEMACH

Published by the RCOG Press at the Royal College of Obstetricians and Gynaecologists, 27 Sussex Place, Regent's Park, London NW1 4RG, UK

www.rcog.org.uk

Registered Charity No. 213280

First published November 2004

ISBN 1-904752-08-X

All correspondence with regard to this Report should be addressed to: CEMACH, Chiltern Court, 188 Baker Street, London NW1 5SD; email: info@cemach.org.uk; website: www.cemach.org.uk

Cover image: Acestock.com

RCOG Press Editor: Jane Moody

Design: Tony Crowley

Production by TechBooks, New Delhi

Printed by Latimer Trend & Co. Ltd, Estover Road, Plymouth PL6 7PL, UK

This work was undertaken by CEMACH and by its predecessor organisation, the Confidential Enquiries into Maternal Deaths (CEMD). The work was funded by the National Centre for Clinical Excellence, the Scottish Programme for Clinical Effectiveness in Reproductive Heath and by the Department of Health, Social Services and Public Safety of Northern Ireland. The views expressed in this publication are those of the Enquiry and not necessarily those of its funding bodies.

Confidential Enquiry into Maternal and Child Health

Improving care for mothers, babies and children

Why Mothers Die 2000–2002

A rene

The Sixth Report
of the Confidential Enquiries into Maternal
Deaths in the United Kingdom

CEMACH Mission Statement

Our aim is to improve the health of mothers,
babies and children by carrying out
confidential enquiries on a nationwide basis
and by widely disseminating our findings
and recommendations

CONTENTS

PREFACE

Fifty years ago, the Preface to the first Report on Confidential Enquiries into Maternal Deaths in England and Wales put the findings into their historical context. Between 1952 and 1954, there were 1,403 "direct" maternal deaths and 2,052,000 "confinements", i.e. a woman faced a 1 in 1500 risk of dying directly as a result of pregnancy or childbirth. This represented an almost five-fold improvement when compared with 1928, when the Minister of Health was Neville Chamberlain and there had been 2,290 maternal deaths in relation to 660,267 live births, i.e. a pregnant woman faced a 1 in 290 risk of dying. The present figures are not entirely comparable. For example, the Enquiry now includes the whole United Kingdom. However, the closest comparison with the data for 50 years ago is provided by the figure of 106 direct maternal deaths in the UK during the 3-year period considered by the present report when there were 2,016,136 live births. This means a pregnant woman in the UK today faces less than a 1 in 19,020 risk of dying from obstetric complications directly related to her pregnant state. In other words, there has been a 12-fold improvement when compared with 50 years ago and an almost 60-fold improvement since the 1920s, which is truly remarkable.

A further 136 women died between 2000 and 2002 as a result of conditions indirectly related to the pregnancy. These include, for example, heart disease and psychiatric illness. This gives a risk of less than 1 in 7,750 of dying of a cause related either directly or indirectly to her pregnancy today. It is sobering to realise that, in some countries in the developing world today, in 2004, this risk is 1 in 16.

While maternal mortality rates remain alarmingly high in many parts of the world, and in some places are actually increasing, the improvement in the rates in the United Kingdom is a major achievement. Nevertheless, outstanding concerns of the 1952 report were the frequency of toxaemia and haemorrhage, the complications of caesarean sections and of anaesthesia, and these also feature in the present report.

This report raises many important health issues that are amenable to intervention. For example, one-third of the women who died were obese. The increases in mortality rates due to haemorrhage and in association with anaesthesia are worrying, but the overall most common cause of maternal death is an indirect one, psychiatric illness. The report highlights inequalities, which continue to cause concern in spite of having been identified by previous reports. The most disadvantaged women are 20 times more likely to die than those from higher socio-economic backgrounds, and women from ethnic groups other than white are three times more likely to die. Mortality rates among refugees and asylum seekers are particularly high. These problems are related to accessing health care and need to be addressed.

This report is the result of hard work and commitment by a great number of people, but special thanks are due to Dr Gwyneth Lewis, Principal Medical Officer at the Department of Health. She collated the data, helped with its interpretation and had the difficult editorial task of pulling this Report together. She has done all this with great dedication and energy.

CEMACH is committed to continuing the programme of maternal enquiries. An achievement of the 1990s and the new century has been improved ascertainment. We will build on this improvement and we will further develop and strengthen this Enquiry by studies of morbidity as well as mortality and by enhancing the methodologies used to conduct these reviews.

Professor Michael Weindling
Chair
CEMACH

ACKNOWLEDGEMENTS

The authors of this Report wish to acknowledge the invaluable contribution of a number of people who are not often thanked in reports of this kind. We owe a huge debt of gratitude to Duncan Hart and Natalie Wilmot, the previous part time secretaries to this Enquiry, whose sensitive and sympathetic manner was greatly appreciated by all who needed their help. We thank Sanjay Patel for his IT skills, without which much of the public health data could not have been analysed. Lesz Lancucki and Mary Grinstead, statisticians in the Department of Health, England, have provided invaluable data, as have Beverley Botting, Nirupa Dattani, Maya Malagoda and Nigel Physick, of the Office for National Statistics (ONS). Carol Abrahams, also of ONS, developed and piloted the record-linkage study that has been used by this Enquiry to great effect and, without the coding clerks at Great Titchfield Street, the social and deprivation analysis would not have been possible. In particular, enormous thanks are due to Alison Macfarlane, who provided assistance with the statistical analysis and provided guidance on the graphs.

The authors also want to thank the staff of CEMACH who have provided unfailing support during the first year of the new Enquiry, and who have made the process of transition painless and pleasant for everyone concerned. In the CEMACH central office particular thanks are due to Richard Congdon, the Chief Executive of CEMACH, and to Mary Humphreys, Alison Miller, Joan Noble and Maureen Wilson. We are also indebted to the hard work undertaken by all the CEMACH Regional Managers, listed in Appendix 2, without whom such a comprehensive Report would not have possible. We look forward to working with them all in the future.

Most of all grateful thanks are due to all the health professionals who assisted with the individual cases. With their help this Enquiry remains an outstanding example of professional self-audit, and will continue to improve the care provided to pregnant and recently delivered women and their families.

ABBREVIATIONS USED IN THIS REPORT

AFE	amniotic fluid embolism
AIDS	acquired immunodeficiency syndrome
ALS	Advanced Life Support
ALSO	Advanced Life Support in Obstetrics
APACHE	Acute Physiology and Chronic Health Evaluation
ARDS	acute respiratory distress syndrome
BLS	Basic Life Support
BMI	body mass index
BP	blood pressure
bpm	beats per minute
CEMACH	Confidential Enquiry into Maternal and Child Health
CEMD	Confidential Enquiries into Maternal Death
CESDI	Confidential Enquiry into Stillbirths and Deaths in Infancy
CIN	cervical intraepithelial neoplasia
CT	computed tomography
CVT	cerebral vein thrombosis
DIC	disseminated intravascular coagulation
DPH	Director of Public Health
DVT	deep vein thrombosis
GHQ	General Health Questionnaire
GP	general practitioner
Hb	haemoglobin concentration
hCG	human Chorionic Gonadotrophin
HDU	high-dependency unit
HFEA	Human Fertilisation and Embryology Authority
HELLP	haemolysis, elevated liver enzymes, low platelets
HES	Hospital Episode Statistics
HIV	human immunodeficiency syndrome
ICD9/10	International Classification of Diseases, Injuries and Causes of Death, revisions 9/10
ICU	Intensive Care Unit
ILS	Intermediate Life Support
IVF	in vitro fertilisation
LSAMO	Local Supervising Authority Midwifery Officers
LMWH	low molecular weight heparin
MDE	Maternal Deaths' Enquiry
MDR(UK)1	Maternal Death Report Form for the United Kingdom (from October 1995)
mm/Hg	millimetres of mercury
MMR	maternal mortality ratio
MOET	Managing Obstetric Emergencies and Trauma
MRI	magnetic resonance imaging
NCEPOD	National Confidential Enquiry into Perioperative Deaths
NCISH	National Confidential Enquiry into Death from Suicide and Homicide by People with Mental Illness
NHS	National Health Service
NICE	National Institute for Clinical Excellence

NSF	National Service Framework
NS SEC	National Statistics Socio-Economic Classification
ONS	Office for National Statistics
PND	postnatal depression
PPH	postpartum haemorrhage
RCOG	Royal College of Obstetricians and Gynaecologists
RM	Regional Manager
SADS	sudden adult death syndrome
SHO	senior house officer
SIGN	Scottish Intercollegiate Guidelines Network
SLE	Systemic lupus erythematosus
SPCERH	Scottish Programme for Clinical Effectiveness in Reproductive Health
SROM	Spontaneous rupture of membranes
SUDEP	sudden unexplained death in epilepsy
SVT	supraventricular tachycardia
TFR	total fertility rate
TTP	thrombocytopenic purpura
UK	United Kingdom
UN	United Nations
VSD	ventricular septal defect
VTE	venous thromboembolism
WHO	World Health Organization

Section

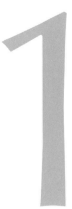

1

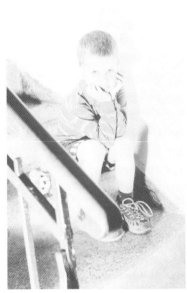 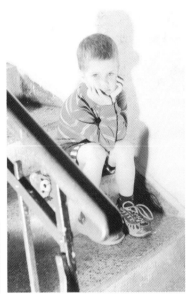 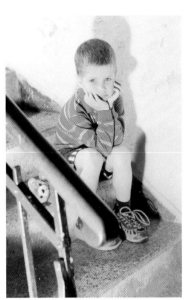

Introduction

BACKGROUND, AIMS AND OBJECTIVES OF THE ENQUIRY

Background to the Enquiry

Over 50 years ago, in 1952, major changes took place in the systems for reviewing maternal deaths in England and Wales. After a discussion on maternal mortality at the 12th British Congress on Obstetrics and Gynaecology in 1949 and representations to the Ministry of Health, the system of local reporting of maternal deaths by Medical Officers of Health directly to the Ministry was replaced by an enhanced national system of regional and national assessment by clinicians. A series of triennial reports was instituted to disseminate the findings and associated recommendations for improving practice to reduce maternal mortality. The first of these triennial reports, covering the years, 1952–54, was published in 1957. Similar systems were instituted in Northern Ireland in 1956 and Scotland in 1965. Since 1985–87, data for all four countries of the UK have been pooled and published in a common Report. This Report is the sixth in the UK series.

For many years, the Enquiry was directly run by the four Health Departments concerned but, in the past few years, this responsibility has been moved to the centrally funded national institutions concerned with reproductive, maternal and child health. The overall organisation and responsibility for producing the final Report rests with the Confidential Enquiries into Maternal and Child Health (CEMACH). CEMACH is commissioned by the National Institute of Clinical Excellence (NICE) to conduct the Enquiry in England and Wales. Northern Ireland does not come under NICE but contributes funds to CEMACH to cover its participation. In Scotland, the Scottish Programme for Clinical Effectiveness in Reproductive Health, acting on behalf of the NHS Quality Improvement for Scotland (NHSQIS), conducts its own enquiry programme but sends its cases to be included in the triennial report and contributes funds towards its participation in the Enquiry.

CEMACH

The Confidential Enquiry into Maternal and Child Health for England and Wales came into being on 1 April 2003. CEMACH reports to, and is primarily funded, by the National Institute for Clinical Excellence. It is, however, an independent body with its own Board, including members nominated by the Royal Colleges of Obstetricians and Gynaecologists, Midwives, Anaesthetists, Pathologists, Paediatrics and Child Health and the Faculty of Public Health Medicine of the Royal College of Physicians. The remit of CEMACH includes the improvement of maternal and child health as well as mortality reviews and it covers babies and children in addition to mothers.

This Report, covering maternal deaths for the UK in the period 2000–02, is the first to be produced under the auspices of CEMACH. The methodology used for its preparation has followed the same pattern as previous Reports. CEMACH intends that the ongoing Enquiry into maternal deaths for the triennium 2003–05 should continue with broadly the same approach as used in earlier Reports. CEMACH is, though, currently working to strengthen the processes underpinning the maternal deaths' Enquiry using its regional network. These are considered to be a vital part of the Enquiry.

The Enquiry Reports have played an important part in the reduction in deaths attributable to pregnancy since 1952. CEMACH is determined to play its part ensuring that this achievement is sustained. The new Enquiry will be reviewing how it can best undertake the continuous monitoring of maternal deaths, in addition to more specific projects aimed at improving maternal health more widely. The professional bodies which previously contributed to the Enquiry, along with those represented on the CEMACH Board, will all continue to play an important part in the further development of the maternal enquiry.

The use of vignettes

The past Enquiry Reports have been characterised by the use of a significant number of vignettes, which broadly described the circumstances surrounding an individual woman's death and the lessons which could be drawn from this. Recognising that ensuring that everyone, including family members and professional staff, require reassurance about the guiding principle of maintaining confidentiality out of respect for those who have died, CEMACH uses vignettes to help in the identification of lessons learned for the improvement of future professional practice or overall service delivery. Vignettes used in this Report do not include the full circumstances of any individual case. They neither provide nor imply a complete overall assessment or judgement of the totality of care provided in a case, although they may point to where general lessons may be learned from particular aspects of care. Individual details in vignettes may be changed to protect the anonymity of the patient and may represent a composite of several cases. CEMACH cannot confirm or deny the identity of any individual woman, aspects of whose care may be included within a vignette, since all records used in the Enquiry are destroyed before publication of the Report. Further details on the method of enquiry are included in Appendix 1 of this Report.

The aims and objectives of the Enquiry

The **aim** of the Enquiry is to form part of the Government's agenda for clinical governance, to help ensure that all pregnant and recently delivered women receive the best possible care delivered in appropriate settings and taking account of their individual needs.

The objectives are:

- to assess the main causes of and trends in maternal deaths

- to identify any avoidable or substandard factors

- to promulgate these findings to all relevant health care professionals

- to improve the care that pregnant and recently delivered women receive and to reduce maternal mortality and morbidity rates still further, as well as the proportion of deaths due to substandard care

- to make recommendations concerning the improvement of clinical care and service provision, including local audit, to purchasers of obstetric services and professionals involved in caring for pregnant women

- to suggest directions for future areas for research and audit at a local and national level

- to produce a triennial report for the funding bodies in four all countries.

**The Enquiry's role in setting clinical standards
and contributing to clinical governance**

The Enquiry is the longest running example of national professional self evaluation in the world. While much has changed since its inception in 1952, the lessons to be learned remain as valid now as in the past. While the Enquiry has always had the support of professionals involved in caring for pregnant or recently delivered women, it is also a government requirement that all maternal deaths should be subject to this confidential Enquiry and all health professionals have a duty to provide the information required. This represents, to a large part, a continuation of current practice.[1-4]

In participating in this Enquiry, all health professionals are asked for two things:

- If they have been caring for a woman who died, health professionals are asked to provide the Enquiry with a full and accurate account of the circumstances leading up to the woman's death, with supporting records.

- Irrespective of whether they have been caring for a woman who died, or not, health professionals are asked to reflect on and take any actions that may be required, either personally or as part of their wider institution, as a result of the recommendations and lessons contained within this Report.

At a **local level** healthcare Trusts can use the findings of the Enquiry to:

- ensure all *Direct* and *Indirect* deaths are subject to a local review and critical incident report

- develop or regularly update multidisciplinary guidelines for the management of complications during or after pregnancy

- review and modify, where necessary, the existing arrangements for the provision of maternity or obstetric care

- promote local audit and clinical governance.

At a **national level**:

In England and Wales, the findings of the Enquiry are used:

- to help inform government policy

- to inform NICE or other guideline or audit development

- to inform guideline and audit development by the relevant Royal Colleges

- to set minimum standards of care, for example as set out in the criteria for the management of maternity services by the Clinical Negligence Scheme for Trusts (CNST)

- as part of the postgraduate training and continuous professional self-development syllabus for all relevant health professionals

- to identify areas for further research.

In Scotland, the findings of the Enquiry inform the work of equivalent bodies responsible for national quality initiatives. These include the Clinical Resource and Audit group (CRAG), the Scottish Intercollegiate Guidelines Network (SIGN), the Clinical Standards

Board for Scotland (CSBS) and the Clinical Negligence and Other Risks Indemnity Scheme (CNORIS). Similar arrangements exist in Northern Ireland.

Study methodology

The findings of this Report demonstrate the contribution of such an observational study to both maternal and child health and the overall public health, and emphasise the need for it to continue in the future.

Some people describe the Enquiry as a form of clinical audit that could be used for performance monitoring. It is not. It is an observational and self-reflective study which identifies patterns of practice, service provision and public health issues that may be causally related to maternal deaths.

This method of reviewing individual deaths has been described as 'sentinel event reporting'. Rutstein et al.,[5] over 25 years ago, stated: "Just as the investigation of an aeroplane accident goes beyond the immediate reasons for the crash to the implications of the design, method of manufacture, maintenance and operation of the plane, so should the study of unnecessary undesirable health events yield crucial information on the scientific, medical, social and personal factors that could lead to better health. Moreover, the evidence collected will not be limited to the factors that yield only to measure of medical control. If there is clear cut documented evidence that identifiable social, environmental, "life-style", economic or genetic factors are responsible for special varieties of unnecessary disease, disability, or untimely death, these factors should be identified and eliminated whenever possible". It is this that the Enquiry aims to achieve.

Some question whether the Reports are 'evidence based'. The highest level of evidence of clinical effectiveness comes from systematic reviews of randomised controlled trials. The most comprehensive and up-to-date systematic reviews of relevance to these Enquiries are produced by the Cochrane Pregnancy and Childbirth Group, whose editorial structure is funded by the NHS Central Programme for Research and Development. The Co-ordinating Editor of the Group is a member of the editorial board of this Enquiry.

Some Cochrane reviews are of direct relevance to topics highlighted by deaths described in recent Reports and have been cited to support recommendations. These include treatments for eclampsia and pre-eclampsia, and antibiotic prophylaxis before caesarean section. However, many problems tackled in successive Reports have not been addressed by randomised trials including prevention of thromboembolic disease and treatment of amniotic fluid embolism, and of massive obstetric haemorrhage.

An important limitation of randomised trials is that, unless they are very large, they may provide little information about rare, but important, complications of treatments. Safety issues are, therefore, sometimes better illuminated by observational studies than by controlled trials.

Many causes of maternal death are very rare (e.g. Ogilvie's syndrome or cervical pregnancy) and treatment options for these may never be subjected to formal scientific study. Inevitably, recommendations for care to avoid such deaths in the future rely on lesser levels of evidence, and frequently on 'expert opinion'. This does not mean that the Report is not evidence based, merely that, necessarily, the evidence cannot be in the form of a randomised control trial or case–control study, owing to the relative rarity of the condition.

Beyond the numbers

The work of this Enquiry has long been recognised as a 'gold standard' in professional self-audit and has started to be replicated by other countries. To date, 15 countries, mainly in the developing world, are now adopting this methodology to help to plan services to improve maternal and child health. This concept of looking "beyond the numbers" to understand the real reasons why women die, through the use of a number of audit methodologies including confidential enquires, is now being promoted by the World Health Organization (WHO) as a key component of its Making Pregnancy Safer strategy. This strategy is designed to assist countries with a large number of maternal deaths to reduce their Maternal Mortality Ratios (MMR) and so work towards the United Nations Millennium Development Goal to reduce maternal deaths by 75% by 2015.[6] WHO has recently published the audit manual *Beyond the Numbers; Reviewing Maternal Deaths and Disabilities to Make Pregnancy Safer*, which includes a chapter based on the practical steps for undertaking similar confidential enquiries into maternal deaths.[7]

References

1. The Department of Health. *A First Class Service: Quality in the NHS.* London: The Department of Health; 1998.
2. The Scottish Office Department of Health. *Clinical Governance.* Management Executive Letter number 29. Edinburgh; 1998.
3. Welsh Office. *Quality Care and Clinical Excellence.* Cardiff: Welsh Office; 1998.
4. Department of Health, Social Services and Public Safety, Northern Ireland. *Best Practice: Best Care. A framework for setting standards, delivering services and improving monitoring and regulation in the HPSS.* Belfast: Department of Health, Social Services and Public Safety; 2001.
5. Ruststein D, Berenberg W, Chalmers T, Child C, Fishman A, et al. Measuring the quality of care; a clinical method. *N Engl J Med* 1976; 582–8.
6. Joint WHO/UNFPA/UNICEF/World Bank statement on the reduction of maternal mortality. Geneva: World Health Organization; 1999.
7. World Health Organization. *Beyond the Numbers; Reviewing Maternal Deaths and Disabilities to Make Pregnancy Safer.* Geneva: WHO; 2004 [www.who.int/reproductive-health].

Other relevant publications and websites

Clinical Resource and Audit Group. *Clinical Outcome Indicators.* Edinburgh; 2000.
Department of Health. *Building a Safer NHS for Patients.* London: Department of Health; 2001 [www.doh.gov.uk/buildsafenhs].
Department of Health. *An Organisation with a Memory.* London: Department of Health; 2000.
National Patient Safety Agency [www.npsa.org.uk].

Scottish Executive Health Department. *A Framework for Maternity Services Scotland.* Edinburgh: Tactica Solutions; 2001.

Scottish Executive Health Department. *Clinical Risk Management Strategy Standards. Clinical Negligence and Other Risks Indemnity Scheme.* Glasgow: Willis; 2001.

Scottish Executive Health Department. *Goals for Clinical Effectiveness.* Edinburgh; 1999.

Scottish Executive Health Department. *Management Executive Letter number 75.* Edinburgh; 2000.

Scottish Executive Health Department. *Non Clinical Risk Management Standards. Clinical Negligence and Other Risks Indemnity Scheme.* Glasgow: Willis; 2001.

Scottish Executive Health Department. *Our National Health: A Plan for Action, a Plan for Change.* Edinburgh; 2001.

Scottish Office Department of Health. *Acute Services Review Report.* Edinburgh: SODOH; 1998.

Scottish Office Department of Health. White Paper. *Designed to Care – Renewing the National Health Service in Scotland.* Edinburgh: SODOH; 1997.

DEFINITIONS OF MATERNAL MORTALITY

The ninth and tenth revisions of the *International Classification of Diseases, Injuries and Causes of Death* (ICD9/10)[1,2] define a maternal death as "the death of a woman while pregnant or within 42 days of termination of pregnancy, from any cause related to or aggravated by the pregnancy or its management, but not from accidental or incidental causes".

This means that there was both a temporal and a causal link between pregnancy and the death. When the woman died, she could have been pregnant at the time (that is, she died before delivery) or within the previous six weeks have had a pregnancy that ended in a live or stillbirth, a spontaneous or induced abortion or an ectopic pregnancy. The pregnancy could have been of any gestational duration. In addition, the death was caused by the fact that the women was or had been pregnant. Either a complication of pregnancy or a condition aggravated by pregnancy or something that happened during the course of caring for the pregnancy caused her death. In other words, if the woman had not been pregnant, she would not have died at that time.

Maternal deaths are subdivided into further groups as shown in Table 1. **Direct** maternal deaths are those resulting from conditions or complications or their management that are unique to pregnancy, occurring during the antenatal, intrapartum or postpartum period. **Indirect** maternal deaths are those resulting from previously existing disease or disease that develops during pregnancy and which were not due to direct obstetric causes but which were aggravated by physiologic effects of pregnancy. Examples of *Indirect* deaths include epilepsy, diabetes, cardiac disease and, in the UK only, hormone-dependent malignancies. The Enquiry also classifies most deaths from suicide as indirect deaths, as they were usually due to puerperal mental illness, although this is not recognised in

Table 1 Definitions of maternal deaths

Term	Definition
Maternal deaths*	Deaths of women while pregnant or within 42 days of the end of the pregnancy, from any cause related to or aggravated by the pregnancy or its management, but not from accidental or incidental causes
Direct*	Deaths resulting from obstetric complications of the pregnant state (pregnancy, labour and puerperium), from interventions, omissions, incorrect treatment or from a chain of events resulting from any of the above
Indirect*	Deaths resulting from previous existing disease, or disease that developed during pregnancy and which was not due to direct obstetric causes, but which was aggravated by the physiologic effects of pregnancy
Late**	Deaths occurring between 42 days and 1 year after abortion, miscarriage or delivery that are due to *Direct* or *Indirect* maternal causes
Coincidental (Fortuitous)**	Deaths from unrelated causes which happen to occur in pregnancy or the puerperium
Pregnancy-related deaths**	Deaths occurring in women while pregnant or within 42 days of termination of pregnancy, irrespective of the cause of the death

* = ICD 9
** = ICD 9/10 classifies these deaths as *Fortuitous* but the Enquiry prefers to use the term *Coincidental* as it a more accurate description. The Enquiry also considers deaths from *Late Coincidental* causes
*** = ICD 10

the ICD coding of such deaths. The UK Enquiry assessors also classify some deaths from cancer in which the hormone-dependant effects of the malignancy could have led to its progress being hastened or modified by pregnancy as *Indirect*, although these also do not accord with international definitions. Only *Direct* and *Indirect* deaths are counted for statistical purposes, as discussed in the next section.

ICD10 also introduced two new terms related to maternal deaths. One of them is **Pregnancy-related death**, defined as the death of a woman while pregnant or within 42 days of termination of pregnancy, irrespective of the cause of the death. Like maternal deaths, pregnancy-related deaths can be associated with any pregnancy outcome and can occur at any gestational age. The difference is that pregnancy-related deaths include deaths from all causes, including accidental and incidental causes. The latter deaths, which would have occurred even if the woman had not been pregnant, namely those from accidental or coincidental causes, are not considered true maternal deaths. However, they often contain valuable lessons for this Enquiry; for example, providing messages and recommendations about domestic violence or road traffic accidents. Therefore, this Enquiry reviews all deaths up to 6 weeks after delivery and within 1 year if possible. From the assessments of these cases it is often possible to make important recommendations. The ICD coding classifies these cases as *Fortuitous* maternal deaths. However, in the opinion of the UK assessors, the use of the term fortuitous could imply a happier event and this Report, as did the last, has renamed these deaths as **Coincidental**.

The other new term introduced in ICD10 is **Late** maternal death, defined as the death of a woman from *Direct* or *Indirect* causes more than 42 days but less than 1 completed year after the delivery or any other event that led to the interruption of the pregnancy. Identifying *Late* maternal deaths enables lessons to be learned from deaths in which a woman had problems that began with the pregnancy, even if she survived for more than 42 days after its end. However, although this category has only been recently recognised in the ICD10 codes, and then only for deaths from *Direct* or *Indirect* causes, the previous three Enquiry Reports had already included all *Late* deaths notified to the assessors (including *Coincidental* deaths) occurring up to 1 year after delivery or abortion, as does this Report.

Estimating maternal mortality ratios and rates

The international definition of the maternal mortality ratio (MMR) is the number of *Direct* and *Indirect* deaths per 100,000 live births. In many countries of the world this is difficult to measure, owing to the lack of death certificate data (should it exist at all) as well as a lack of basic denominator data, as baseline vital statistics are also not available or unreliable. The recent World Health Organization publication, *Beyond The Numbers: Reviewing Maternal Deaths and Disabilities to Make Pregnancy Safer*,[3] contains a more detailed examination and evaluation of the problems in both determining a baseline MMR or interpreting what it actually means in helping to address the problems facing pregnant women in most developing countries. Maternal mortality definitions used in this Report are shown in Table 2.

Conversely, the UK has the advantage of accurate denominator data, including both live and still births, and has defined its MMR as the number of *Direct* and *Indirect* deaths per 100,000 maternities. Maternities are defined as the number of pregnancies that result

Table 2 Maternal mortality definitions used in this Report

Maternal mortality definitions	Reasons for use
UK Enquiry maternal mortality rates; *Direct* and *Indirect* deaths per 100,000 maternities	The most robust figures available for the UK and used for 50 years trend data in this Report
The internationally defined Maternal Mortality Ratio (MMR); *Direct* and *Indirect* causes per 100,000 live births	For international comparison although care needs to be taken in its interpretation due to more accurate case ascertainment in the UK though the use of this Enquiry
Deaths from obstetric causes per million women aged 15–44 years	This enables comparison with the other causes of deaths in this age group
Deaths from obstetric causes per 100,000 maternities	Maternities are the number of mothers delivered of registrable live births at any gestation or stillbirths of 24 weeks of gestation or later; i.e. these are the majority of women at risk of death from obstetric causes
Deaths from obstetric causes per 100,000 estimated pregnancies	Because the data from spontaneous abortions and ectopic pregnancies are unreliable, this denominator is only used when calculating rates of death in early pregnancy

Precise details of these definitions, together with background figures and tables for the United Kingdom 2000–02 can be found in Chapter 21

in a live birth at any gestation or stillbirths occurring at or after 24 weeks of completed gestation and are required to be notified by law. This enables a more detailed picture of maternal death rates to be established and is used for the comparison of trends over time.

Furthermore, in the United Kingdom, maternal mortality rates can be calculated in two ways:

- through official death certification to the Registrars General (the Office for National Statistics [ONS] and its equivalents), or

- through deaths known to this Enquiry. The overall maternal death rate is calculated from the number of *Direct* and *Indirect* deaths.

ONS data are based on death certificates where the cause of death is directly or secondarily coded for a pregnancy-related condition such as postpartum haemorrhage, eclampsia, etc. Chapter 21 contains a summary table of ONS-derived maternal death rates.

For the past 50 years, the Enquiry has calculated its own maternal mortality rate, which, as stated before, includes cases of maternal death from suicides due to perinatal mental illness, as well as some malignancies, as *Indirect* deaths. However, in addition to the inflation of the ONS maternal mortality rate caused by the inclusion of these additional *Indirect* deaths, the overall number of other *Direct* and *Indirect* deaths identified by the Enquiry has always exceeded those officially reported. This is because a large proportion of women known to the Enquiry die of pre-existing medical conditions influenced by their pregnant state; for example, cardiac disorders, epilepsy and some malignancies, but these are excluded from the official statistics. Also excluded are women who require long-term intensive care and whose final cause of death is registered as a non-pregnancy condition, such as multiple organ failure, even though the initiating cause was an obstetric event. Conversely, the maternal deaths known to the Registrars General may include *Late* deaths, as it is not possible to identify from the death certificate when the delivery or termination occurred.

This Report, to aid the international comparison with the ICD-defined MMR, has also calculated the overall UK MMR, as well as the more complete Enquiry MMR. The findings are given in Chapter 1. However, when making such comparisons, it is important to note two points:

- The criteria used by the UK assessors for *Indirect* deaths are far more inclusive than those used in other countries. For example, in this Enquiry, all cases of cardiac disease, asthma and epilepsy are coded as *Indirect,* as are cases of suicide unless obviously occurring in women with a longstanding previous psychiatric history.

- Case ascertainment is lower in the vast majority of other countries because they do not undertake such comprehensive enquiries.

Case ascertainment

The role of the Office for National Statistics

Since the introduction of a new ONS computer program in 1993, all conditions given anywhere on the death certificate are now coded, enabling a more extensive search of death draft entry information to identify all conditions listed which suggest a maternal death. In the past, this has helped in improving case ascertainment, with a number of previously unreported deaths being identified. Fortunately, the record linkage study described in Chapter 1 of this Report has identified very few cases of *Direct* or *Indirect* deaths that were not reported to the Enquiry. This is a reduction in the already small degree of under-ascertainment calculated for previous Reports.

ONS has also devised a record linkage study, described in Chapter 1, designed to identify all deaths in women within one year of delivery.

The role of the CEMACH Regional Managers

Since the Enquiry became part of the new Confidential Enquiry into Maternal and Child Health in April 2003, the day-to-day running of the Enquiry has been taken over by the CEMACH central and regional offices. The CEMACH Managers, apart from their other duties, have assumed the responsibility for ascertainment of maternal deaths in their regions, as well as collecting the relevant clinical information and organising the regional assessment of each case, a process undertaken by the old District Directors of Public Health. The Managers' local knowledge and commitment has already led to more timely case reviews as well as to enhanced notifications of cases, *Indirect* deaths in particular. Although this change occurred after the end of this triennium, they were still able to identify some cases from 2000–02 which had either not been reported on or whom details were missing. This has also had an effect on the case ascertainment for this triennium.

The result of this improved case ascertainment probably is one of the main factors in the increase the numbers known to the Enquiry and, hence, the overall and specific maternal mortality rates reflected in the data given in Chapter 1.

Denominator data used for calculating mortality rates

Number of maternities

It is impossible to know the exact number of pregnancies that occurred during this or any preceding triennium, since not all pregnancies result in a registrable live or still birth. Because of the unreliability of these data, and the lack of appropriate denominators, the most common denominator used throughout this and previous Reports is the number of maternities rather than the total number of pregnancies. Maternities are the number of pregnancies that result in a live birth at any gestation or stillbirths occurring at or after 24 weeks of completed gestation and required to be notified by law. The total number of maternities for the United Kingdom, 2000–02, was 1,997,472.

Estimated pregnancies

This denominator is used for calculating the rate of early pregnancy deaths. It is a combination of the number of maternities, together with legal terminations, hospital admissions for spontaneous abortions (at less than 24 weeks of gestation) and ectopic pregnancies, with an adjustment to allow for the period of gestation and maternal ages at conception. The estimate for the United Kingdom 2000–02 was 2,791,800. However, the resulting total is still an underestimate of the actual number of pregnancies, since these figures do not include other pregnancies which miscarry early, those where the woman is not admitted to hospital or indeed those where the woman herself may not even know she is pregnant. Further details are available in Chapter 21.

Deaths from obstetric causes per million women aged 15–44 years

This denominator, used for some tables in Chapter 21 Trends in epidemiology and women's health, assumes that all women of childbearing age are at risk of becoming pregnant. It lacks the rigour of confining the rate calculated to women who actually were pregnant but has the advantage of enabling comparison with other causes of women's deaths.

References

1. World Health Organization. *International Statistical Classification of Diseases and Related Health Problems, Ninth Revision.* Geneva: WHO; 1977.
2. World Health Organization. *International Statistical Classification of Diseases and Related Health Problems, Tenth Revision.* Geneva: WHO; 1992–1994 [www.who.int/whosis/icd10/].
3. World Health Organization. *Beyond the Numbers; Reviewing Maternal Deaths and Disabilities to Make Pregnancy Safer.* Geneva: WHO; 2004 [www.who.int/reproductive-health].

THE INTERNATIONAL CONTEXT

Although pregnancy and childbirth are not entirely risk free, even in developed countries, every day around 1,600 women and over 5,000 newborn babies die due to complications that could have been prevented.

The discrepancies faced by pregnant women in different parts of the world are extreme. More than 99% of all maternal deaths occur in the developing countries of the world, where a woman's lifetime risk of dying from a pregnancy-related complication can be up to 200 times higher than in many developed countries.[1] More than 50% of the women in the world give birth without a skilled attendant to help, neither do they receive any antenatal care. Overall, the average risk that a woman will die during pregnancy, childbirth or from an unsafe abortion is 1 in 65 in developing countries and in some countries is as high as 1 in 16, compared with 1 in 9,000 for the United Kingdom.

These figures represent the largest public health discrepancy in the world. Each death or long-term complication represents an individual tragedy for the woman, her partner, her children and family. More tragically, most deaths are avoidable. It is estimated that more than 80% of maternal deaths could be prevented or avoided through actions that are proven to be effective and affordable, even in resource-poor countries.[2]

Death is not the only problem that pregnant women face. It is estimated that around 20 million women a year are left with serious ill health or disability as a result of pregnancy and childbirth.[3] Additionally, every year, millions of children are left motherless and an estimated one million young children die as a result of the death of their mother. The risk of death for children under five years is doubled if their mother dies in childbirth. Babies who survive the death of their mother seldom reach their first birthday. The loss of the mother is especially risky for girl children.[4] Furthermore, surviving children are more at risk of long-term health and social problems.

While the largest numbers of maternal deaths, and consequently also pregnancies that result in severe morbidity, are to be found in countries with very high population and fertility rates, such as India, the highest mortality rates are in Africa, followed by Asia and Latin America. However, intra-regional differences are also high, especially in Asia.

The most recent world estimate of the overall maternal mortality ratio (MMR) is around 400 per 100,000 live births[1] compared with 12 per 100,000 for the UK. The maternal mortality rate is calculated as the number of *Direct* and *Indirect* deaths per 100,000 live births. The maternal mortality estimates by the Regions of the World Health Organization (WHO) and United Nation (UN) are shown in Table 3. The MMR is highest in Africa followed by Asia, Oceania, Latin America and the Caribbean. These figures hide wide inter-country variations and even within countries major discrepancies exist between the rich and poor and urban and remote areas. With the exception of Afghanistan and Haiti, all of the 22 countries with MMRs in excess of 1,000 are in sub-Saharan Africa.

Causes of maternal deaths and disabilities

Around 80% of maternal deaths are due to *Direct* obstetric causes and 20% due to *Indirect* causes.

Table 3 Maternal mortality estimates by WHO/UN Regions: 2000

Region	Maternal mortality ratio (maternal deaths per 100,000 live births)	Number of maternal deaths	Lifetime risk of maternal death
World total	400	529,000	74
Developed regions*	20	2,500	2,800
Europe	24	1,700	2,400
Developing regions	440	527,000	61
Africa	830	251,000	20
Northern Africa	130	4,600	210
Sub-Saharan Africa	920	247,000	16
Asia	330	253,000	94
Eastern Asia	55	11,000	840
South-Central Asia	520	207,000	46
South-Eastern Asia	210	25,000	140
Western Asia	190	9,800	120
Latin America & the Caribbean	190	22,000	160
Oceania	240	530	83

* Includes UK, Canada, USA, Japan, Australia and New Zealand, which are excluded from the regional totals

The major causes of *Direct* deaths are shown in Table 4. WHO has developed estimates of mortality and morbidity related to just the five leading *Direct* causes: postpartum haemorrhage, puerperal sepsis, pre-eclampsia and eclampsia, obstructed labour and abortion. Overall, these comprise around 80% of the global deaths due to direct complications of pregnancy. The other 20% comprise deaths from conditions such as ectopic pregnancies, anaesthetic complications and thrombosis. These are very different from the leading cause of maternal death in the UK where, for this triennium, the five global leading causes of death only comprise of 39% of all such cases combined. In the UK, the leading cause of *Direct* death is thromboembolism, which accounts for 28% of these deaths.

Indirect causes account for some 20% of the maternal deaths worldwide. Infectious or vector born diseases aside, the causes of *Indirect* deaths are similar to those in the UK. Countries such as Sri Lanka, who have made major gains in reducing maternal mortality through the introduction of national safe motherhood programmes report that, as with the UK, cardiac disease is the leading cause of *Indirect* deaths. However, infectious disease is a rising cause of maternal death and in certain parts of the world these death rates are rising, reversing the gains made in the last few decades. HIV/AIDS is now the

Table 4 Estimated incidence of major global causes of *Direct* maternal deaths: 2000[4]*

Cause	Incidence of complication (% of live births)	Number of cases (2000)	Case fatality rate	Maternal deaths (*n*)	Percentage of all *Direct* deaths (%)
Haemorrhage	10.5	13,795,000	1.0	132,000	*28*
Sepsis	4.4	5,768,00	1.3	79,000	*16*
Preeclampsia,/ Eclampsia	3.2	4,152,000	1.7	63,000	*13*
Obstructed labour	4.6	6,038,000	0.7	42,000	*9*
Abortion	14.8	19,340,000	0.3	69,000	*15*

* These estimates have been developed for WHO calculations of the global burden of disease and are based upon both literature review and expert consensus; the full results will be published in future issues of the World Health Report

leading cause of maternal death in most African countries. In addition, more than 30 million women in Africa who become pregnant in malaria-endemic areas are at risk of malaria infection,[5] which increases the risk not only of dying from severe malaria or from malaria-related severe anaemia, the presence of which also contributes to death from haemorrhage. Although *Indirect* deaths comprise a small proportion of maternal deaths overall, in the UK the picture is different and *Indirect* deaths are now the leading cause of death, comprising around 60% of maternal deaths.

Why do mothers really die?

While the numbers of maternal deaths and severe complaints are stark, they tell only part of the story. In particular, they tell nothing about the individual stories of suffering and distress and the real underlying reasons why particular women died. Most of all, they tell nothing about why women continue to die in a world where the knowledge and resources to prevent such deaths are available or attainable. While it is important to keep monitoring overall levels of maternal mortality at global, regional and national levels, for both identification and advocacy purposes, statistics about the level of maternal mortality do not help identify what can be done to prevent or avoid such unnecessary deaths.

Today, with a better understanding of the difficulties involved in measuring levels of maternal mortality, and the cost of conducting full scale exercises to determine overall MMRs, there is increasing interest in directing a larger share of limited resources into efforts to understand why the problem persists and what can be done to avert maternal deaths and cases of severe morbidity. Answering these questions is vital for programme planners, managers and service providers. In order to help address this, the WHO's Making Pregnancy Safer initiative has recently published *Beyond the Numbers*,[6] a practical guide which describes a number of strategies and approaches to review cases of maternal death or disability to help understand why mothers really die to enable the necessary actions to be taken on the results.

The methodologies for understanding why women die or suffer long-term complications, described in *Beyond the Numbers*, are designed to be a first step in the process of planning, implementing and evaluating strategies to helping reduce maternal deaths and disability. As with any life-threatening clinical condition, a diagnosis needs to be made before the appropriate treatment can be provided. It is this crucial first step that has often been lacking in the design of well-meaning but eventually partially ineffective programmes for maternal ill-health reduction. The use of these techniques can help with the diagnosis of the underlying causes; for example, are women dying because:

- they were unaware of the need for care, or unaware of the warning signs of problems in pregnancy?

  or

- the services did not exist, or were inaccessible for other reasons such as distance, cost or sociocultural barriers?

  or

- are women dying because the care they receive in traditional or modern health services is inadequate or actually harmful?

Answering such questions and taking positive action on the results is often more important than knowing the precise level of magnitude of maternal mortality. The various approaches described in *Beyond the Numbers* will enable, and empower, health professionals and authorities to act on the answers to these and other important questions about why women die during pregnancy and childbirth. In planning any such review it is important to build in sustainability from the beginning so that such activities become a routine part of clinical practice and health information systems.

The role of this Enquiry

The work of this Enquiry has long been recognised as a gold standard in professional self-audit and is one of the methodologies described and promoted in *Beyond the Numbers*. The manual includes a chapter based on the practical steps for undertaking similar confidential enquiries into maternal deaths based on the UK experience. Some of the authors and assessors of this Enquiry have now helped more than 15 countries, many in the developing world, to adapt this methodology to help plan services to improve maternal and child health. To date, these programmes have been started mainly in Africa and Asia but there are increasing number of requests also coming from the countries of Eastern Europe, including several Central Asian Republics. As a result, the Enquiry Director now works part time for the World Health Organization's Making Pregnancy Safer Programme to continue to support, promote and implement maternal death and disability audits and reviews around the world.

References

1. World Health Organization. *Maternal Mortality in 2000: Estimates Developed by WHO, UNICEF and UNFPA*. Geneva: World Health Organization; 2003 [www.who.int].
2. World Health Organization Regional Office for Africa. *Reducing Maternal Deaths: The Challenge of the New Millennium in the Africa Region*. Brazzaville, Congo: WHO Regional Office for Africa; 2002 [www.afro.who.int/drh].
3. Pittrof R, Cambell O, Filippi VGA. What is quality maternity care? An international perspective. *Acta Obstet Gynecol Scand* 2002; 81:277–83.
4. UNICEF. *The Progress of the Nations 2001*. New York: United Nations Children's Fund; 2001.
5. World Health Organization. *Strategic Framework for Malaria Control During Pregnancy in the WHO Africa Region*. Geneva: WHO; 2002.
6. World Health Organization. *Beyond the Numbers; Reviewing Maternal Deaths and Disabilities to Make Pregnancy Safer*. Geneva: WHO; 2004 [www.who.int/reproductive-health].

SUMMARY OF OVERARCHING RECOMMENDATIONS

Each chapter of this Report contains a number of general and specific recommendations. Many of these are inter-related and, when taken as a whole, certain key themes and general recommendations can be identified. The purpose of this summary, therefore, is not to repeat the recommendations made in each chapter but to synthesise these into a shorter list of key themes and overarching recommendations together with a brief synopsis of the underlying rationale.

1. Planning local maternity services

Rationale

Many women who died, particularly the vulnerable and socially excluded, found it difficult to access or maintain access with the services, and follow-up for those who failed to attend was poor. Inadequate translation services for those who could not speak English were also a recurring feature.

Some women known to be at higher risk of complications were delivered in isolated maternity units without access to blood banks, intensive care, advanced imaging or skilled anaesthetic backup. A very few women died of administrative delays while waiting for therapeutic terminations of pregnancy that might have saved their lives.

The provision of specialist psychiatric services and multidisciplinary care for women with complex mental health or social problems including problem substance misuse and domestic violence was, in many cases, poor, as was interagency working with social and other services for women and children at risk.

Recommendations

- Maternity services should be designed to be approachable and flexible enough to meet the needs of all women, including the vulnerable and hard to reach. These services should be such that all women are then motivated to re-attend throughout their pregnancy. Asylum seekers and refugees are a particularly vulnerable group and services need to respond to their needs.

- The importance of seeking antenatal care early in pregnancy should be part of health education and promotion materials prepared for all groups in society.

- Professional interpreters should be provided for women who do not speak English. The use of family members, including children, should be avoided if at all possible.

- Coordinated multidisciplinary or multi-agency care should be available for all women with medical, mental health or social problems, including substance abuse and domestic violence, who may require specialist advice or support in pregnancy. Women with complex pregnancies and who receive care from a number of specialists or agencies should receive the support and advocacy of a known midwife throughout their pregnancy.

- Women known to be at risk of developing clinical problems should not be delivered in isolated maternity units. This needs to be addressed both in terms developing an overall strategy for maternity services provision as well as developing local protocols for the referral of women with problems, or potential problems, in pregnancy and childbirth.

- Dedicated obstetric anaesthesia services should be available in all consultant obstetric units.

- A specialist perinatal mental health team with the knowledge, skills and experience to provide care for women at risk or, or suffering from, serious postpartum mental illness should be available to every woman. Women who require psychiatric admission following childbirth should be admitted to a specialist mother and baby unit, together with their infant. In areas where this service is not available then admission to the nearest unit should take place.

- Termination of pregnancy services should be readily available and accessible for women with medical conditions precluding safe pregnancy. Women referred for a termination of pregnancy, who have a potentially life-threatening condition, should be given an appointment as quickly as possible and certainly no longer than 3 weeks.

2. Clinical care

Rationale

More than 50% of the women who died had some aspect of substandard clinical care. Some died because their condition was not diagnosed or they received ineffective or the wrong treatment. Not all care was consistent with current national clinical guidelines or provided by experienced staff.

Poor or non-communication between different specialists and groups of staff was a recurrent feature in this Report. Some staff in accident and emergency departments misdiagnosed pregnant women with severe complications, underestimated the degree of urgency of the situation, did not liaise with maternity colleagues or discharged women without referral.

Some midwives and obstetricians, usually the more junior, failed to pick up and act on warning signs of common medical conditions unrelated to pregnancy.

Recommendations

- Each Trust should implement, audit and regularly update multidisciplinary guidelines for the management of women at risk of, or who develop, complications in pregnancy. Where possible, these must be based on any relevant guidelines from the National Institute for Clinical Excellence (NICE) or other country equivalents. Where national guidelines do not exist, there may be evidence-based guidelines from the relevant Royal Colleges. This Report also contains examples of such guidelines in a number of areas.

- The development of locally agreed multidisciplinary and, in some cases, inter-agency protocols will help to place clinical guidelines into the local health service delivery framework. Local protocols should not only include the relevant clinical guidelines but also identify clear and agreed pathways of care and referral mechanisms for women who develop complications.

- As a minimum, and based upon the most up-to-date authoritative clinical evidence, protocols and local referral pathways, including transport in emergencies, should be developed and audited for:
  - the multidisciplinary management of women with pre-existing medical conditions, including cardiac disease, epilepsy and diabetes
  - the management of women who are at risk of a relapse or recurrence of a serious mental illness
  - the management and local support strategies for women who use drugs and/or alcohol or who disclose domestic violence
  - the management of pregnant women who attend accident and emergency departments
  - the management of sepsis, pre-eclampsia and eclampsia, obstetric haemorrhage, and of women who decline blood products
  - the use of thromboprophylaxis.

- Clinical guidelines and local protocols should be prominently placed in all antenatal and postnatal wards, the delivery suite and in accident and emergency departments, and should be given to all new members of staff.

- All pregnant women attending accident and emergency departments with anything other than minor complaints should be seen quickly and in conjunction with an obstetrician or senior midwife. If these people are not available on site then arrangements should be made to discuss their care with the local maternity unit.

- Where possible, an autopsy should be performed for all maternal deaths. If the autopsy cannot be performed by a pathologist with a special interest in these deaths, then help and advice should be sought from a pathologist with expertise in this area.

3. The booking visit

Rationale

The booking visit is crucial in helping assess the specific needs of newly pregnant women, identifying any significant current or past medical, psychiatric or social problems and helping her to plan and make choices for her maternity care and where to give birth. This opportunity was lost to many of the women who died. A recurrent theme in this Report is that highly relevant information was not passed on from the GP to the maternity staff in the referral letter.

Booking also offers an ideal opportunity for maternity staff to identify any current or potential problems that may require more specialist advice or investigation. For the women who died, this does not appear to have been done in a systematic way and, in some cases, vital information was not ascertained or recorded.

At booking, a risk and needs assessment should take place to ensure every woman will be offered the type of care that most suits her own particular requirements. Some women in this Report were offered midwifery-led care that did not meet their more complex needs.

- Clear, relevant and complete information, which accurately details any past current or past medical, psychiatric, social or family history, must be passed from the GP to the antenatal care team at booking.

- A standard national "booking referral letter" should be developed that contains a checklist of medical, social factors and family history, which need to be included to enable the most appropriate care plan for each woman to be developed.

- At the booking visit a clear, systematic history should be recorded and the woman's care plan discussed within a risk assessment framework.

- The systematic enquiries should include:

  o a complete social history

  o any personal or family medical history, including thromboembolism

  o any personal or family psychiatric history, its severity and management

  o the use of drugs, prescribed and non-prescribed, legal and illegal, and tobacco and alcohol.

- A national guideline for a booking clinic 'risk assessment' chart should be developed to identify those pregnant women for whom midwifery-led antenatal care and birth can be advised, and those for whom specialist or joint care is more appropriate.

- Once local multi-agency support services are in place, this Enquiry recommends that routine enquiries should be made about domestic violence, either when taking a social history at booking or at another opportune point in the antenatal period. Where possible, all women should be seen alone at least once during the antenatal period to enable disclosure more easily if they wish.

- Pregnant women with known medical or mental health problems, including complex social problems, substance misuse and domestic violence, should be offered shared multidisciplinary and, if appropriate, multi-agency care in a supportive environment.

- Women with a body mass index of 35 or more are at higher risk of developing problems and, in the opinion of this Enquiry, should be referred for care shared with an obstetrician and advised to deliver in a consultant led obstetric unit.

- If women who are considered to be at higher risk choose midwifery-led care, their midwife should receive support and advice from an experienced superior.

4. Complicated pregnancies

Some women who died who had known obstetric or other complications did not have integrated care. Some had serious medical problems managed by physicians or cardiologists without referral to their obstetrician. Liaison between general practitioners, accident and emergency and oncology services and obstetric services was also poor. Some women with significant symptoms or severe pain were not adequately investigated or referred for a medical or surgical opinion.

- All pregnant women with medical or psychiatric conditions requiring treatment or care by other specialists should have an integrated care plan developed and agreed between all specialities involved. For some more common medical conditions such as cardiac disease, diabetes and epilepsy, joint clinics should be provided.

- Regular communication between specialties is crucial and this should be monitored and ensured by the woman's lead maternity care provider, who will usually be her midwife.

- Women who have a past history of serious psychiatric disorder, postpartum or non-postpartum, should be assessed by a psychiatrist in the antenatal period. A management plan, regarding the high risk of recurrence following delivery, should be agreed with the woman, her family, her maternity team and GP and placed in her handheld records.

- Pregnancy is not a contraindication for radiological investigations for women with severe and unremitting pain or other symptoms.

5. Birth

Rationale

Women with known or anticipated problems that might have affected their delivery were not always delivered in a consultant-led unit. Even when this did occur, some units lacked the appropriate facilities or experienced staff to provide the full range of emergency services required.

- Women known to be at higher risk of developing problems during labour or birth should be advised to deliver in a consultant obstetrician-led unit.

- When presented with problems requiring special skills or investigations, midwives, obstetricians and obstetric anaesthetists should have the authority and should not hesitate to call for assistance from senior colleagues in their own or other disciplines.

- Women known to be at high risk of bleeding should be delivered in centres with facilities for blood transfusion, intensive care and other interventions, and plans made in advance for their management.

- A multidisciplinary massive haemorrhage protocol must be available in all units and should be updated and rehearsed regularly in conjunction with the blood bank. All grades of staff should participate in these 'fire drills'.

- Intensive care should start as soon as it is needed and does not need to wait for admission to an intensive care unit. It is possible to provide the majority of immediate intensive care in an obstetric theatre. Where available, outreach staff should be used.

6. Health professionals

Rationale

There were instances where, in the compiling of the reports for this Enquiry, unwitting staff prejudices were revealed that may have had an effect on the care they provided.

An unexpected maternal death is devastating for the staff who cared for her. Some staff, doctors and midwives appeared to blame themselves inappropriately when a mother for whom they had been caring died. These staff appeared to have been left to shoulder the guilt they felt alone and were not offered counselling or support. A few left their profession as a result.

The Report also identified a number of areas in which all health and other professions caring for pregnant women could benefit from regular and updated training.

- Health professionals who work with disadvantaged clients need to be able to understand a woman's social and cultural background, act as an advocate for women with other colleagues and address their own personal and social prejudices and practice in a reflective manner.

- All healthcare professionals should consider whether there are unrecognised but inherent racial prejudices within their own organisations, in terms of providing an equal service to all women.

- Trusts must make provision for the prompt offer of support and/or counselling for all staff who have cared for a woman who has died, individually and as the whole team who cared for the mother.

Training

- All health professionals should receive regular and updated training on the signs and symptoms of critical illness, from both obstetric and non-obstetric causes.

- All medical and midwifery staff should be trained in basic life support to a nationally recognised level. Emergency drills for maternal resuscitation should be regularly practised in clinical areas in all maternity units.

- All health professionals should received regular and updated training on the impact of domestic violence, mental illness and substance misuse on the lives and health of pregnant women, their babies and families. This should also include the identification, management and local service provision for these women. Such training is essential before any routine enquiries are commenced.

- Obstetricians and midwives should be aware of the laws and issues that relate to child protection and when and to whom to refer if they are concerned.

7. Areas for further research

The findings of this Report have identified many areas for further research, of which the following appear to be the most pressing:

- To identify the barriers which prevent women from seeking care or maintaining contact with the maternity services in order to help plan more appropriate service provision.

- To estimate more robustly what, if any, is the degree of increased risk of maternal deaths associated with caesarean section particularly for those undertaken without a clinical indication.

- To investigate the incidence of postpartum haemorrhage in relation to previous caesarean section.

8. Reporting maternal deaths and assisting with the Enquiry

Rationale

Although case reporting for the women who died of *Direct* causes of deaths was virtually complete, the deaths of some women who died of *Indirect* or *Coincidental* causes of deaths were not reported. In the main, these included *Late* deaths from suicide and others which occurred some months after delivery. It is important that these deaths, too, are reported to this Enquiry.

Although the vast majority of staff willingly complied with the requirements of assisting with this Enquiry, some, particularly from those groups of professionals for whom the enquiry process is relatively new, questioned the need to be involved. These included some GPs, accident and emergency staff and those working in community-based services such as psychiatry or substance misuse. Their input is crucial if a full assessment of the totally of care the women received can be made and future lessons learned.

- Any healthcare professional who is aware of the death, from any cause, of a woman who is either pregnant or within 1 year following delivery, termination of pregnancy, ectopic pregnancy or miscarriage is required to report it to their CEMACH Regional Manager.

- All health professionals are required to participate in the work of the Confidential Enquiry. Full case notes must be made available to the Enquiry Assessors and are treated in strict confidence. All professional staff who cared for the woman must provide information on request. Reports must be completed within 3 months of the death.

- Given the importance of the provision of multi-agency care for pregnant or recently delivered women living in complex social circumstances, it is recommended that social service staff and other be encouraged to contribute to this Enquiry in future.

CHAPTER 1

Introduction and key findings 2000–2002

GWYNETH LEWIS on behalf of the Editorial Board

Introduction

This Report marks the first 50 years of national triennial Reports on Confidential Enquiries into Maternal Deaths. During this time these Reports have aimed to save mothers' lives by underpinning good obstetric and maternity practice in the UK. Huge improvements have been made, as demonstrated in the individual chapters in this book as well as in Chapter 22, which gives an overview of the major changes made to the enquiry process in 1952 and developments up to 2002. The risk of a woman in the United Kingdom dying today of a pregnancy-related cause is extremely small and has been reduced, in some measure, by the impact these Reports have had on clinical practice over the past five decades. However, the additional new and wider public health focus, first seen in the last Report and expanded in this, shows that maternal mortality rates are significantly higher for the most disadvantaged women compared with these from the most advantaged. It has also been estimated that during 2000–02, the period of this Report, over 1,000 existing or newborn children lost their mothers and faced a consequently bleaker start in life. This message is reinforced by the choice of picture used for the cover of this Report.

A very high proportion of the women who died during 2000–02 were economically and socially disadvantaged and are described in this Report as 'vulnerable' or 'socially excluded'. These definitions encompass diverse groups of women who may face a number of similar or different problems. These groups included women living in extreme poverty and those with multiple social problems, women from some minority ethnic groups and those who did not speak English, homeless or travelling women and refugees and asylum seekers. There were also those who believed they had stigmatising conditions such as previous mental illness, being under age or HIV positive, or who misused drugs, alcohol or other substances and those who experienced domestic violence.

The challenges posed by the findings in this Report are therefore not just clinical but, as the findings in this chapter starkly demonstrate, are also around reconfiguring services that meet the needs of women from all groups in society, particularly the socially excluded. By doing so, not only should maternal health outcomes improve, for the greater benefit of all pregnant women, but the number of children growing up without a mother and facing a poor start in life will also be reduced. The recommendations made in this Report therefore offer an opportunity for all involved in planning services and caring for pregnant and recently delivered women to make a real and lasting difference to their lives and those of their families.

Summary of key findings for 2000–02

Mortality rates and main causes of death

- The maternal mortality rate for both *Indirect* and *Direct* causes of death shows a slight increase for this triennium as compared with the last Report, although this is not statistically significant.

- As with the previous Report, the overall maternal death rate for *Indirect* causes of death is higher than for deaths from *Direct* causes.

- The most common cause of *Direct* deaths was again thromboembolism, the rates for which remain largely unchanged since 1997–99. There have been increases in the mortality rates from haemorrhage and those associated with anaesthesia and no significant decreases in deaths from other causes. There was no under-reporting of these deaths.

- The most common cause of *Indirect* deaths and the largest cause of maternal deaths overall was psychiatric illness, although not all of these were reported to the Enquiry and many were identified from linkage with the Office for National Statistics (ONS), as discussed later in this chapter. Cardiac disease remains the second most common cause and most of these cases were reported to the Enquiry.

Risk factors for maternal deaths

- **Social disadvantage:** Women living in families where both partners were unemployed, many of whom had features of social exclusion, were up to 20 times more likely to die than women from the more advantaged groups. In addition, single mothers were three times more likely to die than those in stable relationships.

- **Poor communities:** Women living in the most deprived areas of England had a 45% higher death rate compared with women living in the most affluent areas.

- **Minority ethnic groups:** Women from ethnic groups other than White were, on average, three times more likely to die than White women. Black African women, including asylum seekers and newly arrived refugees had a mortality rate seven times higher than White women and had major problems in accessing maternal health care.

- **Late booking or poor attendance:** 20% (50) of the women who died from *Direct* or *Indirect* causes booked for maternity care after 22 weeks of gestation or had missed over four routine antenatal visits.

- **Obesity:** 35% (78) of the all women who died were obese: 50% more than in the general population.

- **Domestic violence:** 14% (51) of all the women who died self-declared that they were subject to violence in the home.

- **Substance abuse:** 8% (31) of all the women who died were substance misusers.

- **Suboptimal clinical care:** 67% of the 261 women who died from *Direct* and *Indirect* causes were considered to have some form of suboptimal clinical care.

- **Lack of inter-professional and/or inter-agency communications:** In many cases, the care provided to the women who died was hampered by a lack of cross-disciplinary working. There were a number of cases in which crucial clinical information, which may have affected the outcome, was not passed from the general practitioner to the midwifery or obstetric services at booking or shared between consultants in other specialties, including staff in accident and emergency departments and the obstetric team. There were also cases where significant information, particularly regarding a risk of self-harm and child safety, were not shared between the health and social services.

Maternal mortality rates

In the United Kingdom, maternal mortality rates can be calculated in two ways:

- through official death certification to the Registrars General (the Office for National Statistics and its equivalents), or

- through deaths reported to this Enquiry. The overall maternal death rate for the Enquiry is calculated from the number of deaths assessed as being due to *Direct* and *Indirect* deaths.

As described in the section on Aims and Methodology and in Chapter 21 Trends in reproductive epidemiology, the numbers of *Direct* and *Indirect* deaths identified by this Enquiry always exceeds those identified from an examination of the cause of death given on death certificates. The Office for National Statistics (ONS) death certificates are examined to select deaths where there is a mention anywhere on the certificate of a pregnancy-related condition, such as eclampsia. Women who die while pregnant but where no mention of the pregnancy is made on the certificate will not be identified in this way. In Scotland, however, there is a box on the certificate that can be ticked to identify that a woman was pregnant, or had recently given birth, at the time of her death.

The overall number of *Direct* and *Indirect* deaths identified by the Enquiry has always exceeded those officially reported. This is because a large proportion of women known to the Enquiry die of pre-existing medical conditions influenced by their pregnant or recently delivered state; for example, cardiac disorders, epilepsy, hormone-dependent malignancies and deaths from suicide, but these are excluded from the official statistics. Also excluded are women who require long-term intensive care and whose final cause of death is registered as a non-pregnancy-related condition, such as multiple organ failure, even though the initiating cause was an obstetric event. Conversely, the maternal deaths known to the Registrars General may include *Late* deaths, as it is not possible to identify from the death certificate when the delivery or termination occurred.

In 2000–02, 148 deaths in the UK were identified from death registrations as having a pregnancy-related condition mentioned on their death certificate. This Enquiry identified 106 *Direct* maternal deaths and 155 *Indirect* maternal deaths, suggesting that only 57% of maternal deaths mention the pregnancy at death registration. Work is currently being undertaken to assess the feasibility of identifying further deaths by linking women's death certificates with recent birth registrations.

The maternal mortality rates derived by both methods of estimation are shown in Table 1.1.

Table 1.1 *Direct* and *Indirect* maternal deaths and mortality rates per 100,000 maternities as reported to the Registrars General (ONS) and to the Enquiry; United Kingdom 1985–2002

Triennium	Maternal deaths known to Registrars General (ONS)		Direct deaths known to the Enquiry		Indirect deaths known to the Enquiry		Total Direct and Indirect deaths known to the Enquiry		Total maternities	95% confidence intervals
	n	Rate	n	Rate	n	Rate	n	Rate	n	
1985–87	174	7.7	139	6.1	84	3.7	223	9.8	2,268,766	8.6–11.2
1988–90	171	7.2	145	6.1	93	3.9	238	10.1	2,360,309	8.8–11.5
1991–93	149	6.4*	128	5.5	100	4.3	228	9.8	2,315,204	8.6–11.2
1994–96	175	8.0***	134	6.1	134	6.1	268	12.2	2,197,640	10.8–13.8
1997–99	142	6.7**	106	5.0	136	6.4	242	11.4	2,123,614	10.0–12.9
2000–02	148	7.4**	106	5.3	155	7.8	261	13.1	1,997,472	11.5–14.8

* Final ONS revised figures for 1991–93; the rate available at the time for the publication of the 1991–93 Report was 6.0
** England and Wales figures for 1994 onwards now include underlying cause and mentions (ICD9 630–676)
*** The rate for 1994–96 in the previous Report was 7.4
Sources: Office for National Statistics; General Register Office – Scotland; General Records Office – Northern Ireland

Cases known to the Enquiry 2000–02

During this triennium 391 maternal deaths were reported to the Enquiry, a slight increase on the 378 cases reported in 1997–99. There were very limited data for 38 cases but it was still possible to code these deaths according to type. Complete data were available for all but two *Direct* deaths.

Of the 391 deaths, 106 were classified as *Direct* and 155 as *Indirect* deaths, representing 27% and 40% of reported cases, respectively. Thirty-six (9%) were classified as *Coincidental* and 94 (24%) as *Late*. The total number of *Direct* and *Indirect* maternal deaths reported to the Enquiry, 261, is higher than the 242 reported in the previous triennium. As was first seen in the last Report, the number of *Indirect* deaths now exceeds the number of *Direct* deaths, as shown in Table 1.2 and Figure 1.1. The overall maternal mortality rate for the United Kingdom for this triennium from deaths due to both *Direct* and *Indirect* causes is 13.1 maternal deaths per 100,000 maternities.

Table 1.2 The number, type and maternal mortality rates notified to the Enquiry per 100,000 maternities; United Kingdom 1985–2002

Type of death	Triennium											
	1985–87		1988–90		1991–93		1994–96		1997–99		2000–02	
	n	Rate	n	Rate	n	Rate	n	Rate	n	Rate	n	Rate
Direct	139	6.1	145	6.1	128	5.5	134	6.1	106	5.0	106	5.3
Indirect	84	3.7	93	3.9	100	4.3	134	6.1	136	6.4	155	7.8
Direct and Indirect total	223	9.8	238	10.1	228	9.8	268	12.2	242	11.4	261	13.1
Coincidental	26	1.1	39	1.7	46	2.0	36	1.6	29	1.4	36	1.8
Late	16*	0.7	48	2.0	46	2.0	72	3.3	107	5.0	94	4.7
Total	265	11.7	339**	14.4**	320	13.8	376	17.1	378	17.8	391	19.6
95% CI	(10.3–13.2)		(12.9–16.0)		(12.4–15.4)		(15.4–18.9)		(16.1–19.7)		(17.7–21.6)	
Total maternities	2,268,766		2,360,309		2,315,204		2,197,640		2,123,614		1,997,472	

* *Late* deaths not routinely notified during this triennium;
** 14 cases with no information

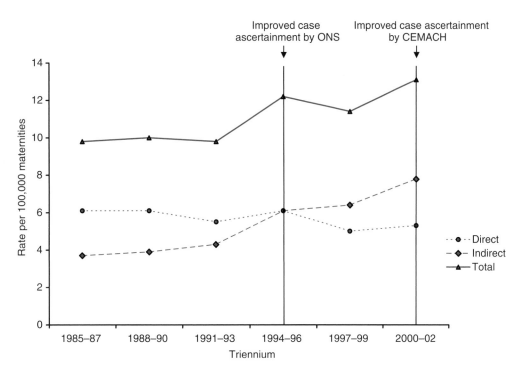

Figure 1.1 *Direct* and *Indirect* maternal mortality rates per 100,000 maternities and the effect of improved systems for case ascertainment; United Kingdom 1985–2002

As described in the earlier section on the definition of maternal mortality, Table 1.3 shows, for purposes of international comparison, the UK Maternal Mortality Ratio (MMR), as defined by the World Health Organization.[1] This is defined as the number of *Direct* and *Indirect* deaths per 100,000 live births. In the UK, maternal death rates have been calculated by using maternities, not just live births, after 24 weeks of gestation, as the denominator. The UK maternal death rate also includes causes of death, which, in the opinion of the Assessors, were related to pregnancy, such as suicide from postnatal mental illness, which are not internationally coded as being maternity related. Thus, the UK MMR is lower than the UK maternal mortality rate.

Table 1.4 gives the actual numbers of deaths and Table 1.5 shows the UK maternal death rates per million maternities by specific cause of death for the last six triennia.

Table 1.3 UK maternal mortality ratio (MMR) 2000–02* compared with UK maternal mortality rate calculated for this Report

Type of death	UK maternal mortality ratio*		UK maternal mortality rate**		
	n	Ratio	*n*	Rate	95% CI
Direct	106	5.3	106	5.3	4.3–6.4
Indirect	136	6.7	155	7.8	6.6–9.1
Total	242	12.0	261	13.1	11.5–14.8

 * International definition; the MMR is defined as the number of *Direct* and *Indirect* deaths (identified by ICD10 codes) per 100,000 live births. The denominator here used is the UK total live births for 2000–02 = 2,016,136. Source: ONS. In this calculation the number of *Indirect* deaths are those which are identified as maternal deaths according to ICD10 definitions only.
** The UK maternal mortality rate is defined as the total number of *Direct* and *Indirect* deaths per 100,000 maternities over 24 weeks of gestation. The denominator here used is all maternities registered in the UK (estimated to be 24 weeks of gestation or more). UK 2000–02 = 1,997,472.
Source: ONS. The number of *Indirect* deaths are those deaths considered by the UK assessors to be indirectly related to pregnancy.

Table 1.4 Number of maternal deaths reported to the Enquiry by cause; United Kingdom 1985–2002*

Chapter	Cause	1985–87	1988–90	1991–93	1994–96	1997–99	2000–02
Direct deaths (occurring during pregnancy and up to and including 42 days inclusive after delivery)							
2	Thrombosis and thromboembolism	32	33	35	48	35	30
3	Hypertensive disease of pregnancy	27	27	20	20	15	14
4	Haemorrhage	10	22	15	12	7	17
5	Amniotic fluid embolism	9	11	10	17	8	5
6	Deaths in early pregnancy total	22	24	18	15	17	15
	Ectopic	16	15	8	12	13	11
	Spontaneous miscarriage	5	6	3	2	2	1
	Legal termination	1	3	5	1	2	3
	Other	0	0	2	0	0	0
7	Genital tract sepsis	6**	7**	9**	14***	14***	11***
8	Other *Direct* total	27	17	14	7	7	8
	Genital tract trauma	6	3	4	5	2	1
	Fatty liver	6	5	2	2	4	3
	Other	15	9	8	0	1	4
9	Anaesthetic	6	4	8	1	3	6
Total number of *Direct* deaths		139	145	128	134	106	106
Indirect deaths (up to and including 42 days after delivery)							
10	Cardiac	22	18	37	39	35	44
11	Psychiatric	N/A	N/A	N/A	9	15	16
12	Other *Indirect*	62	75	63	86	75	90
13	*Indirect* malignancies	N/A	N/A	N/A	N/A	11	5
Total number of *Indirect* deaths		84	93	100	134	136	155
14	*Coincidental* deaths	26	39	46	36	29	36
15	*Late* deaths (42–365 days after delivery)						
	Direct	N/A	13	10	4	7	4
	Indirect	N/A	10	23	32	39	45
	Coincidental	N/A	25	13	36	61	45
Total number of *Late* deaths		16	48	46	72	107	94

N/A = Not available;
 * deaths reported to the Enquiry only and excluding other deaths identified by ONS;
 ** Excluding early pregnancy deaths due to sepsis;
 *** Including early pregnancy deaths due to sepsis

Overall findings 2000–02

- There was an increase in the combined overall maternal mortality rates (*Direct* and *Indirect* deaths) known both to the Registrars General and to this Enquiry. The maternal mortality rate for this triennium, derived from the CEMD data, is 13.1 compared with the 11.4 deaths per 100,000 maternities described in the last Report. There are four factors that could explain this rise:

  - the introduction of the CEMACH Regional Managers and a greater awareness among health professionals in general to report such cases that may not be obviously linked to pregnancy; this appears to have led to a further improvement in case ascertainment, particularly for *Indirect* deaths, which has had the effect of increasing the *Indirect* mortality rate from 6.4 per 100,000 maternities in the last Report to 7.8 in this one

  - the increase in numbers of newly arrived refugees or asylum seekers who did not seek care

Table 1.5 Mortality rates by major cause of maternal death per million maternities; United Kingdom 1985–2002

Chapter	Cause	Rate per million maternities					
		1985–87	1988–90	1991–93	1994–96	1997–99	2000–02
2	Thrombosis and thromboembolism	14.1	14.0	15.1	21.8	16.5	15.0
3	Hypertensive disease of pregnancy	11.9	11.4	8.6	9.1	7.1	7.0
4	Haemorrhage	4.4	9.3	6.5	5.5	3.3	8.5
5	Amniotic fluid embolism	4.0	4.7	4.3	7.7	3.8	2.5
6	Deaths in early pregnancy	7.9*	7.6*	5.2*	6.8	8.0	7.5
7	Genital tract sepsis	4.4	5.5	6.4	6.4*	6.6*	5.5*
8	Total uterine trauma/other *Direct*	11.9	7.2	6.0	3.2	3.3	4.0
	Genital tract trauma	2.6	1.3	1.7	2.3	1.0	0.5
	Other *Direct*	9.3	5.9	4.3	0.9	2.3	3.5
9	Anaesthetic	2.6	1.7	3.5	0.5	1.4	3.0
10	Cardiac *Indirect*	9.7	7.6	15.9	17.7	16.5	22.0
11	Psychiatric *Indirect***	–	–	–	4.1	7.1	8.0
12	Other *Indirect*	27.3	31.0	27.0	39.1	35.3	45.6
13	*Indirect* maligancies	–	–	–	–	5.1	2.5
2–13	Total *Direct* and *Indirect*	98.3	100.1	98.1	121.9	114.0	131.1
14	*Coincidental (Fortuitous)*	11.3	16.5	19.9	16.4	10.8	18.0
15	*Late*	7.1	20.3	19.9	32.8	50.3	47.0

* Including sepsis in early pregnancy;
** until 1993–96 counted as *Coincidental* and note that these are only for suicides which occur during the first 6 weeks. A further explanation of actual death rates from suicide can be found in the text. This table excludes cases identified by ONS but not notified to the Enquiry.

○ numbers increasing by chance; this is likely since the increase in the maternal mortality rate is not statistically significant

○ an increase in the numbers of pregnant women who received substandard care.

• The *Direct* maternal mortality rate, 5.3 deaths per 100,000 maternities, is also higher than the last triennium, but still lower than in any of the other three preceding triennia for which UK data have been collected. By removing the number of *Direct* deaths of recently arrived refugees or asylum seekers this figure is reduced to 5.1 per 100,000 maternities, which is similar to the rate in the last Report.

Specific causes of death

Figure 1.2 shows the major causes of maternal deaths reported to the Enquiry by rate per million maternities. The rate for suicide includes deaths reported to the Enquiry that occurred after the first 6 weeks following delivery, as this is a more accurate reflection of the disease profile of severe puerperal illness. Figure 1.3 gives a breakdown of the main causes of the other *Indirect* deaths.

The ONS birth and maternal death linkage study

In 2001, at the request of this Enquiry, ONS undertook a pilot study to test the feasibility of matching death records of women of fertile age living in England and Wales with birth registrations up to 1 year previously. The aim was to identify deaths of all women

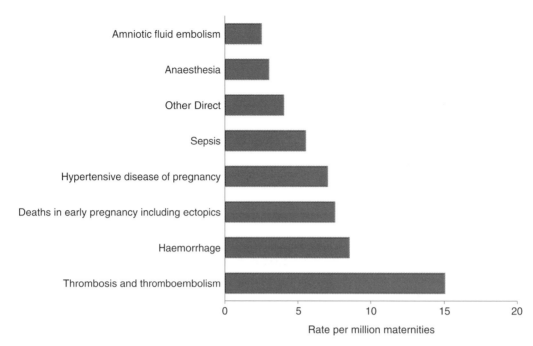

Figure 1.2   Mortality rates per million maternities of leading causes of *Direct* deaths as reported to the Enquiry; United Kingdom 2000–02

in England and Wales who died within 1 year of giving birth and to see how many additional cases would be found. The methodology was reproduced for this triennia and yet again shows that the majority of these deaths occurred some months after delivery. Over 90% (211) of the extra 230 deaths identified through the survey occurred after the first six weeks following delivery and are classified as *Late* deaths. It is not surprising that these deaths were not reported since, by the time they died, these women would have lost contact with their maternity health professional, the person who reports these

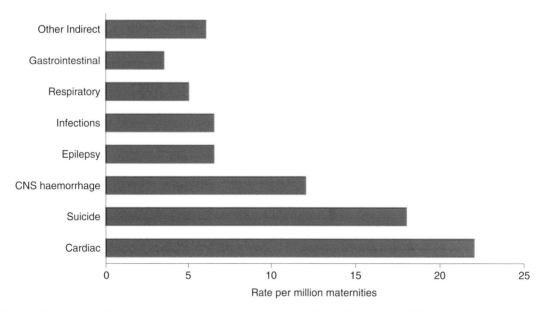

Figure 1.3   Maternal mortality rate from leading causes of *Indirect* deaths per million maternities as reported to the Enquiry; United Kingdom 2000–02

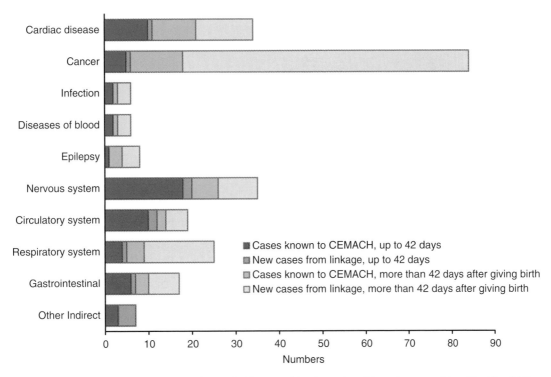

Figure 1.4 Numbers of maternal deaths, excluding psychiatric and accidental causes, identified by ONS record linkage from *Coincidental* or *Indirect* causes: England and Wales 2000–02

cases. The vast majority of these *Late* deaths were due to *Coincidental Late* causes, mainly cancer as shown in Figure 1.4. However, a significant number were due to psychiatric causes and are discussed in the following paragraph.

Suicide is the leading cause of maternal death

As in the last Report, the majority of women who committed suicide after childbirth but within 1 year of delivery were not known to the Enquiry. In all, around 50 women in England and Wales were known to have died of suicide or whose deaths were recorded under an open verdict; only 18 of these were known to the Enquiry. The other 32 deaths all took place some months after delivery. Further, another 14 women had verdicts of deaths due to accidental causes or misadventure and another ten died from drugs and/or alcohol and, in both categories, some of these too would have probably been self-inflicted. All of these groups of women would have not been in contact with the maternity healthcare professionals who would have automatically reported these cases, but they may have been in touch with their general practitioner or local psychiatric services. Figure 1.5 shows the additional cases identified for England and Wales from the record linkage study and Figure 1.6 demonstrates the effect that these additional cases have on the overall UK maternal mortality rate if suicides after 42 days after delivery are included. It is important to note that many women who die as a result of puerperal psychosis do so following the first 6 weeks of delivery, the timeframe usually taken to define a maternal death. Although these cases are classed as *Late Indirect* deaths, they are still counted in the overall maternal mortality rate from suicide. Deaths from psychiatric causes, including suicide drug misuse, are discussed in Chapter 11 Deaths from psychiatric causes.

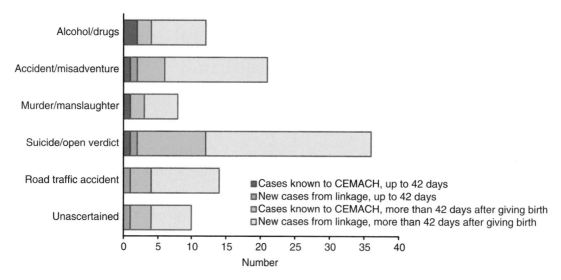

Figure 1.5 Number of maternal deaths identified by ONS record linkage from psychiatric, accidental, violent or unascertained causes; England and Wales 2000–02

Such is the importance that these Enquiries place on learning lessons from deaths from psychiatric causes that CEMACH has now introduced a system of Regional Psychiatric Assessors to enable better and more detailed case assessment.

The children left behind

In the 2000–02 triennium, at least 543 known existing children lost their mother to a reported maternal death. In addition, 209 singleton pregnancies resulted in a live birth and of the ten twin pregnancies and one triplet pregnancy there were 20 live births. This

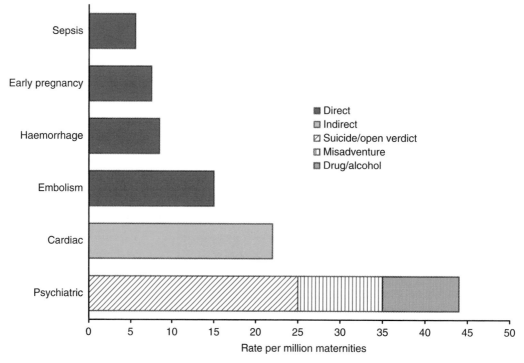

Figure 1.6 Maternal mortality rate per million maternities from leading causes of death as identified by ONS linkage study for England and Wales; 2000–02

Table 1.6 Numbers of maternal deaths by gestation, type of death and the fetal/neonatal outcome; United Kingdom 2000–02

	Undelivered > 24 weeks*	Undelivered < 24 weeks	Live birth**	Stillbirth**	Early neonatal death**	Total
Direct	27	1	64	8	6	106
Indirect	34	24	67	21	9	155
Subtotal Direct and Indirect deaths	61	25	131	29	15	261
Coincidental	17	12	6	1	0	36
Late Direct	0	0	3	1	0	4
Late Indirect	4	0	39	0	2	45
Late Coincidental	3	0	40	1	1	45
Total	85	37	219	32	18	391

* includes ectopic pregnancies, miscarriages and termination of pregnancy
** twins and higher order pregnancies counted as one birth event

gives a total of 229 live babies born to women known to this Enquiry who subsequently died. In all, nearly 800 existing and living newborn children lost their mothers during this triennium. The actual number of children who lost their mothers will undoubtedly be higher, as many of the women who comprise the 230 additional *Late* maternal deaths, not notified to this Enquiry but captured through the ONS record linkage study, will also have had existing children as well as their newborn baby. A perhaps conservative estimate is that over 1,100 children lost their mothers within a few months of pregnancy or giving birth.

Deaths before delivery

As shown in Table 1.6, 86 women died of *Direct* or *Indirect* causes before delivery, 33% of all such maternal deaths. In this group, the main causes of *Direct* deaths were ectopic pregnancy and pulmonary thromboembolism. There were a wide variety of causes of *Indirect* deaths among undelivered women, with deaths from cardiac disease and malignancies among the largest groups.

Delivery of care

Antenatal care

Table 1.7 shows the type of antenatal care received by the women described in this Report. In 37% of cases, care was shared between the GP, community or clinic midwife and the obstetrician – so-called traditional 'shared care'. In many of these cases the woman saw the obstetric staff only once or twice during her antenatal period. For *Direct* and *Indirect* deaths, 61 women (16%), mainly perceived to have been at higher risk of complications, in most instances due to underlying or pre-existing disease, had care provided by the obstetric unit, although they too were often seen at the hospital clinic by the midwife. Sixty-three (16%) women had community-based shared care between midwives and/or GPs, going to the hospital only for scans and other tests. Seventeen percent of women who died from *Direct* or *Indirect* causes did not see an obstetrician until their final admission. In 25 cases, the woman received community-based midwifery-only care, a roughly equal number to the women whose deaths were

Table 1.7 Maternal deaths by type of antenatal care; United Kingdom 2000–02

Type of antenatal care	Classification of death					Total (n)	Overall (%)
	Direct (n)	*Indirect* (n)	*Direct* and *Indirect* (%)	*Coincidental* (n)	*Late* (n)		
Consultant-led unit only	18	26	17	1	16	61	16
Traditional 'shared care'	32	62	36	11	41	146	37
Midwife/GP*	9	13	8	4	12	38	10
Midwife only	7	9	6	2	7	25	6
Concealed pregnancy	2	2	2	1	0	5	1
No antenatal care	4	5	3	3	1	13	3
Late booker/poor attender	11	27	15	4	9	51	13
Death before booking or after miscarriage or TOP	22	7	11	8	5	42	11
Not stated	1	4	2	2	3	10	3
Total	106	155	100	36	94	391	100

* See text

recorded in the last Report but a substantial rise from the eight cases in the 1994–96 Report.

The characteristics of the 25 women who received midwifery-led care are shown in Table 1.8. In ten cases, the women had no known risk factors or significant past medical or psychiatric history, and were appropriate for low-risk midwifery-led care. In these cases, the midwifery-led care appeared excellent, with problems detected early and appropriate transfers made for specialist care. However, in 15 cases (60% of women receiving midwifery-led care) risk factors were clearly present and the women should have been referred for obstetric or multidisciplinary care either at booking or as soon as potential problems became apparent. Several women with known domestic violence, previously involving social services support, also elected for midwifery-led care but failed to access social service or other local support networks and advice. In two cases of midwifery-led care, the woman declined to be referred to the obstetricians and the midwife providing care, in very difficult circumstances, was supported throughout by her local supervisor of midwives and through regular contact with the local obstetric team.

Eighteen (47%) of the women who had joint midwifery- and GP-led care were also at higher risk of developing a significant medical, obstetric or puerperal mental health problem and should have been referred, at least for assessment, to the local multidisciplinary medical, obstetric or perinatal mental health team.

Table 1.8 Characteristics of women receiving midwifery only or joint midwifery and GP care; United Kingdom 2000–02

Characteristic	Midwifery-led care	Joint GP/midwifery care
No known risk factors of past history: appropriate care (n)	10	20
Severe domestic violence and known to social services (n)	4	2
Severe previous or concurrent mental illness (n)	4	6
Known pre-existing cardiac disease (n)	3	2
Obstetric complications with no/late referral (n)	1	4
Significant concurrent medical disorder (n)	3	4
Total women with one or more characteristic (n)	16	22
Total all women (n)	25	38
Overall inappropriate antenatal care (%)	60	47

Table 1.9 Maternal deaths by place of delivery over 24 weeks of completed gestation; United Kingdom 2000–02

Type of death	Consultant unit	Midwife-led unit	A&E	ICU	Hospital other	Home	Total
Direct	74		1			3	78
Indirect	78	1	14	1	3		97
Coincidental	6				1		7
Late	89	2				3	94
Total	247	3	15	1	4	6	276

A&E = accident and emergency department; ICU = intensive care unit

Place of delivery

The place of delivery for women dying of all causes of death is shown in Table 1.9.

Two women who delivered at home died of postpartum haemorrhage. In both cases they had not sought any care during pregnancy, had delivered and died on their own, and were found later by their relatives. One baby survived. Another woman who died of a coincidental cause some months after delivery had also not sought any antenatal care and delivered at home on the toilet; the baby drowned. There were no other instances where the circumstances of the home birth or delivery in a midwifery-led unit had a direct bearing on the eventual outcome. The 13 women who delivered in accident and emergency departments or elsewhere in the hospital were either brought in undergoing cardiopulmonary resuscitation, had collapsed or had a precipitate delivery.

Type of delivery

Table 1.10 shows the type of delivery for all maternal deaths occurring after 24 weeks of completed gestation.

The types of caesarean section were classified according to the definitions from the Royal College of Obstetrics and Gynaecology (RCOG) and these are given in Box 1.1.

Table 1.10 Number of maternal deaths by mode of delivery; United Kingdom 2000–02

Type of delivery	Direct	Indirect	Coincidental	Late	Total
Spontaneous vaginal	19	36	3	53	111
Induced vaginal	2	4	1	7	14
Ventouse	2	3		2	7
Forceps	3	3		3	9
Vaginal breech	2	1			3
Caesarean section					
Emergency	24	13		9	46
Urgent	2	5		5	12
Elective	15	14	3	15	47
Perimortem	5	14			19
Postmortem	4	4			8
Caesarean section total	50	50	3	29	132
Total delivered	78	97	7	94	276

Box 1.1   RCOG Definition of type of caesarean section

Type	Definition
Emergency	Immediate threat to life of woman or fetus
Urgent	Maternal or fetal compromise which is not immediately life threatening
Scheduled	Needing early delivery but no maternal or fetal compromise
Elective	At a time to suit the patient and the maternity team
Perimortem	Carried out in extremis while the mother is undergoing active resuscitation
Postmortem	Carried out after the death of the mother in order to try to save the fetus

Caesarean section

Previous Reports have sometimes included a specific chapter on deaths after caesarean section. The balance of maternal and fetal risks between caesarean section and vaginal delivery is a controversial topic. The 2004 guideline on caesarean section from the National Collaborating Centre for Women's and Children's Health on behalf of the National Institute of Clinical Excellence (NICE) does not support planned caesarean sections without clear clinical indications.[2] Others have argued that, within the agenda of maternal choice in maternity care, this is a legitimate option. The risk of maternal death is one of the factors included in estimates of risk–benefit and death rates calculated in previous Reports which have been used to inform this debate.

However, in considering these deaths, it is almost impossible to disentangle the consequences of caesarean section from the indication for the operation. True, there are occasional deaths from anaesthesia or haemorrhage that result directly from the procedure. There are also deaths that may well have been made more likely by the method of delivery, for example from pulmonary embolism. There were several cases in this triennium in which the caesarean section itself may well have contributed to the fatal outcome but, in these cases, the caesarean section itself was undertaken as a possible life-saving measure for the mother and/or her baby. For the large majority of deaths that followed caesarean section, however, there were serious prenatal complications or illness that, in many cases, precipitated the caesarean section. Perimortem caesarean section is the starkest example of this.

Because of these difficulties of interpretation, the authors of this Report decided not to include a separate chapter on caesarean section because of the undue weight this might place on the findings presented here. The caveats discussed here mean that **the simple mortality rates calculated according to method of delivery, shown in Table 1.11, should be interpreted with caution and require further study and interpretation before any meaningful conclusion can be drawn**. It is important to note that, during this triennium, no women died from the direct effects of anaesthesia for a caesarean section undertaken at her request and for which there was no clinical indication.

Table 1.11 was calculated by using Hospital Episode Statistics (HES) data to estimate the overall number of caesarean sections that took place in the United Kingdom between 2000 and 2002. Unfortunately, information on the RCOG classification of the denominator of type of caesarean section is not available. An assumption has been made that

Table 1.11 Estimated case fatality rates per 100,000 maternities over 24 weeks of gestation and relative risk by type of delivery for *Direct* and *Indirect* deaths; United Kingdom 2000–02

Type of delivery	Total number (000s)	Delivered *Direct* and *Indirect* deaths (*n*)	Death rate per 100,000 maternities	95% CI for death rate	Relative risk (RR)	95% CI for RR
Vaginal	1571	75	48	3.8–6.0	1.0	–
All Caesarean section	426	73	172	13.4–21.6	3.7	2.6–5.0
Emergency and urgent	212	44	208	15.1–27.9	4.3	3.0–6.3
Scheduled and elective	214	29	136	9.1–19.5	2.8	1.9–4.4

Source: Derived from the Department of Health Hospital Episode Statistics data for 2000–02

the relative proportion of each type is identical to the previous triennium. This means that the estimates are even less secure.

Further, from the reports available to this Enquiry, there were problems in identifying the correct coding of deaths according to type. For example only seven cases were recorded as urgent and 35 were classified as an emergency. No caesarean sections were classified as scheduled, yet 29 were classified as being elective procedures. In this Report, all the elective caesarean sections were undertaken for clinical reasons but did not need to be performed urgently. These categories have therefore been combined in Table 1.11, which estimates the crude relative risk of the type of caesarean section against all vaginal deliveries where the relative risk of maternal death is taken to be one. Women who had already died or who were undergoing active cardiopulmonary resuscitation are excluded form this table, as the indication for the procedure in their case was a maternal death.

Such is the difficulty in interpreting the data available to the Enquiry that it is recommended urgent further research, in the form of a prospective study, be undertaken in this area. This will help to estimate more robustly what, if any, is the degree of increased risk associated with all types of caesarean section but particularly for those undertaken without urgent or immediate need to save the life of the mother or baby.

Table 1.12 shows the fetal outcomes for peri- or postmortem caesarean sections carried out either while the mother was undergoing active cardiopulmonary resuscitation or after her death had been confirmed. No babies survived a postmortem caesarean section but eight of nineteen babies survived a perimortem caesarean section, including five undertaken in an accident and emergency department. These findings yet again show that, in this and all previous triennia, no baby has survived a postmortem caesarean section. On the other hand, the eight babies who survived a perimortem section represent a significant increase compared to previous Reports. These findings underscore the futility of attempting a postmortem section but indicate that, with improved

Table 1.12 Outcomes of peri- or postmortem caesarean sections by place of delivery; United Kingdom 2000–02

	A&E	Delivery room or operating theatre	ICU or hospital other	Total
Live birth	1	4	3	8
Still birth	12	3	0	15
Early neonatal death	2	1	1	4
Total	15	8	4	27

resuscitation techniques, more babies are surviving perimortem caesarean sections, particularly where the woman has collapsed in an already well-staffed and equipped delivery room or operating theatre.

Risk factors for maternal deaths

Access to care

Poor attendance

Table 1.13 shows that 19% of the women who died of *Direct* or *Indirect* causes did not receive optimum antenatal care, in that they booked late (after 22 weeks of gestation), did not attend for antenatal care at all or were described as poor attenders at the antenatal clinic. As with the 20% of such women identified in the last Report, in the vast majority of cases these women were not actively followed up when they failed to attend the clinic. A disproportionate number of these women came from non-White ethnic groups.

Characteristics of women who booked late or who were poor attenders at antenatal clinic.

From Table 1.13 it can be seen that, if *Late* deaths are used as a control, with 11% of these women overall attending for antenatal care less than optimally advised, women who died of *Direct, Indirect* or *Coincidental* causes were twice as likely to book late or to be poor attenders for antenatal care. Further analysis by the type of *Late* death (*Direct, Indirect* or *Coincidental*) shows no variation in their attendance patterns by type of death for this group of women.

The predominant characteristics of women who booked late or who were poor attenders at clinic are shown in Table 1.14. Virtually all of the women who died from *Direct* or *Indirect* causes were socially excluded. By contrast, an average of eight percent of women who died from *Coincidental* or *Late* causes appeared to be socially excluded.

It can be seen from Table 1.14 that the majority of women who died and who were homeless, refugees or asylum seekers, known to social services or who had previous children in care, were very poor attenders for care. Further, the majority of women

Table 1.13 Antenatal attendance by type of death; United Kingdom 2000–02

	Total deaths	Late booker > 22 weeks	Late booker > 28 weeks	Poor attender at ANC	No antenatal care at all*	Total of late, non or poor attenders (n)	Percentage of all deaths (%)
Direct (n)	106	6	2	4	6	18	18
Indirect (n)	155	7	8	10	7	32	22
Total Direct and Indirect (n)	261	13	10	14	13	50	19
Total Direct and Indirect (%)		5	4	5	5	19	19
Coincidental (n)	36	1	1	2	4	8	22
Late (n)	94	2	1	6	1	10	11
Total (n)	391	16	12	22	18	68	17

* excluding early deaths; ANC = antenatal clinic

Table 1.14 Analysis of women who were late bookers (more than 22 weeks of gestation) or poor or non-attenders by predominant characteristics*; United Kingdom 2000–02

Predominant characteristics	Direct	Indirect	Coincidental	Late	All	Total number of women in this group	Characteristic for all women in this group (%)
Homeless/constant change of address	2	2		1	5	5	100
Children in care	2	3	1	1	7	8	88
Refugee/asylum seeker	5	4		2	11	14	79
Known to social services	4	5	2	3	14	19	74
Domestic violence	12	9	11	7	39	55	71
Little/no English	4	5			9	15	60
Substance misuse	4	5	2	3	14	32	45
Extreme poverty	4	5		2	11	25	44
Past or ongoing severe psychiatric illness	3	6		3	12	60	20
Ethnic Group *(for England only see later section)*							
Indian/Pakistani	4	5		1	10	17	59
Black African	7	6		1	17	30	57
Black Caribbean		4	1	1	6	13	46
Asian/other		1			1	4	25
White	10	10	6	4	30	151	20

* many had more than one characteristic

experiencing domestic violence found it hard to keep in touch with antenatal services, as did almost 50% of the women whose lives were characterised by extreme poverty or substance misuse.

More than 50% of the women who died and who came from ethnic groups other than White or Asian also found it difficult to book at the appropriate time or attended clinics rarely.

HES data show that, in general, women from non-White ethnic groups are twice as likely to book later than 20 weeks of gestation. Late bookers constitute about 11% of the White pregnant population and 20% of the non-White pregnant population. In this Report, 40% of the women from the non-White groups who died from *Direct* causes and 24% of those women who died from *Indirect* causes had not booked by 24 weeks of gestation.

Women who concealed their pregnancies or who did not attend for any care and were unknown to the antenatal maternity services

Five women who actively concealed their pregnancies and a further 12 women who did not attend for any antenatal care at all died. The major characteristics of these women are shown in Table 1.15. Four of the five women who concealed their pregnancies were known to social services and three had had their previous children taken into care. Being previously known to social services and having other children in care was the highest risk factor for poor attendance (56%). Fifty percent of the women who did not seek care at all also suffered from partner violence. The lessons to be drawn from the deaths in this group of women are discussed in more detail in Chapter 11 Deaths from psychiatric causes.

All of the women who concealed their pregnancies were White, whereas five of the eleven women who did not attend for antenatal care were from non-White ethnic minority groups. Three were refugees or asylum seekers who did not speak English.

Table 1.15 Characteristics of women who concealed their pregnancies or who did not attend for antenatal care; United Kingdom 2000–02

	Concealed	Did not attend	Total (*n*)	All deaths (%)
Type of death				
Direct	2	4	6	*6*
Indirect	1	5	6	*4*
Coincidental	2	2	4	*11*
Late	0	1	1	*0.3*
Total	5	12	17	*4*
Predominant characteristics (most had had more than one)				
Domestic violence	3	5	8	*50*
Little/no English	1	3	4	*24*
Substance misuse	1	4	5	*31*
Extreme poverty	4	4	8	*50*
Refugee/asylum seeker	1	3	4	*24*
Homeless/constant change of address	2	2	4	*24*
Grande multipara (more than 4 previous births)	2	0	2	*12*
Always concealed pregnancies	2	0	2	*12*
Previous children in care	3	3	6	*36*
Known to social services	4	5	9	*56*
Ethnic group other than White	0	5	5	*31*

Substandard care

Substandard care was difficult to evaluate in some of the cases in this Report, owing to the lack of key data from some records and case notes. While it is clear that many of the cases received less than optimum care, it has not always been possible to quantify these with certainty. Box 1.2 gives the definitions of substandard care used in this Report for those cases it was possible to completely assess.

Box 1.2   Definitions of substandard care used in this Report

Major   Contributed significantly to the death of the mother i.e. different management would reasonably have been expected to alter the outcome

Minor   It was a relevant contributory factor. Different management might have made a difference but the mother's survival was unlikely in any case

---

Despite the limitations, the assessors classified 67% of *Direct* deaths as having some form of substandard care, as shown in Table 1.16. This compares with 60% in the last Report. Forty-seven percent of *Direct* deaths had major substandard care in which different treatment may have affected the outcome. Forty-one percent of cardiac deaths were associated with some degree of substandard care, as were 62% of psychiatric deaths and 28% of deaths from *Other Indirect* causes. These figures are shown in Table 1.17 and are all increased from the last Report. By contrast, only about 10% of both *Coincidental* and *Late* deaths had substandard care with 7% in each category being classified as major. The concerns about the care of these cases were a lack of liaison and communication between the health and social services in providing support for vulnerable young girls and in lack of multidisciplinary or coordinated care.

Table 1.16 Numbers and percentage of *Direct* deaths assessed as having substandard care; United Kingdom 2000–02

Cause of death and chapter number	Major substandard care (*n*)	Minor substandard care (*n*)	Total cases in chapter (*n*)	Overall substandard care (*n*)	(%)
2. Thrombosis	12	5	30	17	57
3. Hypertension	6	1	14	7	50
4. Haemorrhage	10	2	17	12	71
5. Amniotic fluid embolism	0	3	5	3	60
6. Early pregnancy	10	0	15	10	67
7. Sepsis	2	8	13	10	77
8. Other *Direct*	4	2	8	6	75
9. Anaesthetic	6	0	6	6	100
Total	50	21	106	71	67

The specific cases and lessons to be learned are discussed in the relevant chapters of this Report and lessons are highlighted and reflected in the recommendations.

With the introduction of the new CEMACH Regional Managers it is anticipated that more complete case notes will be available for the next Report, thus enabling a greater degree of accuracy in the assessment of these cases.

Table 1.18 gives the percentage change of cases with substandard care compared with the last Report. The increase, particularly in the proportion of cases of *Indirect* deaths with substandard care, is worrying and requires more detailed consideration and assessment in future Reports. Several assessors were concerned that, in their opinion, there appeared to have been an increase in some healthcare professionals failing to identify and manage common medical conditions or potential emergencies outside their immediate area of expertise. This message is repeated in several chapters in this Report.

Overall, many of the main causes of substandard care remain unchanged from previous Reports and while they are discussed in more detail in the individual chapters in this Report, they are also summarised below. Some are due to problems in the system of healthcare delivery, such as lack of intensive care beds or problems with blood supplies, but in the main the faults lie at the professional level within facilities. The four bullet

Table 1.17 Numbers and percentage of *Indirect* deaths assessed as having substandard care; United Kingdom 2000–02

Cause of death and chapter number	Major substandard care (*n*)	Minor substandard care (*n*)	Total cases in chapter (*n*)	Overall substandard care (*n*)	(%)
10. Cardiac	9	9	44	18	41
11. Psychiatric*	5	5	16	10	62
12. Other *Indirect*	15	10	90	25	28
13. Cancer**	2	1	5	3	60
Total	31	25	155	56	36

* Only includes deaths from suicide and drug overdose classified as *Indirect*
** Only includes deaths from cancer classified as *Indirect*

Table 1.18 Percentage change in cases of *Direct* and *Indirect* deaths associated with substandard care; United Kingdom 1997–2002

	1997–99 (%)	2000–02 (%)
Direct		
Major	50	47
Minor	10	20
Total	60	67
Indirect		
Major	13	20
Minor	9	16
Total	22	36
Coincidental	10	10
Late	10	10

points in bold are new findings relating to this Report:

- **failure of some obstetric and midwifery staff to recognise and act on medical conditions outside their immediate experience**

- **failure of accident and emergency staff to recognise the severity of the illness in sick pregnant women and to ask for obstetric or midwifery assessment**

- **lack of active follow-up of women who were known not to attend for antenatal care, particularly for those women with known high risk conditions**

- **failure of GPs and other medical specialists to pass on relevant past or current medical information in referral letters or by telephone to the booking clinics or to maternity health care staff during pregnancy**

- lack of communication and teamwork, both within the obstetric and midwifery teams and in multidisciplinary team working

- failure to appreciate the severity of the illness, suboptimal treatment or to call for senior assistance

- wrong diagnoses or treatment

- failure of junior staff or general practitioners to diagnose or refer the case to a senior colleague or hospital

- failure of consultants to attend and inappropriate delegation of responsibility

- lack of immediate access to intensive care or high dependency beds or to blood supplies

- in some units, the continuing lack of a clear policy for the prevention or treatment of conditions such as pulmonary embolism, eclampsia or massive haemorrhage.

Care in accident and emergency departments

While, in some cases, the standard of care or resuscitation that women received from accident and emergency departments was excellent, regrettably 14 women with significant obstetric or medical problems in pregnancy were mismanaged by the staff of the departments they attended. A number of other women had more minor incidences of substandard care. Concerns over the lack of appropriate diagnosis and care in some accident and emergency departments has been a growing trend over the previous two Reports but is now significant enough to warrant a separate section as a possible risk factor for maternal deaths. Many of the lessons from these cases are discussed in the relevant chapters of this Report but the overall lessons to be learned are drawn together here. Examples of poor care include:

> An obviously pregnant woman who could not speak English was taken by her friends to the local accident and emergency department with a history of what seemed liked fits; an unequivocal symptom of an obstetric emergency. She was seen by the triage nurse who, despite a recording a raised blood pressure, assessed her as not to be an urgent case and placed her in a side ward. She was not reviewed again and was found dead some hours later.

> A woman with abdominal pain that proved to be an ectopic pregnancy was classed as a low priority by another triage nurse. She, too, waited for several hours without seeing a doctor and collapsed and died.

> A woman with a suspected pulmonary embolism in pregnancy was left on a trolley in the accident and emergency department for more than 24 hours and was then discharged, having been shown how to inject herself with low-molecular-weight heparin. She was neither admitted nor seen by or referred to an obstetrician.

Box 1.3   Accident and emergency department recommendations

- All pregnant women attending accident and emergency departments should be seen quickly, by a doctor, and those with anything other than very minor physical injuries should be seen in conjunction with an obstetrician or senior midwife. If these are not available on site then arrangements should be made with the local maternity unit to discuss these cases.

- The care of pregnant women with medical conditions requiring treatment, and particularly hospital admission, should be discussed and planned in conjunction with the local obstetric team.

- All women of childbearing age who present with unexplained abdominal pain should have ectopic pregnancy excluded as part of their diagnostic work up. Dipstick testing for hCG is now quick, easy, and sensitive.

- Clinicians and staff in primary care and accident and emergency departments, in particular, need to be aware of atypical clinical presentations of ectopic pregnancy and especially of the way in which it may mimic gastrointestinal disease.

- Individual obstetric units should develop protocols for the management of pregnant women who are acutely ill/collapsed for non-obstetric reasons. This must involve liaison with emergency services and accident and emergency departments regarding the most appropriate site (accident and emergency departments, local delivery suite or another hospital) to ensure women receive speedy resuscitation.

The general failings in accident and emergency departments can be summarised as:

- failure by the triage nurses to recognise warning symptoms of obstetric emergencies, including ectopic pregnancies, resulting in a few women being assessed as low risk and not being seen by any medical staff before they collapsed and died

- failure by junior accident and emergency staff and senior medical staff to recognise the warning symptoms of obstetric emergencies, including ectopic pregnancies, resulting in failure of accident and emergency department senior staff and other consultants to involve the obstetric department over planning care for very sick women; pregnant women were discharged home or admitted and treated, sometimes for a week or longer, without their obstetrician or midwife ever being informed

- excessively long waits for clearly ill pregnant women to be seen by medical staff or be admitted.

As a result of the current findings, the recommendations made in previous Reports have been strengthened; restated here and given in Box 1.3. CEMACH is also appointing an assessor for accident and emergency departments to be part of this Enquiry.

Ethnicity

As ONS data for the ethnic group of the mother are confined to country of birth, it is not possible to calculate directly the maternal death rates by ethnic group, as many mothers will be second- third or more generation women born in the UK. Ethnic group information is now being collected as part of the HES system for England, but it is not complete for the years covered by this Report. There was 67% HES coverage of births by ethnic group for the period 2000–02.

Using the 2000–02 distribution by ethnic group as a best estimate for the period covered by this Report leads to the estimates of maternal death rates by ethnic group for England only. Unlike the last Report where the specific coding was often incomplete and the ONS codes for Black African, Black Caribbean, Black Other and Black Mixed were grouped together, in this Report the category Black African has been separated out, as these women have by far the greatest risk of maternal death. Table 1.19 shows the estimated rate of maternal death by major ethnic group classifications for 2000–02.

Table 1.19   Number and estimated rates of maternal deaths by type and ethnic group: *England only* 2000–02

Ethnic group	Estimated number of maternities	*Direct* deaths* (*n*)	*Indirect* deaths* (*n*)	Total *Direct* and *Indirect* deaths (*n*)	Estimated rate per 100,000 maternities	95% CI for death rate	Relative risk	95% CI for RR
White	1,407,352	58	93	151	*10.7*	9.1–12.6	1.0	
Black African	41,615	13	17	30	*72.1*	48.6–102.9	6.7	4.5–9.9
Black Caribbean	50,463	7	6	13	*25.8*	13.7–44.1	2.4	1.4–4.2
Pakistani	81,052	7	3	10	*12.3*	5.9–22.7	1.2	0.6–2.2
Indian	45,157	2	5	7	*15.5*	6.2–31.9	1.4	0.7–3.1
Bangladeshi	35,626	3	5	8	*22.5*	9.7–44.2	2.1	1.0–4.3
Asian and Others	70,136	3	1	4	*5.7*	1.6–14.6	0.5	0.2–1.4
Non white	231,971	35	37	72	*31.0*	24.3–39.1	2.9	2.2–3.9
Total	1,639,323	93	130	223	*13.6*	11.9–15.5		

* includes 10 Black African refugee/asylum-seeking women; excluding these women gives a maternal deaths rate for Black African women in England of 48 per 100,000 maternities

As Table 1.19 shows, there was a statistically increased risk of maternal mortality for women from the Black African and Black Caribbean ethnic groups. Of these, by far the largest proportion of deaths was in Black African women. These women are seven times more likely to die than White women and three times more likely to die than Black Caribbean or other Black women and those of Bangladeshi origin. Excluding deaths from Black African refugees and asylum seekers reduces the overall risk to four-fold, still the highest risk group in terms of ethnicity for maternal death. These are discussed further below. While rates for women from India, Bangladesh and Pakistan appear to be slightly increased when compared with the rates for White women, these are not statistically significant.

These findings need to be interpreted with some caution, owing to the small numbers involved and coding difficulties. However, from the other data available to this Enquiry, the relative risk of death among all groups of women appears to be related to their health-seeking behaviour, with women who did not access care, from whatever ethnic background, being at most risk. Cultural differences also appeared to have played a part.

Asylum seekers and recent immigrants

Fourteen women were recently arrived in the UK, of whom ten could be classified as refugees or asylum seekers. Of these, only three were known to be pregnant on arrival. Among this group there were seven *Direct* deaths, five *Indirect* deaths and two *Late* deaths. Four of these women did not access antenatal care at all, five booked after 28 weeks of gestation and another two were very poor attenders for care. Eight did not speak English and only three received timely and appropriate care. Of the women who had little or no access to antenatal care, all but one presented late with an acute obstetric emergency which, in the main, was treated appropriately. However, in two cases care was substandard.

Translation

Fifteen women did not speak English and only two had access to translation services. In the other cases, family members were used as interpreters. Several of these were the woman's own children, who may have been the only family members who could speak English, having learned it at school. As with the last Report, the use of family members as translators causes concern because:

- the woman may be too shy to seek help for intimate concerns

- it is not clear how much correct information was conveyed to the woman, as the person who was interpreting did not have a good grasp of the language or may have withheld information in those cases where the woman's pre-existing medical condition meant she was at significant risk

- in some cases, the translator was a perpetrator of domestic violence against his partner, thus not enabling her to ask for advice or help

- it is not appropriate for a child to translate intimate details about his or her mother and unfair on both the woman and child.

National Statistics Socio-Economic Classification

From 2001, the National Statistics Socio-Economic Classification (NS SEC) has replaced social class in all official statistics in the United Kingdom. To calculate the NS SEC, the occupational code of either the husband or partner of the woman was classified into the three-class version of NS SEC. Single mothers were identified as having no partner.

The United Kingdom maternity denominators have been derived by using a 10% sample of live births for England and Wales coded by NS SEC (based on father's occupation) and 100% of live births coded by NS SEC from Scotland and Northern Ireland. Similar maternity denominators for single mothers were derived using sole registration live births data. The proportions for NS SEC and single mothers were then applied to the 2000–02 UK maternity total (1,997,472).

The results, for the cases for which information was available, are shown in Table 1.20. A true comparison with the findings in the previous Report 1997–99 is not possible. However, women in the lower NS SEC categories still have a higher risk of maternal death. Women from the 'Not Classified' group appear to have almost a 20 times greater risk of dying of *Direct* and *Indirect* causes compared with women in 'Managerial and Professional occupations'. The "Not Classified" group includes all those who were described as unemployed. Single mothers have a three times greater risk of maternal death than women with a husband or partner. Although not directly statistically comparable with the last Report, findings by NS SEC are remarkably similar to those calculated using the old social class definitions given in the last Report. This inequality could be seen for all causes of maternal death apart from suicide, which showed little gradient.

Deprivation classification

For the first time, maternal deaths that occurred to residents of England have been analysed using the 2004 English Indices of Multiple Deprivation. This is a measure of multiple deprivation that is experienced by individuals living in an area (for further details, see: www.odpm.gov.uk/stellent/groups/odpm_urbanpolicy/documents/page/odpm_urbpol_

Table 1.20   Maternal deaths by National Statistics Socio-Economic Classification (NS SEC); United Kingdom 2000–02

NS SEC	Direct deaths (*n*)	Indirect deaths (*n*)	Total (*n*)	Maternal mortality rate*	95% CI
Based on husband's/partner's occupation					
Managerial and professional occupations	10	18	28	4.1	2.7–5.9
Intermediate occupations	11	18	29	8.3	5.5–11.8
Routine and manual occupations	27	24	51	7.0	5.2–9.2
Not classified**	24	41	65	76.7	59.2–97.7
Total	72	101	173	9.3	7.9–10.7
Single mothers	18	25	43	29.7	21.5–40.0
Total	90	126	216	10.8	9.4–12.3

* per 100,000 maternities
** includes the following pseudo code definitions: Inadequately described conditions; Retired; Students; Independent means; Permanently sick; Full-time care of the home and/or dependent relatives, voluntary workers; No previous job; Unemployed person with no other information

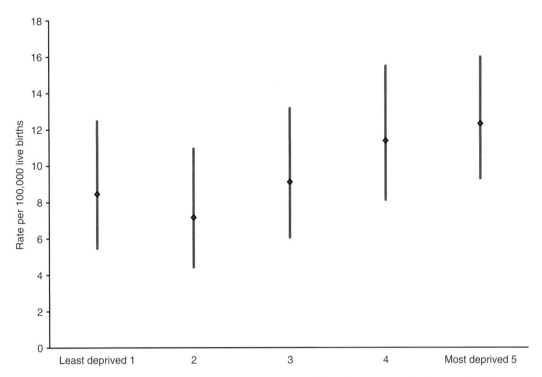

Figure 1.7 Maternal death rates and 95% confidence intervals by deprivation quintiles; England 2000–2002

029534.pdf). There were 187 maternal deaths in England and 170 of these had a valid postcode at the time of death. A deprivation score was assigned to each woman using the postcode. The scores were then grouped into quintiles.

Figure 1.7 shows the maternal (*Direct* and *Indirect*) mortality rate in England by deprivation quintiles. This shows that there is a strong correlation between deprivation and maternal deaths. Women living in the most deprived areas of England had a 45% higher death rate compared with women living in the most affluent areas.

Domestic violence

Fifty-one (13%) of the 391 women whose deaths were assessed had either self-reported a history of domestic violence to a healthcare professional caring for them or the abuse was already known to health and social services. Domestic violence was fatal for 12 women. Thirty-two of the other 39 deaths where the women were known to have suffered violence were due to either *Direct* or *Indirect* causes. Among *Coincidental* and *Late* deaths, 6% and 10%, respectively, were in women known to be subject to domestic violence. This percentage is undoubtedly an underestimate of the true prevalence of violence among this group of women, as in none of the 391 cases was a history of violence actively sought through routine questioning as part of the social or family history at booking.

Seven of the nine girls or young women aged less than 18 years who died were in violent, dependent relationships and four had been sexually abused in the past. Three of the girls who had suffered sexual abuse were aged 16 years or under. Five of these women were living in or had recently lived in refuges.

The characteristics of domestic violence in relation to pregnancy are discussed in more detail in Chapter 14 but, as in the last Report, one of the major findings was that 64%

Table 1.21 Deaths in women known to be suffering domestic violence (DV) and who were delivered or 22 weeks pregnant or more; United Kingdom 2000–02

	Total deaths in women with DV (n)	Late booker > 22 weeks (n)	Poor attender at ANC (n)	No antenatal care at all (n)	Total of late or non attenders (n)	Total poor or non-attendance in women with known DV (%)
Direct	13	4	4	2	10	77
Indirect	12	3	2	1	6	50
Murdered	11	4	3	3	10	90
Other						
Coincidental	2	1			1	50
Late	9	1	4		5	55
Total	51	13	13	6	32	64

of women in abusive relationships found it difficult to access or maintain contact with antenatal care services. Table 1.21 shows more detailed characteristics of this. This table also shows that the rates for late booking, poor or no attendance at all were even higher among women who were murdered or who died of *Direct* causes.

Substance misuse

Thirty-one women died during 2000–02 whose deaths were known to be associated with problem drug and/or alcohol use, although this may not have been the final cause of their death. Their deaths and the lessons to drawn from these are discussed in Chapter 11B Drug and/or alcohol misuse in pregnancy.

Fifteen of these women were known by maternity services to have a drug and/or alcohol problem. Only three women were managed within integrated multidisciplinary services according to best practice guidelines. The remainder appeared to have been managed within mainstream services. In three cases, it was recorded that a specialist midwife contributed to care with inputs that ranged from regular support to a single consultation. These women also attended addiction and/or social services but did so in parallel with no inter-agency liaison. Some other women attending mainstream services were also referred to addiction services.

Obesity

Seventy-eight women (35%) who died from *Direct* or *Indirect* causes were classified by the assessors as obese with a body mass index (BMI) of 30 or more and, of these, over 20 were morbidly obese (BMI 35 or greater). Thirty-five percent of women who died from *Direct* causes were obese as were 26% of those who died from *Indirect* deaths. On average, 29% of women who suffered a *Direct* or *Indirect* maternal death were obese. This compares with 23% of the general female population of childbearing age in England as described in Chapter 21 Trends in reproductive epidemiology.

Several of these women were so obese that they required special equipment to help at their delivery and, in a few cases, caesarean sections had to be performed on normal beds, as the weight of the woman exceeded the maximum weight for the operating table. This is discussed more in Chapter 18 Midwifery practice.

Table 1.22 Maternal mortality rate for multiple births; United Kingdom 1997–2002

| | Maternities (*n*) | Direct and Indirect deaths | | |
		(*n*)	Rate per 100,000 maternities	95% CI
Singleton				
1997–99	2,093,965	234	11.2	9.8–12.7
2000–02	1,967,834	255	13.0	11.5–14.6
Multiple				
1997–99	30,578	8	26.2	13.3–51.6
2000–02	29,638	6	20.2	9.3–44.2

Multiple pregnancies

Eleven women had multiple pregnancies: ten sets of twins and one set of triplets. Five deaths were due to *Direct* causes, three were *Coincidental* and three *Late*. One of the three *Late* deaths was *Indirect*. In the previous Report, eight of the eleven deaths associated with multiple pregnancy were considered to be directly or indirectly associated with pregnancy. Table 1.22 shows that these differences are compatible with random variation, but this may be a consequence of the small numbers of women with multiple pregnancies.

Infertility

Eight women were known to have undergone in vitro fertilisation (IVF) for infertility, four resulting in a multiple pregnancy. Each of these deaths was from a different cause. Five were from *Direct* and three were from *Indirect* causes of deaths. Thus, all eight deaths were considered to be directly or indirectly associated with pregnancy. Figures from the Human Fertilisation and Embryology Authority (HFEA), which are published on a financial year basis, show that for the three financial years April 1999 to April 2002, there were 21,424 IVF maternities. Using these data as a proxy for January 2000 to December 2002, the period of this Report, gives an estimated maternal mortality rate of 37.3 per 100,000 IVF maternities with 95% confidence limits from 18.9 to 73.7 per 100,000 IVF maternities. The estimated rate for the last Report was 48.4 per 100,000 maternities, with 95% confidence limits from 26.3 to 89.1 per 100,000 maternities. Thus, no difference was detected between the mortality rates for women undergoing IVF in the two triennia but, in both triennia, the rates were well above the overall rates of *Direct* and *Indirect* maternal deaths and those for singleton pregnancies.

Age

Maternal mortality is closely related to maternal age, as shown in Table 1.23 and Figure 1.8. For more robust analysis, the rates have been calculated for all maternal deaths by age between the years 1985 and 2002. In this triennium, the youngest woman was 15 years and the oldest 54 years of age.

Parity

While there is a strong association between maternal deaths and age, the association with parity is now much less clear. This may be due to the smaller number and proportion

Table 1.23 Total number of *Direct* and *Indirect* deaths by maternal age; United Kingdom 1985–2002, and rate per 100,000 maternities*

Age (years)	1985–87	1988–90	1991–93	1994–96	1997–99	2000–02	Overall 1985–2002		
							Total	Rate	95% CI
< 20	15	17	7	15	19	16	89	8.6	6.9–10.6
20–24	47	38	30	40	34	30	219	7.3	6.4–8.3
25–29	53	74	87	71	60	70	415	8.6	8.5–10.4
30–34	60	57	61	70	66	79	393	11.7	10.6–13.0
35–39	35	31	35	53	50	47	251	19.6	17.4–22.2
40+	13	18	7	11	13	19	81	35.5	28.5–44.1
Not stated	0	0	1	8	0	0	12		
Total	223	238	228	268	242	261	1460	11.0	10.5–11.6

of women having four or more children in the 21st century. The apparent relationship reported in the last Report, suggesting that increasing death rates with increasing parity were sustained, was based on an incorrect analysis. The figures for the current triennium and for each of the three previous triennia show that the lowest maternal death rates occur for women who have had one previous maternity. Over the whole 12-year period, the mortality rate for women with one previous maternity has been about three-quarters of the overall rate. The rates for women whose parity is three or more have been about one-third higher than the overall rate during this period, but these rates are based on very small numbers and vary considerably between triennia. The findings for 2000–02 are shown in Figure 1.9.

Marital status

Fifty percent of the women who had a *Direct* or *Indirect* maternal death in 2000–02 were known to be married at the time of death and a further 32% were living in a stable relationship. Of the 18% of deaths that occurred in women who did not have a partner,

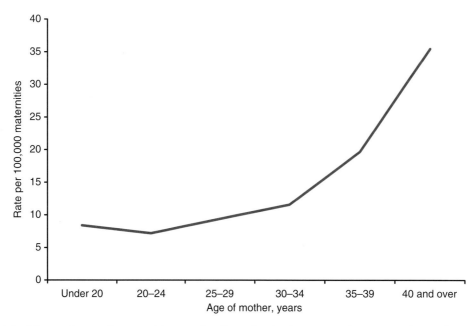

Figure 1.8 Maternal mortality rate, *Direct* and *Indirect* deaths, by maternal age; United Kingdom 1985–02

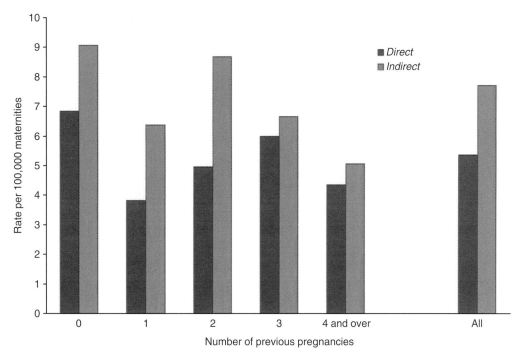

Figure 1.9 Maternal mortality rates by parity; United Kingdom 2000–02

more than 50% were in women who lived alone and appeared to be unsupported by their families.

The healthcare workers who helped report cases

It is easy to forget, when reviewing these sad events, that every healthcare worker who knew or was involved in providing care for these women would have been affected by their death. The individual comments made by many professionals in the course of this Enquiry bear this out. Many had never come across a maternal death before in the course of their career and all hope they would not do so again. A very few had to manage more than one in their Trust, due entirely to the play of chance, and the impact of several deaths in a short period of time was immensely distressing for them.

These are rare events that have a huge and long-lasting impact on the staff involved. Many professionals in this triennium reported having changed local protocols or personal practice as a result, particularly in relation to deaths from *Indirect* causes, and others say that they have learned valuable personal lessons as well:

> "She taught me the true meaning of maternal choice."

> "I never really understood the importance of "just being there" before. Holding the hand of such a brave woman was a true privilege."

> "I have struggled to cope with the death of X and her baby. I have learnt only that sometimes things go wrong unexpectedly. My care of X was good and I do not feel I could have done anything differently. But this thought does not make me feel any better."

Sadly, other health professionals appeared to have taken the blame for events outside their control. For example:

> "I did my best but it just wasn't good enough. I am wondering if I am in the right job."

> "I decided as a result to give up my career. I was not suitable for the job and she died as a result. I blame myself constantly. I did not have the necessary knowledge and I am now looking for less stressful work."

In both of these cases, but particularly the latter, the Assessors were greatly saddened, as they considered the care these professionals had provided was exemplary and that the failings in the system were totally outside the control of these workers. Nevertheless, these and others have reported taking unwarranted blame and feeling guilt without being offered support and counselling to help them come to terms with their own reactions. Chapter 9 Anaesthesia also reports that:

> "Supportive counselling of anaesthetic personnel involved in a maternal death is essential. It should be remembered that such an event represents a tragedy not only for the mother's family but also for the anaesthetist involved who commonly assumes full responsibility for the death."

Some staff who cared for women who declined help or who had to watch a woman bleed to death while refusing blood products, also reported significant personal distress. These findings have the following recommendation in Box 1.4.

Sadly, there were other comments from healthcare professionals that showed how very little they had learnt from these circumstances.

> "It went well. I just followed my usual practice."

> "It was a normal uneventful delivery."

The first comment relates to a member of staff working without reference to the Trust protocol for the management of an obstetric condition. The second relates to the death of a woman who arrested and died during an emergency caesarean section requiring massive amounts of blood during which the baby also died.

The Assessors were also concerned by the apparently culturally dismissive or insensitive remarks made by a very few professionals during the course of the reviews. This extended even to the appalling standard of some autopsies for women from the more vulnerable communities:

> "The system, having let her down in life, let her down in death as well."

Box 1.4   Recommendation: Staff support

Trusts must make provision for the prompt offer of support and/or counselling for all staff who have cared for a woman who has died.

Discussion and conclusions

The stark findings in this chapter on risk factors for maternal deaths highlight yet again that a disproportionate number of women who died were from the vulnerable and more excluded groups of our society. The findings also show that these women were less likely to access or continue to remain in contact with maternity services.

Excluded women also tend to have a multiplicity of problems in conjunction with their pregnancies.

Sir Donald Acheson highlighted good maternal health as one of the five key areas for action in his influential 1998 report on reducing health inequalities.[3] Care for mother and baby throughout pregnancy and the early postnatal period can have a marked effect on achieving a good start to family life, to the child's healthy development and on their resilience to problems encountered later in childhood.

It is also known that those who are likely to suffer poorer maternal or child outcomes, not just associated with death, are often the more excluded women in our country. Women and girls from the most vulnerable groups of society are not only embarking on pregnancy from possibly poorer overall general health but are also more likely to delay seeking care when pregnant, and/or fail to attend clinics regularly. Some, such as teenage or minority ethnic parents and drug users may feel that the current services are inappropriate for them or take little notice of their particular needs or concerns. Others, who fear that they have stigmatising conditions such as being victims of partner abuse, obese women and those who smoke often seek care later, possibly because they are concerned about judgmental attitudes from the healthcare staff.

A 2002 survey of patterns of booking for antenatal care in nine maternity units in England and Wales found that first-time mothers at high obstetric risk were 13% more likely to fail to book for antenatal care by ten weeks of gestation than the low-risk reference group.[4] Further, they were 34% more likely to not have 'booked' for antenatal care by 18 weeks of gestation. High obstetric risk included coexisting medical illness, previous poor psychiatric history, obesity, substance misuse and teenage motherhood. The following characteristics were also associated with failure to book early: maternal age, smoking status, ethnicity, the planned pattern of antenatal care and planned place of delivery. These associations were exacerbated between the clinical and sociodemographic characteristics for women who had failed to book by 18 weeks of gestation. The study also found that women from ethnic minority groups were up to five times as likely to fail to initiate care by 18 weeks, the numbers increasing if the woman had previous children. Although the findings are not directly comparable with this Report, this study adds value to these findings, in that it shows that women who were already at higher risk of obstetric or medical complication were more likely to book late and thus more likely to suffer adverse health outcomes.

Once women have sought care, many vulnerable women found it difficult to maintain access to the services. Again, they tended to be the socially excluded, with an over-representation of women from ethnic minority groups. A 2001 study of the sociodemographic determinants of the number of antenatal visits has shown that women from minority ethnic groups make 9% fewer antenatal visits than women of white British origin. As with women who 'book' late, other factors included social deprivation, pre-existing disease, psychiatric ill health and substance misuse and domestic violence.

In order to address the findings in this Report, there is an urgent need to identify and then provide services that help overcome the barriers that prevented many of the women who died from seeking care or maintaining contact with the maternity services.

Women should have their consultation in a medium or language with which they are comfortable, without the need for a relative interpreting. Women may also need to be put in touch with voluntary organisations that provide the sort of social network that will assist and support them while they are pregnant. The midwife must know to whom to go to get them the help they need.

It is vital that modern maternity services ensure that women from all groups of society have easy and equal access to the full range of high quality antenatal, intrapartum and postnatal services to ensure the needs of the most vulnerable are treated with equal importance. This means enabling every woman to seek care she feels happy with early in pregnancy and to continue to maintain regular contact throughout her pregnancy.

High-quality maternity care does not just include providing a supportive clinical environment to ensure a healthy pregnancy that is progressing well but also provides a gateway to other services that will help to achieve the best possible start to family life. These services include not only birth and parenting classes but also the provision of multidisciplinary support for women with particular medical, social or psychiatric needs and for those from the more vulnerable groups of our society.

Antenatal care must therefore be inclusive and flexible enough to meet the needs of all women. The needs of those from the most vulnerable and less articulate groups in society are of equal, if not more, importance and may need to be met through different patterns and places of care than have been traditionally provided. When required, care should be integrated with social services support and education services for women and their partners. Supportive midwifery and obstetric care should be based on providing good clinical and psychological outcomes, but also recognise the equal importance of helping the parents prepare for parenthood.

References

1. The Millennium Development Goals can be found on the World Health Organization website, at www.who.int/reproductive-health.
2. National Collaborating Centre for Women's and Children's Health. *Caesarean Section*. Clinical Guideline. London: RCOG Press; 2004 [www.nice.org.uk or www.rcog.org.uk].
3. Acheson D. *Independent Enquiry into Inequalities in Health*. London: The Stationery Office; 1999.
4. Kupek E, Petrou S, Vause S, Maresh M. Clinical, provider and sociodemographic predictors of late initiation of antenatal care in England and Wales. *BJOG* 2002;109:265–74.
5. Petrou S, Kupek E, Vause V, Maresh M. Clinical, provider and sociodemographic determinants of the number of antenatal visits in England and Wales. *Soc Sci Med* 2001;52:1123–34.

Key recommendations

Research

In order to address the findings in this Report, there is an urgent need to identify and then provide services which to help overcome the barriers that prevented many of the women who died from seeking care or maintaining contact with the maternity services.

It is recommended that a prospective study be undertaken to help to estimate more robustly what, if any, is the degree of increased risk of maternal deaths associated with caesarean section particularly for those undertaken without a clinical indication.

Further research is required on the incidence of postpartum haemorrhage in relation to previous caesarean section.

Service provision

Current patterns of antenatal care services are not meeting the needs of the women most at risk of maternal death. Services should be flexible enough to meet the needs of all women including the vulnerable and hard to reach. The needs of those from the most excluded and less articulate groups in society are of equal if not more importance. Asylum seekers and refugees are a particularly vulnerable group and services need to respond to their needs.

Many of the women in this Report found it difficult to access or maintain access with the services, and follow-up for those who failed to attend was poor. Services should be such that all women are motivated to attend throughout their pregnancy.

Women who fail to attend for care should be actively followed up. In general, this was not the case in this Report, despite a number of women already being known to be at high risk from obstetric, medical or psychiatric conditions.

When planning new methods of service provision it is helpful to involve the women, or representative from their communities, who might have difficulties in accessing and continuing to use the service. Where this has been done, antenatal clinic attendances have significantly improved. Such flexibility may require imaginative solutions in terms of the timing and setting for antenatal clinics, and the provision of outreach services.

The importance of seeking antenatal care early in pregnancy should be part of health education and promotion materials prepared for all groups in society.

Multidisciplinary care, provided through well-understood clinical and local social services networks, should be available for all women with pre-existing medical, psychological or social problems that may require specialist advice in pregnancy.

Women with complex pregnancies and who receive care from a number of specialists or agencies should receive the support and advocacy of a known midwife throughout their pregnancy. Their midwives will help with promoting the normal aspects of pregnancy and birth as well as supporting and advocating for the women through the variety of services they are being offered.

Interpreters should be provided for women who do not speak English. The use of family members, including children and partners as interpreters, should be avoided if at all possible.

Individual practitioners

General practitioners and other specialists should ensure that all relevant information is passed on the maternity or obstetric team in referral letters to booking clinics or at any other opportunity.

At booking, a risk and needs assessment should take place to ensure that every woman will be offered the type of care that most suits her own particular requirements. Some women in this Report were offered midwifery-led care which did not meet their more complex needs.

Healthcare professionals who work with disadvantaged clients need to be able to understand a woman's social and cultural background, act as an advocate for women, overcome their own personal and social prejudices and practise in a reflective manner.

All healthcare professionals should consider whether there are unrecognised but inherent prejudices within their own organisations, in terms of providing an equal service to all users.

Section

2

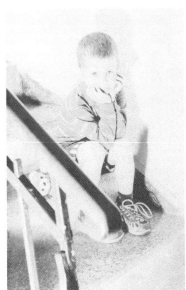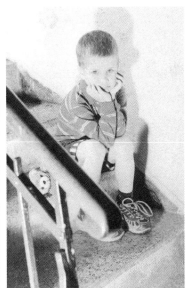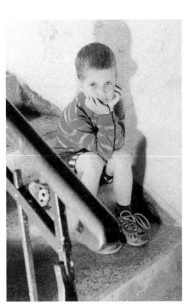

Direct deaths

CHAPTER 2

Thrombosis and thromboembolism

JAMES DRIFE on behalf of the Editorial Board

Thromboembolism: key recommendations

Individual practitioners

All women should undergo an assessment of risk factors for venous thromboembolism (VTE) in early pregnancy. This assessment should be repeated if the woman is admitted to hospital or develops other intercurrent problems.

Pregnant women with a past history of thromboembolism should be tested for thrombophilia, to more accurately define their risk of recurrence and guide thromboprophylaxis.

Acute symptoms suggestive of thromboembolism in known high-risk women are an emergency and anticoagulation may be indicated before the diagnosis is clear.

The RCOG guidelines on thromboprophylaxis, during pregnancy and labour and after normal vaginal delivery and caesarean section, should be followed.[2-4] Particular attention should be paid to the up-to-date guidance on dosages, published in 2004,[2] as this has changed from the older guideline.[3]

New guidelines on thromboprophylaxis for women at risk of thromboembolism during pregnancy, labour and after normal vaginal delivery were issued by the RCOG in January 2004.[2] The key recommendations are given in Annex A to this chapter. A summary of the existing RCOG guidelines for thromboprophylaxis at caesarean section[3] is also repeated in Annex B. **It should be noted that the new guidelines have updated and replaced the previous recommendations on dosages**.

Fifty years ago. . .

In 1952–54, the number of reported antepartum deaths from pulmonary embolism was exactly the same as in the present Report: four. Postpartum deaths, however, were very different, with 104 following vaginal delivery and 30 following caesarean section, contrasting with seven and ten, respectively, in the current report. In 57 of the 138 reported cases, venous thrombosis had already been diagnosed but "the use of anticoagulant preparations was mentioned in only ten of these cases". According to the Report, "the fact that anticoagulants were not prescribed has not been regarded as an avoidable factor . . . since expert clinical opinion is still divided on this question".

Over the next decade, the number of deaths from thromboembolism in each triennium remained virtually unchanged. In 1961–63, the total of 129 was second only to abortion

(139 deaths). This constant total disguised a trend, however: antepartum deaths had steadily risen to 36 while deaths after vaginal delivery had fallen to 66. Seven of the antenatal patients had been confined to bed for at least a week before their embolism but all antenatal deaths were regarded as "unavoidable". The requirement for 'lying in' after delivery was changing and the Report commented that 31 of the 66 women who died after vaginal delivery were "ambulant early". Of all the women who died, only 12 received anticoagulants, the use of which was still regarded as a matter of 'clinical judgement'. Few avoidable factors were identified.

During the 1960s, the total began to fall and in 1973–75 it was 38 (just below the 39 deaths from hypertensive disease). The 1973–75 report noted that 15 of the women were obese and 20% had had lactation suppressed by oestrogens. It drew attention to the risk factors of age, parity and operative delivery, commenting that risks were particularly high in women who were rested in bed because of hypertension and then delivered by caesarean section. As now, the Report concluded: "Attention is again drawn to failure to recognise warning signs and symptoms . . . ".

In 1979–81, there was a further fall to 28 deaths, which probably reflected "greater awareness of the dangers of thromboembolism, greater use of prophylactic therapy and more effective treatment". Subsequently, the picture remained constant, with no more than 30 deaths in each triennium, and the Enquiry increasingly emphasised thromboprophylaxis. The 1979–81 Report commented that: "previous proven deep vein thrombosis or pulmonary embolism warrants serious consideration of prophylactic anticoagulant therapy during pregnancy". The 1988–90 Report suggested that: "wider use of prophylactic anticoagulation or other methods of prophylaxis in high-risk cases could reduce the risk still further".

Successive Reports noted with increasing concern the number of deaths occurring after caesarean section. The 1991–93 Report, published in 1996, included a separate discussion of this topic. It pointed out that the 1991/92 National Confidential Enquiry into Perioperative Deaths (NCEPOD) Report, published in 1993, had highlighted the need for thromboprophylaxis in gynaecological surgery. It also reproduced the RCOG's recommendations on risk assessment and thromboprophylaxis in gynaecology and obstetrics, which had been published in 1995. These applied to caesarean section but not to vaginal delivery.

The RCOG recommendations, stimulated by the 1988–90 CEMD Report and the 1991/92 NCEPOD report, were timely. In 1994–96 deaths from thromboembolism rose sharply to 46, with ten occurring after vaginal delivery and 15 after caesarean section. The RCOG recommendations were widely publicised and in 1997–99 deaths after caesarean section fell sharply again to four. Deaths after vaginal delivery did not fall, however, and the 1997–99 CEMD Report commented: "There is a clear need for national guidelines on thromboprophylaxis after normal delivery". They have now been published and are included as an Annex to this chapter.

This review illustrates the increasing complexity of measures needed to maintain improvement. The first major fall in deaths from pulmonary thromboembolism, between 1963 and 1975, resulted from applying common sense and encouraging women to mobilise early after childbirth. The second fall, from 1996 onwards, has required close cooperation between the Enquiry, which highlighted emerging risk factors, the RCOG, which produced evidence-based guidelines, and the professionals, who read the detailed guidelines and put them into practice.

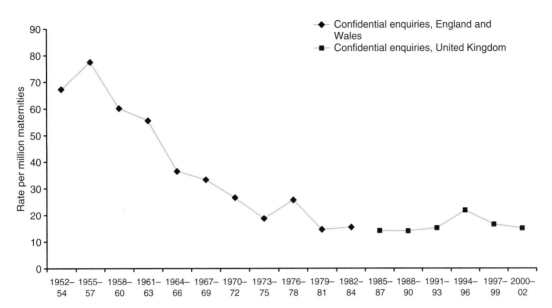

Figure 2.1   Maternal deaths from thrombosis and thromboembolism; England and Wales 1952–84; United Kingdom 1985–2002

Figure 2.1 shows maternal deaths from thrombosis and thromboembolism for England and Wales 1952–84 and for the United Kingdom 1985–2002.

Summary of cases for 2000–02

There are 30 deaths from thrombosis and/or thromboembolism counted in this chapter: 25 from pulmonary embolism and five from cerebral vein thrombosis. In addition, one *Late Direct* death from pulmonary embolism is counted in Chapter 15.

Of the 25 deaths from pulmonary embolism, four occurred during pregnancy; three in the first trimester and one in the third. One further death occurred during labour. Of the 17 postpartum deaths, seven followed vaginal delivery and ten followed caesarean section. Three further deaths followed fetal losses early in pregnancy. The timing of these deaths compared with those in previous triennia is shown in Figures 2.2 and 2.3.

The overall total of 25 deaths from pulmonary embolism this triennium represents a continuing reduction from 31 in 1997–99 and 46 in 1994–96. The previous fall, between 1994–96 and 1997–99, resulted from a drop in postnatal deaths following improved prophylaxis for caesarean section. The fall in deaths during this triennium is due to a reduction in deaths in the antenatal period but the reason for this is unclear.

Nineteen of the 25 women had known specific risk factors for thromboembolism. In the other cases, information about risk factors was not available. Of these six women, three could be described as being at increased general risk because of social factors including alcohol abuse, asylum seeker status, and late booking.

Of the four women who died before delivery, three had a previous deep venous thrombosis (DVT) and no history was available for the fourth. Sixteen of the women who died after delivery had risk factors for thromboembolism. Eight were obese, another described as "overweight", two had had significant bed rest during the pregnancy, one had a previous DVT, one had a previous arterial thrombosis and one had a family history of venous thrombosis. In addition, two women had recently undertaken long journeys, by air or by car.

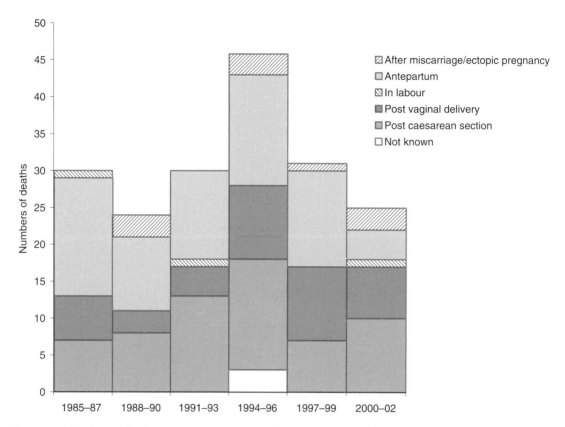

Figure 2.2   Timing of deaths from pulmonary embolism; United Kingdom 1985–2002

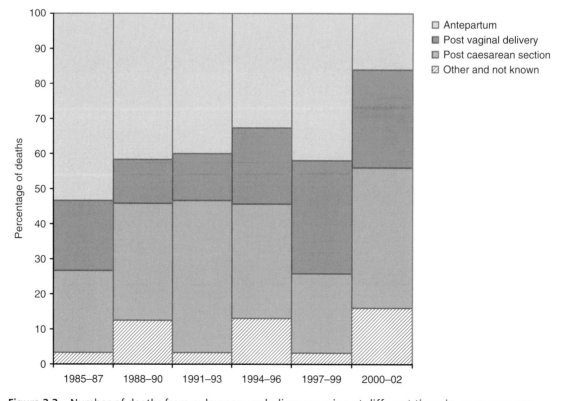

Figure 2.3   Number of deaths from pulmonary embolism occurring at different times in pregnancy as a proportion of the total; Untied Kingdom 1985–2002

Substandard care was identified in 57% of cases. This took the form of delayed diagnosis, delayed or inadequate treatment and inadequate thromboprophylaxis. The significance of symptoms in women who already had obvious risk factors was also sometimes not recognised.

While the fall in deaths from this cause over the last ten years is gratifying, there is still scope for further improvement by implementing the new RCOG guideline on thrombo-prophylaxis during pregnancy, labour and after normal vaginal delivery,[2] particularly in relation to risk assessment and appropriate therapeutic regimens. Continuing effort is needed to ensure that symptoms are taken seriously in women at risk; one way to do this is to educate the public about risk factors for thromboembolism.

Pulmonary embolism

Despite another fall in this triennium, pulmonary embolism is still the leading *Direct* cause of maternal death in the United Kingdom. The total of 25 deaths (excluding one *Late* death) equates to a rate of 1.2 per 100,000 maternities. Table 2.1 shows the comparison with previous triennia.

The most striking change compared with previous triennia is the sharp fall in antepartum deaths.

Cases counted in other chapters

Two women who died from other causes and whose cases are counted in the relevant chapters were initially incorrectly diagnosed and treated for pulmonary embolism. The lesson from both cases is that pulmonary embolism is not the only cause of chest pain. In both cases, once it became clear that thromboembolism was not the cause for the woman's symptoms, there was insufficient urgency about further investigation.

There was only one *Late Direct* death from pulmonary embolism in this triennium, which is counted in Chapter 15.

Risk factors for thromboembolism

Risk factors for VTE were present in 19 of the 25 women. Of the other six, details of possible risk factors were inadequate for the following reasons. No details are available

Table 2.1   Deaths from pulmonary embolism (excluding *Late* deaths) and rates per 100,000 maternities; United Kingdom 1985–99

Triennium	Total	Deaths after miscarriage/ectopic pregnancy	Antepartum deaths	Deaths in labour	Deaths after caesarean section	Deaths after vaginal delivery	Mortaility rate per 100,000 maternities	95% CI
1985–87	30	1	16	0	7	6	1.3	0.9–1.9
1988–90	24	3	10	0	8	3	1.0	0.7–1.5
1991–93	30	0	12	1	13	4	1.3	0.9–1.9
1994–96	46	3	15	0	15	10	2.1	1.5–2.8
1997–99	31	1	13	0	7*	10	1.5	1.0–2.1
2000–02	25	3	4	1	10**	7	1.3	0.8–1.9

* In three of these women collapse occurred before delivery
** In one of these women collapse occurred before delivery

Table 2.2 Mortality rates from deaths from pulmonary embolism (PE) by age; United Kingdom: 1997–2002

| Age (years) | Deaths from PE (n) | Rate per million maternities | | Maternities* (n) |
		Rate	95% CI	
<20	1	3.2	0.1–17.7	313,961
20–24	7	9.4	3.8–19.3	746,506
25–29	14	11.8	6.5–19.8	1,185,785
30–34	18	14.7	8.7–23.2	1,225,584
35–39	14	25.5	13.9–42.7	549,820
40+	2	20.3	2.5–73.5	98,298
Total	56	13.6	10.3–17.7	4,119,955

* Revised figures from the Office for National Statistics

for one woman who died before booking and another who died after delivery. One died after termination of pregnancy and risk factors may not have been enquired about. One booked late and her weight was not recorded. One did not speak English. One had very poor social circumstances, making her at increased overall risk.

Age

Age has been identified in previous Reports as a risk factor for VTE. The mortality rate per million maternities, by age group, for *Direct* deaths due to pulmonary embolism in this and the last triennium is shown in Table 2.2.

Travel

One woman died after a long-haul flight in pregnancy. Another, who had previously had a DVT following a long car journey died from another DVT, which also followed a long car journey.

Although the risks of long-haul air travel are now well known, there is insufficient awareness of the risks of a long car journey. The RCOG's advice on preventing DVT for pregnant women travelling by air points out that thrombosis attributable to prolonged immobility may occur in association with car, bus and rail travel.[4]

Immobility

In at least four cases, embolism occurred after a period of bed rest and, in one of these, the woman's weight was also a risk factor.

Family history

Only one woman was known to have a family history of thromboembolism in a first-degree relative such as a mother or sister.

Previous history

Four women had a previous VTE. Three died before delivery and one (whose social circumstances were particularly poor) died after vaginal delivery. One further woman had a previous arterial thrombosis and, in retrospect, is likely to have had antiphospholipid syndrome.

Maternal weight

Obesity is known to be a risk factor for VTE but maternal weight or body mass index (BMI) is still being poorly recorded in maternity notes. Among the 25 deaths from pulmonary embolism, the woman's weight was recorded in only 16 cases, either in the antenatal notes or elsewhere. In three further cases, a verbal description was available ("obese" or "very obese") but in nine cases there was no indication of the weight. It is regrettable that, in spite of attention being drawn repeatedly to this risk factor, it is still often ignored, as is recording the mother's weight and height or calculating her BMI at booking.

Death from pulmonary embolism does occur in women of normal or low weight but the risk rises with increasing weight. This should be taken into account when thromboprophylaxis is considered.

Oral contraception

One death was reported of pulmonary embolism in an obese woman prescribed the oral contraceptive pill immediately after delivery The importance of weight as a contraindication for the combined oral contraceptive pill was discussed in detail in the 1997–99 Report.

Oral contraception: learning points

The Faculty of Family Planning and Reproductive Health Care of the RCOG advises that women with a BMI above 30 kg/m² should be counselled regarding an increased risk of VTE and should consider alternative contraceptive methods.[5] It is particularly important to bear this in mind when discussing contraception after delivery.

The combined oral contraceptive pill should not be started until 21 days after delivery whatever the woman's weight.[5]

Antepartum deaths

A total of four women died from pulmonary embolism during the antenatal period. Three of the deaths occurred early in pregnancy. In one case, no details of the woman's past history were available but in each of the other three cases there was a previous history of VTE. This high incidence of a positive past history is striking.

None of the three women who had had a previous VTE were given antenatal thromboprophylaxis, apart from compression stockings in one case. None was tested for a possible underlying thrombophilia. Two had consulted a general practitioner about leg pains but had been reassured, despite the known past history. It must be emphasised that clinical diagnosis is unreliable and objective testing is required.[6] Two women who attended accident and emergency departments had long waits and delays in diagnosis and were not seen by an obstetrician.

Deaths after vaginal delivery

There were seven deaths after vaginal delivery and one late death. Six *Direct* deaths followed spontaneous vertex deliveries and one followed a breech delivery. Four of the deaths occurred within 14 days of vaginal delivery and the others were evenly distributed from 15 to 42 days after delivery, as shown in Table 2.3.

Table 2.3 Interval in days between delivery and pulmonary embolism; *Direct* deaths and *Late Direct* deaths, United Kingdom: 2000–02

Type of delivery	0–7	8–14	15–21	22–28	29–35	36–42	43–365	Total
Vaginal delivery	2	2	1	1	0	1	1	8
Caesarean section	5	1	2	0	2	0	0	10
Total	7	3	3	1	2	1	1	18

The women's ages ranged from 21 years to over 50 years. Important risk factors in this group were obesity and immobilisation. Social exclusion was a factor in four cases. Management was substandard with regard to diagnosis in two cases and treatment in two more cases.

Obesity

Three of the women were reported to be obese and the weight was not available for two others. One of the three, a grand multipara with other risk factors, had midwife-only care and also apparently started the combined oral contraceptive immediately after delivery, although it is not clear who prescribed it.

These cases raise the question of thromboprophylaxis in the very obese despite early mobilisation and the absence of other risk factors. In the 2004 RCOG guideline, one of the risk factors is obesity (BMI > 30 kg/m^2 either prepregnancy or in early pregnancy). The guideline advises that in the absence of thrombophilia or previous VTE, a woman with two current or persisting risk factors should be considered for prophylactic low-molecular-weight heparin (LMWH) for 3–5 days after vaginal delivery. It continues: "Clinical judgement is required with regard to the weighting of the above risk factors. There are circumstances were one or two risk factors alone may be sufficient to justify antenatal thromboprophylaxis with LMWH, for example an extremely obese woman admitted to the antenatal ward".[1]

Immobilisation

Prolonged bed rest after delivery is a known risk factor for VTE and was the probable underlying factor in two deaths. In some cultures, women are required to stay indoors for 'one month and one day' of confinement. One woman died because, for her family, this meant actually staying in bed for this period of time. Care must take account of a woman's beliefs and practices and, although the custom is now generally interpreted as staying at home by the younger generation in the UK, if women choose to spend this period of time in bed, they should be treated and advised according to their increased risk of VTE.

Delays in diagnosis

In two cases, the diagnosis was delayed due to failure to appreciate the significance of symptoms suggestive of pulmonary embolism. One was an older woman with prolonged immobilisation who complained of breathlessness and loin pain. The other was a woman with continuing pleuritic pain, lower lobe collapse and reduced oxygen saturation, who was treated with antibiotics without being investigated for pulmonary embolism.

Postpartum chest pain: learning point

Pleuritic pain, reduced oxygen saturation and lower lobe collapse in postpartum women suggest pulmonary embolism and investigations must be undertaken as a matter of urgency to exclude this.

Management

In some cases, when thromboprophylaxis was started it was too late and in too small a dose. The 2004 RCOG guideline recommends that: "Postpartum thromboprophylaxis should be given as soon as possible after delivery, provided there is no postpartum haemorrhage". The recommended doses are given in Table 2.4, towards the end of this chapter.

When one woman collapsed with a clinical diagnosis of pulmonary embolism the high dependency unit considered that the request for a bed was "not urgent". This apparent lack of appreciation for the severity of the illness mirrors the case of another woman who was discharged home having spent a significant period of time on a trolley in the accident and emergency department.

In some cases, the social circumstances or mental health of the women were such that treatment had to be commenced either on an outpatient basis or continued in the community after early self-discharge. Compliance with the prescribed therapeutic regimen was erratic. Maintaining contact with these women can be difficult and, although the hospital teams did their best to try to contact them, it is not clear whether there was any input from the community midwife or GP. These women had also been poor attenders for antenatal care and this should have alerted the community postnatal team to the need for increased support during this period.

Deaths after caesarean section

There were ten deaths after caesarean section. One woman collapsed before the operation, which was then carried out as an emergency, and therefore this thromboembolic event should properly be classified as antenatal rather than postnatal. Two other deaths occurred on day one after delivery and the other seven between 6 and around 34 days postpartum. Eight women had risk factors for VTE and no information was available about the weight of one of the other two women. Care was substandard in seven cases.

Table 2.4 Guidelines for antenatal prophylactic and therapeutic doses of low-molecular-weight heparin (LMWH)[2]

Prophylaxis	Enoxaparin (100 units/mg)	Dalteparin	Tinzaparin
Normal body weight	40 mg daily	5000 units daily	4500 units daily
Body weight < 50 kg	20 mg daily	2500 units daily	3500 units daily
Body weight > 90 kg*	40 mg 12-hourly	5000 units 12-hourly	4500 units 12-hourly
Therapeutic dose	1 mg/kg 12-hourly	90 units/kg 12-hourly	90 units/kg 12-hourly**

*These doses also apply to a woman who has a BMI of > 30 kg/m^2 in early pregnancy
**The manufacturer recommends 175 units/kg once a day

Age

Six of the women were aged 35 years or older.

Obesity

Five of the women were obese or overweight. One of these women was not weighed during the antenatal period. Another woman was not weighed at all. One woman, in addition to her obesity, also had anaemia and haemoglobin sickle cell disease, which are both risk factors for thromboembolism, and had recently travelled on a long-haul air flight. She did not receive thromboprophylaxis.

History

One woman had a family history of VTE, which was missed at booking. Had it been noted, the significance of her repeated episodes of shortness of breath during the pregnancy might have been appreciated. Another woman had a history of arterial thrombosis.

Adequacy of thromboprophylaxis

Thromboprophylaxis was inadequate in seven cases. In two cases, there is no record of any thromboprophylaxis and in two others the dose of LMWH was inadequate according to the guidelines in Table 2.4. In another two cases, the risk assessment was inadequate, so appropriate prophylaxis was not given, and in the seventh case LMWH was stopped too quickly when warfarin was started.

Failure of diagnosis

Two of the women were admitted to the accident and emergency department within 2 weeks of caesarean section, complaining of breathlessness and chest pain, and the diagnosis was not made promptly. In one case, the obstetrician was called only after the woman collapsed. In the other case, the woman was admitted to a medical ward and treated by junior doctors for "asthma" for 2 days before the correct diagnosis was made. She then received an inadequate dose of LMWH. A woman admitted to an accident and emergency department with chest symptoms after a caesarean section should be seen urgently by an obstetrician.

Late deaths

Only one *Late* death related directly to pulmonary embolism is recorded in this triennium and is counted in Chapter 15.

Cerebral vein thrombosis

There were five cases of cerebral vein thrombosis in this triennium. Two of the women were from ethnic minorities.

Three cases were initially misdiagnosed. In two, the woman's symptoms were labelled as "psychiatric": one had a confusional state and the other had convulsions, which were diagnosed as hysteria. In the third, the woman's symptoms of headache and inability to communicate were initially attributed to opiates.

In all but one of the five cases, care was substandard. In addition to the misdiagnoses, there was delay in one case in obtaining a consultant opinion when the woman became ill. In another case, a family history of homocysteinuria (a risk factor) was missed, and in a third case there was failure to involve obstetricians or midwives when a pregnant woman was admitted under the care of a medical team and undue concern about radiation exposure in pregnancy led to a delay in imaging.

Although such tragedies cannot be predicted in the absence of risk factors, after they occur consideration should be given to offering the members of the woman's family testing for thrombophilia, to identify any who are at risk of a similar complication.

Comments

Care was judged to be substandard in 17 of the 30 cases (57%) discussed in this chapter.

With the introduction of clinical governance and critical incident reporting in hospitals, it might be expected that the identification of substandard care by national reports like this one would become less necessary. To date, this is not the case. Although we have evidence that, in many cases, local clinicians have reflected with insight on the cases in this chapter, we have also noted in a few cases that lessons which seem obvious to national assessors have not been learned at local level, particularly when substandard care has been due to pressure on resources.

Thromboembolism; substandard care: learning point

Substandard care took the form of a failure to recognise risk factors, failure to appreciate the significance of signs and symptoms in the light of background risk factors, failure to act promptly enough in implementing either prophylaxis or treatment, and inadequate dosage of thromboprophylaxis. When VTE has been identified, treatment must be begun with minimal delay.[6] Care must also be taken to ensure that both prophylactic and therapeutic anticoagulation is given in the appropriate dosage as given in Table 2.4, which updates and replaces the dosages given in previous guidelines.

There are several reasons why the incidence of VTE might be expected to be increasing. The caesarean section rate has been steadily rising, at least until recently. The average age of childbearing has also been rising, and there is an increase in obesity in the British population. Long-haul air travel remains popular. It is therefore gratifying that the overall number of deaths from VTE has fallen for the last two triennia. The most recent fall has been in antenatal deaths, with the current total of four being less than half that in any triennium since the UK Reports began in 1985.

The reason for this fall in deaths in the antenatal period is unclear. It may be that, with increasing awareness of the risks of thromboembolism among both the public and professionals, cases are being identified and appropriately treated during pregnancy. Women may be more aware of the risks of long-distance travel. The fall may be due to the introduction of the RCOG guidelines for the management of women with thromboembolism.[6] We have no way of confirming or refuting this from the data available to us.

Nevertheless, there is a clear potential for further improvement. Pulmonary embolism remains the major *Direct* cause of maternal deaths in the UK and, in the present chapter, substandard care was identified in over 50% of cases. The most important aspect of substandard care was the failure to recognise risk factors, and we therefore welcome the publication of the new RCOG guideline, which clearly recommends risk assessment for all pregnant women.[2]

The importance of risk assessment is underlined by the fact that a high proportion of the women whose deaths are reported here had at least one risk factor for thromboembolism. Awareness of these risk factors is relevant both to decisions on thromboprophylaxis and to the interpretation of signs and symptoms which might otherwise seem insignificant.

Previous Reports have emphasised the importance of thromboprophylaxis in relation to caesarean section and it is disappointing that the number of deaths after caesarean has risen again in this triennium. Prompt initiation of thromboprophylaxis in the correct dosage after caesarean section may reduce deaths again in the future.

In some cases, VTE had been diagnosed but not treated energetically enough. Appropriate management of VTE is essential and a guideline in the acute management of VTE was issued by the RCOG in 2001.[6] The dosage of prophylactic or therapeutic anticoagulation was inadequate in some cases. Recommended dosages have been updated in the guideline issued by the RCOG in 2004 and are summarised in Table 2.4.

Finally, it should be remembered that women who survive VTE may be left with a painful disability.[7] More than 60% develop deep venous thrombosis and thromboembolic compression stockings reduce this. Effective prevention and treatment is important for survivors as well, although the emphasis in this Report is of course on striving to prevent death.

References

1. Department of Health. *Reports on Public Health and Medical Subjects No.97. Report of Confidential Enquiries into Maternal Deaths in England and Wales. 1952–1954.* London: HMSO; 1957.
2. Royal College of Obstetricians and Gynaecologists. *Thromboprophylaxis during pregnancy, labour and after normal vaginal delivery.* Guideline No. 37. London: RCOG; 2004. Available at www.rcog.org.uk.
3. Royal College of Obstetricians and Gynaecologists. *Report of the RCOG Working Party on Prophylaxis Against Thromboembolism in Gynaecology and Obstetrics.* London: RCOG; 1995.
4. Royal College of Obstetricians and Gynaecologists. *Advice on Preventing Deep Vein Thrombosis for Pregnant Women Travelling by Air.* Scientific Advisory Committee Opinion Paper 1. London: RCOG; 2001. Available at www.rcog.org.uk.

5. Faculty of Family Planning and Reproductive Health Care. FFPRHC Guidance (October 2003): First Prescription of Combined Oral Contraceptives. *J Fam Plann Reprod Health Care* 2003; 29: 209–33. Available at www.ffprhc.org.uk.

6. Royal College of Obstetricians and Gynaecologists. *Thromboembolic Disease in Pregnancy and the Puerperium: Acute Management.* Guideline no 28. London: RCOG; 2001. Available at www.rcog.org.uk.

7. Drife J. Thromboembolism. *Br Med Bull* 2003; 67: 177–90.

CHAPTER 2: ANNEX A
Summary of the key recommendations of the 2004 RCOG Guideline Thromboprophylaxis during pregnancy, labour and after normal vaginal delivery[2]

Risk factors for venous thromboembolism in pregnancy and the puerperium[a]

Pre-existing	New onset or transient[b]
Previous VTE	Surgical procedure in pregnancy or puerperium (e.g. evacuation of retained products of conception, postpartum sterilisation)
Thrombophilia:	Hyperemesis
Congenital	Dehydration
Antithrombin deficiency	Severe infection (e.g. pyelonephritis)
Protein C deficiency	Immobility (> 4 days of bed rest)
Factor V Leiden	Pre-eclampsia
Prothrombin gene variant	Excessive blood loss
Acquired antiphospholipid syndrome	Long-haul travel
Lupus anticoagulant	Prolonged labour[c]
Anticardiolipin antibodies	Midcavity instrumental delivery[c]
Age over 35 years	Immobility after delivery[c]
Obesity (BMI > 30 kg/m² either pre-pregnancy or in early pregnancy)	
Parity > 4	
Gross varicose veins	
Paraplegia	
Sickle cell disease	
Inflammatory disorders (e.g. inflammatory bowel disease)	
Some medical disorders (e.g. nephritic syndrome, certain cardiac diseases)	
Myeloproliferative disorders (e.g. essential thrombocythaemia, polycythaemia vera)	

[a] Although these are all accepted as thromboembolic risk factors, there are few data to support the degree of increased risk associated with many of them.
[b] These risk factors are potentially reversible and may develop at later stages in gestation than the initial risk assessment or may resolve; an ongoing individual risk assessment is important.
[c] Risk factors specific to postpartum VTE only.

Recommendations

All women should undergo an assessment of risk factors for VTE in early pregnancy or before pregnancy. This assessment should be repeated if the woman is admitted to hospital or develops other intercurrent problems. (Grade C) (grade definitions see p.75)

Women with previous VTE should be screened for inherited and acquired thrombophilia, ideally before pregnancy. (Grade B)

Regardless of their risk of VTE, immobilisation of women during pregnancy, labour and the puerperium should be minimised and dehydration should be avoided. (*Good practice point)

Women with previous VTE should be offered postpartum thromboprophylaxis with LMWH. It may be reasonable not to use antenatal thromboprophylaxis with heparin in women with a single previous VTE associated with a temporary risk factor that has now resolved. (Grade C)

Women with previous recurrent VTE, or a previous VTE and a family history of VTE in a first-degree relative, should be offered thromboprophylaxis with LMWH antenatally and for at least 6 weeks postpartum. (Grade C)

Women with previous VTE and thrombophilia should be offered thromboprophylaxis with LMWH antenatally and for at least 6 weeks postpartum. (Grade B)

Women with asymptomatic inherited or acquired thrombophilia may qualify for antenatal or postnatal thromboprophylaxis, depending on the specific thrombophilia and the presence of other risk factors. (Grade C)

Women with three or more persisting risk factors should be considered for thromboprophylaxis with LMWH antenatally and for 3–5 days postpartum. (*Good practice point)

Women should be reassessed before or during labour for risk factors for VTE. Age over 35 years and BMI greater than 30/body weight greater than 90 kg are important independent risk factors for postpartum VTE, even after vaginal delivery. The combination of either of these risk factors with any other risk factor for VTE (such as pre-eclampsia or immobility) or the presence of two other persisting risk factors should lead the clinician to consider the use of LMWH for 3–5 days postpartum. (*Good practice point)

Antenatal thromboprophylaxis should begin as early in pregnancy as practical. Postpartum prophylaxis should begin as soon as possible after delivery (but see precautions after use of regional anaesthesia). (Grade B)

LMWHs are the agents of choice for antenatal thromboprophylaxis. They are as effective as and safer than unfractionated heparin in pregnancy. (Grade B)

Warfarin should usually be avoided during pregnancy. It is safe after delivery and during breastfeeding. (Grade B)

Once the woman is in labour or thinks she is in labour, she should be advised not to inject any further heparin. She should be reassessed on admission to hospital and further doses should be prescribed by medical staff. (*Good practice point)

The **grades of recommendations (B or C)** are as follows:

B	Requires the availability of well-controlled clinical studies but no randomised clinical trials on the topic of recommendations. (Evidence levels IIa, IIb, III)

C   Requires evidence obtained form expert committee reports or opinions and/or clinical experiences of respected authorities. Indicates an absence of directly applicable clinical studies of good quality. (Evidence level IV)

*Good practice points   The other recommendations represent good practice points; i.e., recommended best practice based on the clinical experience of the guideline development group.

For further details, see the full report (Reference 1).

CHAPTER 2: ANNEX B
Prophylaxis against thromboembolism in caesarean section

A risk assessment of all women undergoing elective or emergency caesarean section should be performed and prophylaxis instituted as appropriate.

The table below, taken from the 1995 RCOG Working Party Report on Prophylaxis Against Thromboembolism,[3] is widely used for risk assessment in caesarean section and is reproduced again here. It is important to remember that the 2004 RCOG Guideline[2] updates and replaces previous guidance on dosage of thromboprophylaxis.

RCOG Risk assessment profile for thromboembolism in caesarean section

Low risk: Early mobilisation and hydration
Elective caesarean section: uncomplicated pregnancy and no other risk factors.

Moderate risk: Consider one of a variety of prophylactic measures
- Age > 35 years

- Obesity (> 80 kg)

- Parity 4 or more

- Labour 12 hours or more

- Gross varicose veins

- Current infection

- Pre-eclampsia

- Immobility prior to surgery (> 4 days)

- Major current illness (e.g. heart or lung disease, cancer, inflammatory bowel disease, nephrotic syndrome)

- Emergency caesarean section in labour.

High risk: Heparin prophylaxis with or without leg stockings
- A woman with three or more moderate risk factors from above

- Extended major pelvic or abdominal surgery (e.g. caesarean hysterectomy)

- Women with personal or family history of deep venous thrombosis, pulmonary embolism or thrombophilia, paralysis of lower limbs

- Women with antiphospholipid antibody (cardiolipin antibody or lupus anticoagulant).

Management of different risk groups

Low-risk women

Women undergoing elective caesarean section with uncomplicated pregnancy and no other risk factors require only early mobilisation and attention to hydration.

Moderate risk patients

Women assessed as of moderate risk should receive subcutaneous heparin (doses are higher during pregnancy) or mechanical methods. Dextran 70 is not recommended until after the delivery of the fetus and is probably best avoided in pregnant women.

High-risk women

Women assessed as high risk should receive heparin prophylaxis and, in addition, leg stockings would be beneficial.

Prophylaxis until the fifth postoperative day is advised (or until fully mobilised if longer).

The use of subcutaneous heparin as prophylaxis in women with an epidural or spinal block remains contentious. Evidence from general and orthopaedic surgery does not point to an increased risk of spinal haematoma.

CHAPTER 3

Pre-eclampsia and eclampsia

JAMES P NEILSON on behalf of the Editorial Board

Pre-eclampsia and eclampsia: key recommendations

Service provision

Guidelines and protocols
Clear, written, management protocols for severe pre-eclampsia should guide initial and ongoing treatment in hospital.

Severe, life-threatening hypertension must be treated effectively. Management protocols should recognise the need to avoid very high systolic blood pressures associated with the risk of intracerebral haemorrhage. It is recommended that clinical protocols identify a systolic blood pressure above which urgent and effective antihypertensive treatment is required.

The early involvement of consultant obstetricians in the management of women with suspected or proven pre-eclampsia and eclampsia is essential.

There should be early engagement of intensive care specialists in the care of women with severe pre-eclampsia.

Individual practitioners

Pregnant women with a headache of sufficient severity to seek medical advice, or with new epigastric pain, should have their blood pressure measured and urine tested for protein, as a minimum.

Automated blood pressure recording systems can systematically underestimate blood pressure in pre-eclampsia, to a serious degree. Blood pressure values should be compared, at the beginning of treatment, with those obtained by conventional sphygmomanometers.

In women presenting with potentially severe pre-eclampsia (e.g. symptoms, sudden heavy proteinuria, markedly disordered liver function and/or haematological tests results) but with unexceptional blood pressure measurements, alarming rises in blood pressure should be anticipated. Consideration should be given to early administration of antihypertensive drugs.

Magnesium sulphate is the anticonvulsant drug of choice in the treatment of eclampsia.

To avoid the potentially serious consequences of fluid overload careful monitoring of fluid input and output, fluid restriction, and central monitoring is essential.

Fifty years ago...

The small number of deaths in the current triennium, 14, contrasts starkly with deaths in the early years of the Enquiry. There were 246 in 1952–54 due to pre-eclampsia, eclampsia or placental abruption associated with pre-eclampsia. There was a sharp decline in mortalities in the 1950s and 1960s followed by a steady decrease in deaths since the mid 1960s, as Figure 3.1 shows. Failures of antenatal care were highlighted as the major avoidable factors in early Reports, including a need (a continuing theme today) to make contact with women who fail to attend antenatal clinics.

The ability of phaeochromocytomas to mimic pre-eclampsia was described in the 1964–66 and 1967–69 Reports, which included, respectively, six and two deaths from this cause.

By the 1970s, the number of deaths had decreased substantially from 47 in 1970–72, 39 in 1973–75, and 29 in 1976–78.

The 1979–81 Report resonates with the main theme in this Report's chapter, by highlighting cerebral haemorrhage as the most common cause of death in women with pre-eclampsia and eclampsia and recommending more widespread use of anti-hypertensive drugs. The Report was far-sighted, at a time when subspecialisation in obstetrics and gynaecology was embryonic and written clinical guidelines virtually unknown, in recommending the establishment of regional centres to advise on management of severe pre-eclampsia and provide a lead on education and what we would now recognise as audit.

The 1985–87 Report recorded, with concern, a plateau in the number of deaths. Deaths due to acute respiratory distress syndrome (ARDS) were described for the first time – ascribed to longer survival in severely ill women but perhaps due to increasing recognition of this clinical condition. The dangers of excessive infusion were stressed. Diazepam was criticised as an anticonvulsant and, with prescience, a plea was made to re-evaluate

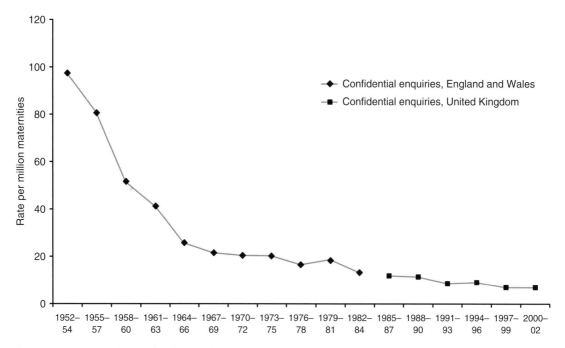

Figure 3.1 Maternal mortality from eclampsia and pre-eclampsia; England and Wales 1952–84; United Kingdom 1985–2002

scientifically the value of magnesium sulphate and phenytoin. Subsequent clinical trials], of course, demonstrated the superiority of magnesium sulphate in the treatment of eclampsia,[1,2] and the Magpie Trial showed the value of magnesium sulphate in pre-eclampsia.[3]

The 1994–96 Report acknowledged that severe pre-eclampsia can develop within days of entirely normal observations at the antenatal clinic. In keeping with greater engagement of users of the health services, the Report stressed the need to educate women about symptoms associated with pre-eclampsia and recommended the educational material produced by the still active lay organisation APEC (Action on Pre-eclampsia).[4]

Summary of findings for 2000–02

Fourteen deaths from eclampsia or pre-eclampsia are counted in this chapter. Nine women died from intracranial haemorrhage, one from ARDS, two from multi-organ failure which included ARDS and two from severe disseminated intravascular dissemination (DIC). The causes of death are compared with figures from recent triennia in Table 3.1. The ages of the women ranged between 17 and 38 years. The gestational age ranged from 24 weeks to 40 weeks with a bimodal distribution, there being no deaths between 30 weeks and 34 weeks, inclusive. In all, seven deaths (50%) occurred before term (37 weeks), with five of these occurring before 30 weeks. Parity ranged from 0 to 6; seven women were primigravid. All the pregnancies were singleton. Six women had eclamptic fits, four antenatally. There was evidence of HELLP syndrome (haemolysis, elevated liver enzymes and low platelets) in eight women. Although there has been a steady trend towards fewer deaths, six of the 13 cases assessed (46%) showed clear features of substandard care and may have been avoidable deaths. Intracranial haemorrhage, as the single largest cause of death, indicates a failure of effective anti-hypertensive therapy. This must be the priority for improved clinical care.

Table 3.1 Number of deaths by cause due to eclampsia and pre-eclampsia; United Kingdom 1988–2002

Cause of death	Triennium				
	1988–90	1991–93	1994–96	1997–99	2000–02
Cerebral:					
Intracranial haemorrhage	10	5	3	7	9
Subarachnoid	2	0	1	0	0
Infarct	2	0	0	0	0
Oedema	0	0	3	0	0
Subtotal	14	5	7	7	9
Pulmonary:					
ARDS	9	8	6	2	1
Oedema	1	3	2	0	0
Subtotal	10	11	8	2	1
Hepatic:					
Rupture	0	0	2	2	0
Failure/necrosis	1	0	1	0	0
Other	2	4	2	5	4
Subtotal	3	4	5	7	4
Overall total	27	20	20	16	14

In some other cases, the course of the illness was so rapid that improving outcome would have been a very major challenge even under optimal circumstances.

All deaths that are recorded in this chapter occurred in hospital. There was some circumstantial evidence to suggest the possibility of eclampsia in a woman who was found dead at home but there was insufficient evidence to be certain, and this death has been classified as 'unascertained' and included in Chapter 12.

In one case, the first indication of clinical concern was the observation of fetal growth restriction, pre-dating signs of pre-eclampsia.

Women with pre-eclampsia whose deaths are discussed in other chapters and are not counted here, include a woman with ARDS and repeated episodes of sepsis who died in the intensive care unit several weeks after delivery and a woman with mild pre-eclampsia who died of subarachnoid haemorrhage a week after delivery. These cases are counted in Chapters 15 and 12, respectively.

Two women who died, and who had been treated with magnesium sulphate for presumed eclampsia, were subsequently diagnosed as having other pathology – primary cerebral haemorrhage and bacterial meningitis.

The single major failing in clinical care in the current triennium was inadequate treatment of hypertension, with subsequent intracranial haemorrhage. In most of these cases the consultant obstetrician was involved too late. An example vignette, representative of a number of the cases counted in this chapter, is given here:

> A woman, whose blood pressure was 110/60 mm/Hg in early pregnancy, was admitted in late pregnancy with a diastolic pressure of 92 mm/Hg and proteinuria +++. Over the subsequent days, blood pressures of 155/95 mm/Hg and 145/100 mm/Hg were noted and a 24-hour urine collection showed greater than 4 g of protein. She was given dexamethasone and induction of labour was planned for the next day. This did not happen because a lack of special care baby unit cots; her blood pressure was 160/105 mm/Hg and there was proteinuria ++++. The following day, she complained of epigastric pain and a puffy face; her blood pressure was 170/105 mm/Hg. Attempts were made to induce labour despite an unfavourable cervix. After her blood pressure rose to 220/120 mm/Hg, antihypertensive treatment was started for the first time (intravenous labetalol); midazolam was also given. Her blood pressure remained elevated at 215/120 mm/Hg and she remained symptomatic. A caesarean section was performed. There was continuing poor control of her blood pressure after delivery. She developed twitching, slurred speech and mouth dropping, and was seen for the first time since admission by a consultant obstetrician. A computed tomography (CT) scan showed a massive intracranial haemorrhage. She was transferred to a neurosurgical unit but died despite craniotomy. Laboratory tests showed HELLP syndrome.

This is one of a number of cases in which there was insufficient weight placed on the rise in systolic blood pressure. In the distant past, obstetricians were often inappropriately fixated on diastolic blood pressure. Calculation of mean arterial pressure (as often required in modern severe pre-eclampsia management guidelines) was an advance, by incorporating both systolic and diastolic blood pressure. However, while diastolic blood pressure is one of a number of useful indices of severity of pre-eclampsia, it is thought to be the pressure during systole which causes intracerebral haemorrhage. Recognition of this concept should be incorporated into clinical guidelines to try to ensure effective reduction of systolic pressure. **It is, therefore, recommended that clinical protocols identify a systolic blood pressure above which urgent and effective antihypertensive treatment is required**. Some would recommend 160 mmHg as a useful guide to treatment.

Two cases are discussed in Chapter 10 of women with essential hypertension in whom insufficient attention was also paid to the systolic pressure, with fatal results.

Consideration should also be made to starting early antihypertensive treatment when the blood pressure is not, in itself, alarming but where the severity of the pre-eclampsia makes a rapid increase in pressure likely.

It is also worth re-emphasising, as in the last Report, the observation that many automated blood pressure monitoring systems systematically underestimate systolic pressure in pre-eclampsia. Mercury sphygmomanometers should be used to establish baseline blood pressure as a reference for automated monitoring in hospital for women with pre-eclampsia, unless the automated system has been validated in pregnancy.[5]

Further substandard elements of care in some cases were inappropriate delay in delivery to allow marginal improvements in fetal outcome, as demonstrated by the following vignette:

> A woman had ineffective treatment of hypertension after delivery. Her 'booking' blood pressure had been 100/50 mm/Hg. At her final antenatal clinic visit, her blood pressure was 120/85 mm/Hg and her urine was not checked for protein. She had a seizure at home several days later. On admission to hospital, her blood pressure was 150/100 mm/Hg and there was proteinuria ++++. She was treated with hydralazine and magnesium sulphate and underwent caesarean section for fetal distress. After delivery, her hypertension was poorly controlled with a maximum pressure of 170/115 mm/Hg. She had a grossly elevated serum urate, raised ALT and lowered platelet count. Her blood pressure rose to 180/120 mm/ Hg and, shortly afterwards, she became unresponsive. A CT scan showed an intracranial haemorrhage, from which she subsequently died.

In some cases, the rapidity of development of the features of pre-eclampsia may be such that blood pressure control remains difficult despite assiduous efforts. This is illustrated by the following case, which did not show substandard care:

> An unbooked woman from out of the country presented to an accident and emergency department with abdominal pain during late second trimester. Her blood pressure was recorded as 155/70 mm /Hg but she had proteinuria ++++. She was admitted to the maternity unit with a provisional diagnosis of urinary tract infection. Shortly after admission, she had eclamptic fits, at which time her blood pressure had risen to 170/120mm/Hg. She was treated with magnesium sulphate and labetalol. Liver function was grossly disordered and she had a coagulopathy. Her blood pressure proved difficult to control despite combined therapy with labetalol and hydralazine. Attempts made to induce labour with misoprostol (the fetus had died) but there was further clinical deterioration and she was transferred to the intensive care unit, where she died.

Although the major challenge is in blood pressure control, there were instances of inappropriate fluid management resulting in pulmonary insult with the development of ARDS:

> A woman was admitted to hospital in late second trimester with pre-eclampsia. Her first pregnancy had been complicated by early severe pre-eclampsia; the second was normal. Her blood pressure was only modestly elevated but she had proteinuria ++++. A decision was made to deliver her the next day by caesarean section after administration of corticosteroids. That night, she had a placental abruption and she was delivered by caesarean section. Postoperatively, she received a massive intravenous fluid overload without any central monitoring. She subsequently died in the intensive care unit, from a combination of ARDS and pneumonia.

The fluid balance charts of another woman with pre-eclampsia (who is counted in Chapter 15 *Late deaths*) are missing but there is evidence to suggest fluid overload in her case as well. The need for careful monitoring of fluid input and output, fluid restriction, and central monitoring must be emphasised.

Pre-eclampsia and eclampsia: learning points

- Early onset pre-eclampsia poses serious threats to the mother as well as the fetus.

- The dangers of high systolic blood pressure leading to intracranial haemorrhage need greater recognition by clinicians and more ready response with antihypertensive treatment.

- The early involvement of consultant obstetricians in the management of women with suspected or proven pre-eclampsia and eclampsia is essential.

- Magnesium sulphate is the anticonvulsant of choice in the treatment of eclampsia and pre-eclampsia.

- To avoid the potentially serious consequences of fluid overload, careful monitoring of fluid input and output, fluid restriction and central monitoring is essential.

- Although most substandard care was seen in the hospital sector, there were examples in primary care of midwives failing to test urine for proteinuria in women who subsequently developed severe pre-eclampsia.

References

1. Duley L, Henderson-Smart DJ. Magnesium sulphate versus diazepam for eclampsia. *Cochrane Database Syst Rev* 2004(2).
2. Duley L, Henderson-Smart DJ. Magnesium sulphate versus phenytoin for eclampsia. *Cochrane Database Syst Rev* 2004(2).

3. Magpie Trial Collaborative Group. Do women with pre-eclampsia, and their babies, benefit from magnesium sulphate? The Magpie Trial: a randomised placebo-controlled trial. *Lancet* 2002;359:1877–90.
4. Action on Pre-eclampsia [www.apec.org.uk].
5. Golara M, Benedict A, Jones C, Randhawa M, Poston L, Shennan AH. Inflationary oscillometry provides accurate measurement of blood pressure in pre-eclampsia. *BJOG* 2002;109:1143–7.

CHAPTER 4

Haemorrhage

MARION H HALL on behalf of the Editorial Board

Obstetric haemorrhage: key recommendations

Service provision

Guidelines and protocols

A multidisciplinary massive haemorrhage protocol must be available in all units and should be updated and rehearsed regularly in conjunction with the blood bank. All grades of staff should participate in these 'fire drills' on site.

Women known to be at high risk of bleeding should be delivered in centres with facilities for blood transfusion, intensive care and other interventions, and plans should be made in advance for their management.

Individual practitioners

Consultant haematologists should be involved in the care of women with coagulopathy.

Placenta praevia, particularly in women with a previous uterine scar, may be associated with uncontrollable uterine haemorrhage at delivery and caesarean hysterectomy may be necessary. A consultant must be in attendance.

On-call consultant obstetricians must consider all available interventions to stop haemorrhage such as B-Lynch suture, embolisation of uterine arteries or radical surgery and they should not hesitate to involve surgical or radiological colleagues as required.

Fifty years ago...

Figure 4.1 shows the change in death rates from haemorrhage over the last 50 years. Looking at the absolute numbers, it is shocking to recall that at least 40 women per annum died from haemorrhage in the early 1950s compared with about three per annum in recent years. The major fall in death rates had occurred by 1975 and this improvement in outcome was thought to have been due to:

- hospitalisation for delivery of women at higher risk (older women, grand multiparae, and those with pre-eclampsia)

- better surveillance of ill women and, for some, major surgery such as hysterectomy

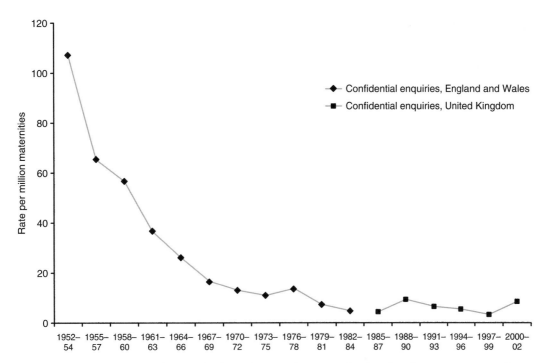

Figure 4.1 Maternal mortality for deaths due to haemorrhage; England and Wales 1952–84; United Kingdom 1984–2002

- using the flying squad to resuscitate women at home or in small hospitals prior to transfer to a large hospital

- the active management of coagulopathy and of women at risk of renal failure.

All of these had been recommendations in earlier Reports of the Confidential Enquiries into Maternal Deaths.

In recent years some possible risk factors for haemorrhage appear to becoming more common, for example:

- the increasing mean age of childbirth

- an increasing number of women with complex medical disorders choosing to become pregnant

- increased numbers of multiple pregnancies following assisted reproduction

- increased caesarean section rates leading to subsequent placenta praevia or accreta.

These risk factors, together with changes in obstetric training, may be relevant to the increase in deaths in this triennium, which are discussed below.

Summary of findings for 2000–02

Of the 17 deaths directly due to haemorrhage counted in this chapter, four were due to placenta praevia, three to placental abruption and ten to postpartum haemorrhage (PPH). The numbers of deaths from abruption and placenta praevia are unchanged from the previous triennium but there has been a striking increase in the numbers of deaths from postpartum haemorrhage, from one case in the last Report to ten in the present triennium.

Table 4.1 Numbers of deaths from haemorrhage by underlying cause and mortality rate per million maternities; United Kingdom 1985–2002

Triennium	Placental abruption	Placenta praevia	Postpartum haemorrhage	Total (n)	Rate per million maternities	
					Rate	95% CI
1985–87	4	0	6	10	4.4	2.1–8.1
1988–90	6	5	11	22	9.3	5.8–14.1
1991–93	3	4	8	15	6.5	3.6–10.7
1994–96	4	3	5	12	5.5	2.8–9.5
1997–99	3	3	1	7	3.3	1.3–6.8
2000–02	3	4	10	17	8.5	5.0–13.6
Total	23	19	41	83	6.3	5.0–7.8

Five other women, whose deaths are counted in other chapters, also had complications in which significant haemorrhage occurred. The underlying causes of these were eclampsia, placenta increta at termination of pregnancy, amniotic fluid embolism and ruptured uterus.

As shown in Table 4.1, haemorrhage is a continuing problem and the mortality rate per million maternities has more than doubled since the last triennium. However, two of the women who died in this triennium had no contact at all with health services and another two declined blood transfusions that would probably have saved their lives. Without these four cases, the death rate would be 6.5 per million, which is similar to the rate over the last decade, although higher than in any triennium since 1998–90, as shown in Figure 4.2.

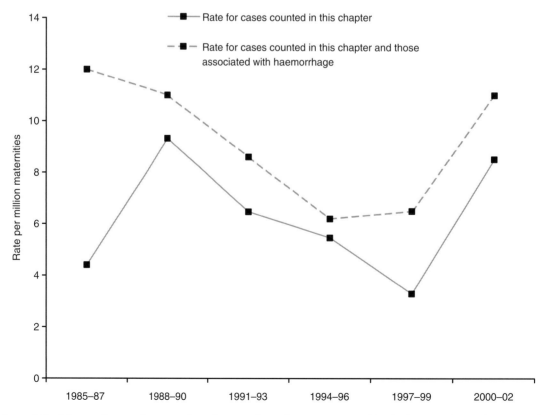

Figure 4.2 Maternal mortality rates from haemorrhage by cases counted in the haemorrhage chapter and by total number of cases associated with haemorrhage; United Kingdom 1985–2002

Substandard care

Fifteen (80%) of the 17 women who died from haemorrhage did seek medical care. Two did not. Two of the 15 women who sought care refused blood products. In 12 of the 15 cases where the woman sought care, this was assessed to have been poor. In seven cases, organisational problems (including inappropriate booking) were identified. In five cases the anaesthetic care was assessed as substandard, and lessons from these cases are discussed in Chapter 9 Anaesthesia.

The quality of resuscitation provided for these women was variable and sometimes poor. Of the 13 women who sought care and were prepared to accept blood products, most did have a transfusion, sometimes massive (range 7–82 units). Acknowledging the fact that death can occur very rapidly, it is nevertheless noteworthy that some women who died of haemorrhage seem to have received remarkably little blood.

Despite repeated recommendations given in successive Reports of this Enquiry, some high-risk women are still being booked for delivery in hospitals with neither blood transfusion nor intensive care facilities on site and with poor lines of communication to the nearest of appropriate facilities. In one case, urgently needed blood had been withdrawn from the refrigerator by the blood transfusion service because it was out of date 30 minutes before it was required. One hospital reported malfunctioning of specimen transport systems, which led to delay in crossmatched blood being available. Another reported a lack of a properly staffed recovery area.

In a few cases the care given was very poorly documented. Antenatal anaemia was not always corrected, although this is not counted as substandard care because anaemia can be refractory. In some cases, there was a failure to identify complex medical problems that would have been evident on careful scrutiny of family history, previous investigations and clinical symptoms as shown in the following vignette:

> A woman had a pre-pregnancy chest X-ray (screening for tuberculosis) that showed atrial enlargement, which was not reported but was evidence of mitral stenosis. Some of her female relatives had had unexplained deaths, but this history was not elicited until after the women herself had died. She also had recurring epistaxis which was not adequately investigated until it was too late. She actually had factor XI deficiency.

It is also important to check obvious antecedent factors, such as partial retained placenta, which was missed in one case.

In most cases, consultant obstetricians and anaesthetists were actively involved, although emergency surgery was sometimes started by non-consultant staff. In one case, however, there was no consultant attendance and no life-saving procedure was attempted. Twelve women had hysterectomies and some also had internal iliac ligation. No deaths were reported of women who had had a B-Lynch suture or radiological embolisation. There are no denominator data to allow interpretation but it may be that these procedures are more effective than heroic surgery.

It is very clear how helpful senior anaesthetic advice can be. In several cases where the woman was undergoing a caesarean section, the consultant anaesthetists had to persuade the obstetricians that physical signs such as oliguria, tachycardia or hypotension were in fact attributable to haemorrhage and that further surgery was required.

The quality of surgical treatment gave rise to concern. There were two cases in which re-suturing had to be undertaken in the operative field. Two women appeared to have had the abdomen closed prematurely after the first surgical procedure.

One woman was extubated prematurely when she had pulmonary oedema. In one woman, the administration of four doses of intramyometrial carboprost (Hemabate®, Pharmacia) was thought to have contributed to her collapse.

Placental abruption

Placental abruption can occur at any gestational age.[1] It is usually treated actively by delivery, by caesarean section if the fetus is alive and viable but vaginally if the fetus is dead. Three deaths occurred in this triennium. All were in relatively young women and all were preterm, one in the second trimester of pregnancy. Care was considered good in one case but substandard in the other two. One was being managed conservatively, which is certainly unusual, although whether active management would have prevented her death is uncertain. One woman had an amniotic fluid embolism after the abruption occurred. The following vignette provides an example of other features that may be associated with abruption:

> A woman had a rupture of the scar from previous caesarean sections. Intrauterine death had occurred from abruption and she was allowed to labour but then collapsed with upper abdominal pain. Dehiscence of the scar was diagnosed at examination under anaesthesia because of postpartum haemorrhage.

Labouring with a known intrauterine death is reasonable, even with previous caesarean section scars, but does present a problem for early diagnosis of scar dehiscence (which is usually diagnosed from fetal distress on cardiotocographic tracing). Special attention should be given to surveillance of women in such circumstances. Dehiscence may be diagnosed by eliciting scar tenderness or pain.

Placenta praevia

When placenta praevia is diagnosed during pregnancy, delivery should be postponed until 14 days before term to improve perinatal outcome. However, death occurred before 38 weeks in three of the four cases in this triennium. In the other case the woman died just before her elective surgery.

All four women who died from placenta praevia presented with bleeding. Previous caesarean section predisposes to placenta praevia and placenta accreta. All four women had at least one previous caesarean and three had previous accreta.

It is increasingly argued that where there is a scan diagnosis of placenta praevia but no bleeding, hospital admission is not necessary. Hospitalisation is preferable where bleeding occurs, however, as illustrated in the following case:

> A woman who had several previous caesarean sections was admitted with antepartum haemorrhage at around 28 weeks of gestation. A scan showed placenta praevia and two units of blood were transfused. She then went home but was readmitted two weeks later with further bleeding and again

was allowed to go home. She was readmitted with bleeding a few weeks later and had an emergency caesarean section. Unfortunately, this was in a unit with neither blood transfusion facilities nor an intensive care unit on site.

Admission is advisable when repeated bleeding occurs. Very close surveillance is even more necessary if placenta accreta has been diagnosed, because of the risk of dehiscence of the scar, as has been already discussed. Such high-risk women should be managed in a hospital which has facilities for embolisation, major surgery, blood transfusion and intensive care.

Postpartum haemorrhage

There was a wide age range in the women who died from postpartum haemorrhage. Five of the ten deaths were in primigravidae, four in women of low parity and only one in a grand multipara, the group usually considered most at risk. One woman had a fundal placenta accreta and there was one death associated with multiple pregnancy.

Two deaths occurred in women who had no antenatal or intrapartum care. One may not have known she was pregnant. The other always avoided acknowledging pregnancy because she expected her children to be taken into care. There does not seem to have been any scope for midwifery or medical intervention.

Women who decline blood transfusion

Two deaths occurred in women who declined blood transfusions. This is not considered as substandard care. Both were delivered by elective section, for reasons which were not clearly documented, and both subsequently required hysterectomy. Delay in carrying out the subsequent hysterectomy in one case may have been due to difficulty in obtaining consent.

There have only been six cases of death in women refusing blood transfusion in the last 21 years (1982–2002) so it is a very uncommon event, although it may well be that those women are over-represented among deaths. Staff find it very difficult to manage such situations. The recommendations for the management of women who decline blood products, made in the 1991–93 Report,[2] have been updated and are annexed to this Chapter. Since these have been published there have been some new developments which will prove helpful for managing these women in future:

a. Interventional radiology for embolisation of the uterine or other vessels[3] may be difficult to deliver where haemorrhage has occurred without warning, where the woman's condition is unstable and she cannot be moved and especially where the delivery hospital is not on a general hospital site. But consideration could be given to arranging for the woman to deliver where there are appropriate facilities and it may sometimes be possible to stabilise the situation using angioplasty balloons prior to embolisation.

b. Cell savers to harvest and wash the blood cells that the woman has lost and return them to her are acceptable to some women who decline blood transfusion and may be useful if the blood loss is intra-abdominal and is not contaminated with amniotic fluid. These conditions may not be met, however, if there is torrential vaginal loss or bleeding in the early stages of caesarean section. There is a risk of iso-immunisation if fetal cells are given to the mother and administration of Anti-D immunoglobulin can reduce this. The risk of causing coagulopathy by returning amniotic fluid into the circulation is thought to be small.[4]

The above procedures may, of course, be used in any case of obstetric haemorrhage, including women who will accept blood transfusion.

Substandard care

Among the eight women who sought care, there were elements of substandard care in seven. Most aspects of substandard care have been discussed earlier in this chapter, but one further point deserves discussion.

Recent changes in medical training may be relevant to the increased numbers of deaths from haemorrhage. Reduction in the overall length of obstetric training and in working hours during training may have reduced the amount of experience gained. There is also a trend towards subspecialisation among consultants and those with a special interest in obstetrics do not necessarily have highly developed surgical skills. The information available to the Enquiry does not permit any firm conclusion as to whether these factors contributed to the recent change in death rates. If they did contribute, this would strengthen the recommendation for regular 'fire drills' or 'skills drills' for the management of obstetric emergencies, including major haemorrhage, for all grades of staff in every unit.

Obstetric haemorrhage: learning points

- Catastrophic haemorrhage is a persisting problem.

- All of the women who died with placenta praevia had previous caesarean sections.

- Women at high risk of haemorrhage are still delivering in isolated or units ill equipped to sudden, life-threatening emergencies. These units may be without immediate access to specialist consultant care, blood products or intensive care.

- Women who decline blood products should be treated with respect and a management plan in case of haemorrhage agreed with them before delivery is anticipated.

- During this triennium, two women who concealed their pregnancies for fear that their babies might be taken into care died of postpartum haemorrhage at home.

- Obstetric care was considered to be substandard in 12 out of 15 (80%) of cases where the woman had sought treatment; anaesthetic care was considered to be substandard for five (see Chapter 9).

- No deaths were reported in women who had had interventional radiology or B-Lynch suture.

References

1. Hall MH, Wagaarachchi P. Antepartum haemorrhage. In: MacLean AB, Neilson JP, editors. *Maternal Morbidity and Mortality*. London: RCOG Press; 2002. p. 227–40.
2. Department of Health. *Report on Confidential Enquiries into Maternal Deaths in the United Kingdom 1991–93*. London: HMSO; 1996.
3. Hong T-M, Tseng H-S, Lee R-C, Wang J-H, Chang C-Y. Uterine artery embolisation: an effective treatment for intractable obstetric haemorrhage. *Clin Radiol* 2004;59: 96–101.
4. Catling SJ, Freites O, Krishnan S, Gibbs R. Clinical experience with cell salvage in obstetrics: 4 cases from one UK centre. I*nt J Obstet Anesth* 2002;11:128–34.

CHAPTER 4: ANNEX A
Guidelines for the management and treatment of obstetric haemorrhage in women who decline blood transfusion

The vast majority of women accept blood transfusion if the clinical reasons for its use are fully explained. However, a few may continue to refuse transfusion because of personal or religious beliefs. Massive obstetric haemorrhage is often unpredictable and can become life threatening in a short time. In most cases, blood transfusion can save the woman's life and very few women refuse transfusion in these circumstances. If it is known in advance that a woman may decline blood products, plans for the management of massive haemorrhage, should it occur, should be made and discussed during her pregnancy.

Management

At booking
1. When women are asked about religious beliefs they should also be asked if they have any objections to receiving a blood transfusion. This discussion should be documented. All relevant information should be given to her in a non-confrontational manner, including the possibility that hysterectomy may be required if massive haemorrhage occurs.

2. If she decides against accepting blood transfusion in any circumstances, she should be booked for delivery in a unit with facilities for prompt management of haemorrhage, such as interventional radiology, cell salvage and surgical expertise.

Antenatal care
3. Her blood group, antibody status and haemoglobin should be checked in the usual way and haematinics given throughout pregnancy to maximise iron stores.

4. The placental site should be identified by ultrasound scan in late pregnancy.

5. Even if it is acceptable to the woman, autologous transfusion should not be suggested to pregnant women, as the amounts of blood required to treat massive obstetric haemorrhage are far in excess of the amount that could be donated during pregnancy. If cell salvage is available, it should be ascertained whether she would agree to this.

Labour
6. The consultant obstetrician and anaesthetist should be informed when a woman who will decline transfusion is admitted in labour or for delivery. Vaginal delivery is usually associated with lower blood loss than caesarean section and caesarean section should be performed only if there is a clear medical indication. In that case it should be performed by a consultant obstetrician.

7. The third stage of labour should be actively managed with oxytocics. The woman should not be left alone for at least an hour after delivery.

Haemorrhage

8. Blood loss must be carefully quantified and clotting status investigated promptly. Delay should be avoided in intervention such as embolisation of uterine arteries, B-Lynch suture, internal iliac ligation or hysterectomy.

9. Pharmacological interventions which may be useful include intravenous vitamin K, and antifibrinolytics such as tranexamic acid.

10. The woman and her partner should be kept fully informed throughout. If the situation is critical, she should be asked again whether she would accept transfusion, in case she has changed her mind. Medical and midwifery staff should try to see her on her own to comfort themselves that she is making her decision of her own free will.

11. If she continues to refuse blood or blood products, her wishes must be respected. Any adult patient who has the necessary mental capacity is entitled to refuse treatment, even if that will result in death. No other person can consent to or refuse treatment on her behalf.

12. If, in spite of all care, the woman dies, her relatives require support like any other bereaved family.

13. It is very distressing for staff to have to watch a woman bleed to death while refusing effective treatment. Support must be promptly available for staff in these circumstances.

CHAPTER 5
Amniotic fluid embolism

ROBIN VLIES on behalf of the Editorial Board

Amniotic fluid embolism: recommendations

Audit

All cases of suspected or proven amniotic fluid embolism, whether fatal or not, should be reported to the National Amniotic Fluid Embolism Register:

UKOSS, National Perinatal Epidemiology Unit, University of Oxford, Old Road Campus, Old Road, Headington, Oxford OX3 7LF.

Service provision

Guidelines, protocols and training
Cardiac arrests are rare in maternity units but they can and do happen and their management may be suboptimal. All medical and midwifery staff should be trained to a nationally recognised level: Basic Life Support, Immediate Life Support or Advanced Life support (BLS, ILS and ALS), as appropriate. Emergency drills for maternal resuscitation should be regularly practised in clinical areas in all maternity units. These drills should include the identification of the equipment required and appropriate methods for ensuring that cardiac arrest teams know the location of the maternity unit and theatres in order to arrive promptly. Specialised courses such as Advanced Life Support in Obstetrics (ALSO) and Managing Obstetric Emergencies and Trauma (MOET) provide additional training for obstetric, midwifery and other staff.

Individual practitioners

All staff should be aware that a sudden change in a woman's behaviour may be an early feature of the onset of hypoxia and a toxic confusional state. The early involvement of senior staff and, in particular, anaesthetists and intensivists, once these or other warning symptoms of amniotic fluid embolism develop is important, as it is with any case of maternal collapse.

Pathology

Fetal elements should be searched for in the pulmonary vasculature at autopsy in any pregnant or recently delivered woman who dies following sudden collapse. If the diagnosis of amniotic fluid embolism is suspected clinically, all attempts should be made to confirm this at autopsy.

Amniotic fluid embolism should only be diagnosed on clinical grounds in the absence of an autopsy or an inadequately investigated autopsy.

50 years ago . . .

Entry of amniotic fluid into the maternal circulation was first described in 1926[1] but it was not until 1941 that death following sudden collapse in late pregnancy was attributed to amniotic fluid embolism.[2] Amniotic fluid embolism was first recorded as a cause of death in the Report in England and Wales 1955–57, when there were 11 cases; only cases confirmed at autopsy were included. The authors suggested that previous deaths attributed to shock may have been caused by amniotic fluid embolism.

There has been a declining rate of death from amniotic fluid embolism over the last 40 years, as shown in Figure 5.1. It should be noted that, from 1991, clinical diagnoses were accepted as well as those confirmed at autopsy.

Summary of findings for 2000–02

There were five cases of amniotic fluid embolism in the United Kingdom reported during this triennium. This compares with eight in 1997–99 and 17 in 1994–95. The details of the five cases are described in this chapter, although there is little information in one case.

For four women, the diagnosis was confirmed at autopsy and one diagnosis made clinically as no autopsy was held. The youngest woman was in her mid-20s, two were nulliparous and all had reached term. Labour was spontaneous for two woman, induced with prostaglandins for a further two, and the other received oxytocin augmentation. At the time of embolism, one woman still had her membranes intact, for two they had spontaneously ruptured (in one, a few minutes before collapse) and they were artificially ruptured for the other two women. All the women were delivered by caesarean section, four being perimortem during maternal resuscitation and one performed before the

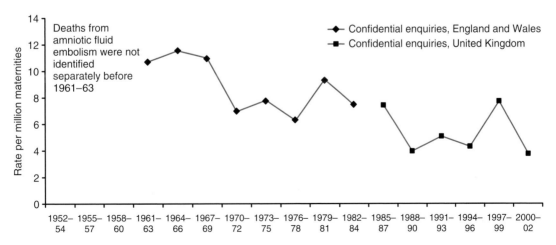

Figure 5.1   Maternal morality from amniotic fluid embolism; England and Wales 1961–84, United Kingdom 1985–2002

woman collapsed. Four of the babies were born alive but two died in the early neonatal period. One was stillborn.

Three women died within 1 hour of collapse and two between 5 and 7 hours later. Two women required hysterectomies after caesarean section because of continued heavy bleeding, with one requiring a subsequent laparotomy. A third woman underwent a laparotomy without hysterectomy. A brief summary of these cases is given in Table 5.1.

Diagnosis

The classical scenario of amniotic fluid embolism involves an older multiparous woman in advanced labour who suddenly collapses, although it can occur following termination of pregnancy, amniocentesis, placental abruption and trauma, during caesarean section and unexpectedly up to 30 minutes after delivery. There may be cardiotocographic abnormalities, uterine hypertonus and an obstetric intervention such as artificial rupture of the membranes. The initial pulmonary symptoms may be minor. Cardiovascular collapse follows due to acute left ventricular failure. Disseminated intravascular coagulation and haemorrhage rapidly follow. Most mortality occurs in the first few hours. Death rates from the major case series vary between 26.4%[3] and 61%.[4]

Diagnosis may be clinical but should be confirmed by the presence of fetal squames and lanugo hair in the pulmonary vasculature at autopsy. Fetal elements have been found however, in pulmonary artery aspirate[5] in living patients with and without the clinical syndrome of amniotic fluid embolism, as well as in maternal sputum.[6] The Report only accepts amniotic fluid embolism as a cause of death if this is confirmed at autopsy or on clinical grounds in the absence of an autopsy or where the autopsy was inadequately performed or investigated.

All the cases described in the present triennium were in their late 20s or 30s and four were in advanced labour at term. Three had some form of uterine stimulation. The relationship between uterine stimulation and amniotic fluid embolism however, has been questioned;[7] indeed, it has been suggested that hypertonus occurs as a result of amniotic fluid embolism.[4]

Speed of collapse

Three women experienced premonitory symptoms before their collapse. In one case, the woman complained of feeling cold and developed stertorous breathing and cyanosis for an unspecified time before collapse. Another woman developed respiratory distress, restlessness and cyanosis, and the third experienced extreme distress and was said to have behaved in an abnormal manner. These symptoms appeared to have developed within the half an hour preceding their collapse.

The time taken to deliver the baby from first symptoms ranged from 15 minutes to 45 minutes. The time from maternal collapse to death was less than 1 hour in three cases and between 5.5 and 7 hours in the other two. Previous Reports have suggested that improved treatment for women who survive long enough to be transferred to the intensive care unit offers hope for better survival. Only one case was admitted to intensive care but she died shortly after admission and the other four cases died rapidly where they had delivered or collapsed.

Table 5.1 Clinical features of amniotic fluid embolism cases; United Kingdom 2000–02

	Case 1	Case 2	Case 3	Case 4	Case 5
Parity	Nulliparous	Multiparous	Nulliparous	Multiparous	Multiparous
Gestation*	Term	Term+	Term	Term+	Term
Uterine stimulation	Induced with PG	Induced with PG	Nil	Oxytocin augmentation	Nil
State of membranes at maternal collapse	Intact	Spontaneous rupture	Artificial rupture	Artificial rupture	Spontaneous rupture
Type of caesarean	Perimortem	Perimortem	Emergency for fetal distress	Perimortem	Perimortem
Premonitory signs/ symptoms	Felt cold, stertorous breathing, cyanosis	Respiratory distress, cyanosis, restlessness	Extreme distress, abnormal behaviour	Nil	N/K
Interval between symptoms and delivery	15–30 minutes	30–45 minutes	15–30 minutes	15–30 minutes	30–45 minutes
Time between collapse and death	30–45 minutes	30–45 minutes	5–7 hours	45–60 minutes	5–7 hours
Neonatal outcome	Early neonatal death	Early neonatal death	Survived	Survived	Stillborn

Term = within 7 days of due date; Term+ = later than 7 days of due date; N/K = information not available

Pathology

Postmortem diagnosis was made in four cases where there was evidence of amniotic fluid embolism in the pulmonary vasculature. One autopsy, however, was barely adequate. Details of these cases are discussed in Chapter 16 Pathology. One diagnosis was made on clinical grounds. The clinical criteria for diagnosis of amniotic fluid embolism, in the absence of autopsy findings, include:

- acute hypoxia (dyspnoea, cyanosis or respiratory arrest)
- acute hypotension or cardiac arrest
- coagulopathy
- no other clinical condition or potential explanation for the symptoms and signs.

Substandard care

It appears that maternal death was inevitable in all of these cases. There was no substandard care in two cases and, although there are some more general lessons around the provision of anaesthesia in the other cases, these would not, in all probability, have affected the outcome. These issues are discussed in Chapter 9 Anaesthesia. However, it is disconcerting that, in one case, the arrival of the cardiac arrest team was delayed because they apparently did not know where the obstetric theatre was.

Comment

The number of maternal deaths due to amniotic fluid embolism has fallen significantly over the last three triennia. Amniotic fluid embolism is rare. It remains unpredictable, unpreventable and is rapidly progressive. Management is supportive (oxygenation, correction of cardiovascular collapse, blood transfusion and replacement of clotting factors) and maternal outcome is improved if she has rapid access to an intensive care unit.

Premonitory signs and symptoms (restlessness, abnormal behaviour, respiratory distress and cyanosis) may occur before collapse. There may be associated hypertonic contractions and fetal distress. Early recognition of the possibility of amniotic fluid embolism could lead to earlier involvement of the resuscitation team, as well as consultant input in obstetrics, anaesthetics, intensive care and haematology.

All the cases described here involved resuscitation and advanced life support. All relevant staff should keep up to date their basic and advanced life support skills and be encouraged to attend appropriate courses, such as Advanced Life Support in Obstetrics (ALSO) and Managing Obstetric Emergencies and Trauma (MOET). Resuscitation protocols should be kept up to date. MOET recommends caesarean section delivery of the infant within five minutes of cardiac arrest.[8]

Amniotic fluid register

All cases of suspected or proven amniotic fluid embolism, be they fatal or not, should be reported to the National Amniotic Fluid Embolism Register. Contact details are given in the recommendations at the start of this Chapter. Comparison of fatalities and survivors may help to identify treatment strategies that improve survival.

In 2000–02, 19 cases were reported to the Register, including four of the five deaths discussed here. This gives a 21% case mortality rate in cases reported to the Register. If the unreported case were included, mortality would be around 25%. This confirms that the condition should not be thought of as universally fatal and that early recognition should be encouraged. Early consideration of the diagnosis seems more common in survivors than in deaths. The early involvement of anaesthetists once symptoms develop is also be important.[9]

Amniotic fluid embolism: learning points

- Amniotic fluid embolism is not universally fatal but, despite improved resuscitation techniques, in some cases death is still inevitable.

- Only 25% of the known or suspected cases reported to the Amniotic Fluid Embolism Register died.

- Women with symptoms suspicious of amniotic fluid embolism should be transferred to intensive care as soon as possible, as these women may have a better chance of survival.

- Significant premonitory signs and symptoms, i.e. respiratory distress, cyanosis, restlessness and altered behaviour, may give the first clue to diagnosis before collapse and haemorrhage occur.

Acknowledgements
This Chapter has been seen and commented on by Derek Tuffnell FRCOG.

References

1. Meyer JR. Embolis pulmonar-caseosa. *Bras Med* 1926;2:301–3.
2. Steiner PE, Lushbaugh CC. Maternal pulmonary embolism by amniotic fluid as a cause of obstetric shock and unexpected deaths in obstetrics. *JAMA* 1941;117:1245–54, 1340–5.
3. Gilbert WM, Danielsen B. Amniotic fluid embolism: decreased mortality in a population-based study. *Obstet Gynecol* 1999;93:973–7.
4. Clarke SL, Hankins GD, Dudley DA, Dildy GA, Porter TF. Amniotic fluid embolism: analysis of the national registry. *Am J Obstet Gynecol* 1995;172:1158–69.
5. Clark SL, Pavlova Z, Greenspoon J, Horenstein J, Phelan JP. Squamous cells in the maternal pulmonary circulation. *Am J Obstet Gynecol* 1986;154:104–6.
6. Zipser G. Amniotic fluid embolism. *Med J Aust* 1971:2:953–6.
7. Morgan M. Amniotic fluid embolism. *Anaesthesia* 1979;34:20–32.
8. Grady K, Prasad BGR, Howell C. Cardiopulmonary resuscitation in the non-pregnant and pregnant patient. In: Johanson R, Cox C, Grady K, Howell C, editors. *Managing Obstetric Emergencies and Trauma*. London: RCOG Press; 2003. p. 24.
9. Tuffnell DJ. Amniotic fluid embolism. In: MacLean AB, Neilson JP, editors. *Maternal Mortality and Morbidity*. London: RCOG Press; 2002. p. 190–200.

CHAPTER 6

Early pregnancy deaths

JAMES P NEILSON on behalf of the Editorial Board

Early pregnancy deaths: recommendations

Service provision

All pregnant women presenting with abdominal pain to an accident and emergency department should be reviewed by staff from the obstetrics and gynaecology department.

No woman should wait longer than 3 weeks from initial referral to the time of her termination. Women referred for a termination of pregnancy who have a potentially life-threatening condition should be given an appointment as quickly as possible.

Individual practitioners

Clinicians in primary care and accident and emergency departments, in particular, need to be aware of atypical clinical presentations of ectopic pregnancy and especially of the way in which it may mimic gastrointestinal disease. This needs to be taught to undergraduate medical and nursing students and highlighted in textbooks.

Dipstick testing for human chorionic gonadotrophin (hCG) should be considered in any woman of reproductive age with unexplained abdominal pain. The test is now quick, easy, and sensitive.

Training

The presentation and management of ectopic pregnancy, especially the atypical symptoms, needs to be taught to undergraduate medical and nursing students and highlighted in textbooks, and reinforced in medical postgraduate education.

---

50 years ago...

The most striking change during the first 50 years of this Report has been the disappearance of unsafe, illegal abortion as a cause of early pregnancy *Direct* deaths which followed the passage of the Abortion Act in 1967.

The first Enquiry Report, covering the years 1952–54, described 153 deaths from 'abortion', of which 108 at the least had been procured illegally.[1] No social class was exempt. "Of cases ... in which domestic circumstances were noted in reports, the majority of

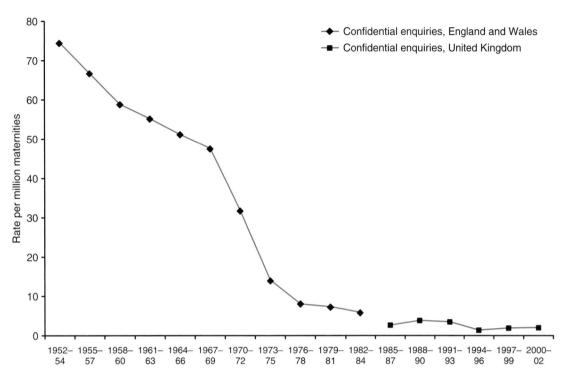

Figure 6.1 Maternal mortality rate from all maternal deaths from miscarriage (embryonic deaths) and terminations of pregnancy; England and Wales 1952–84, United Kingdom 1985–2002

single women were noted to be living in comfortable circumstances, whereas one-third of married women were noted to be living in poor circumstances and many had families of considerable size." Around 30 deaths per year from illegal abortion continued through the rest of the 1950s and the 1960s. The first full working year of the Abortion Act was 1969 and the number of deaths "clearly due to illegal abortion" fell, that year, to 17. It is interesting that several further years passed before deaths from illegal abortion disappeared completely, demonstrating presumably that legislative changes do not necessarily equate with availability. There were four such deaths during the triennium 1976–78 and one in 1979–81. It was not until 1982–84 that no deaths from illegal abortion were recorded (Figure 6.1).

It is quite possible that the number of deaths from illegal abortion were underestimated. The 1979–81 Report noted that the number of deaths attributed to spontaneous miscarriage had decreased from 1970, in parallel with those from illegal abortion.

The success of the Abortion Act in Britain, and of similar legislation in other countries, is still to be mirrored in many parts of the world, where the scourge of unsafe abortion is still responsible for a large proportion of maternal deaths. In the international context, it is essential that renewed efforts are made to address this continuing challenge.

In the early years of legalised termination of pregnancy, this procedure was very far from innocuous. In 1970–72, the number of deaths from legal and illegal abortion were virtually identical (37 and 38). Termination of pregnancy has, since, become much safer, as shown in Figure 6.2.

The main challenge in reducing deaths in early pregnancy is now the diagnosis and management of women with an ectopic pregnancy.

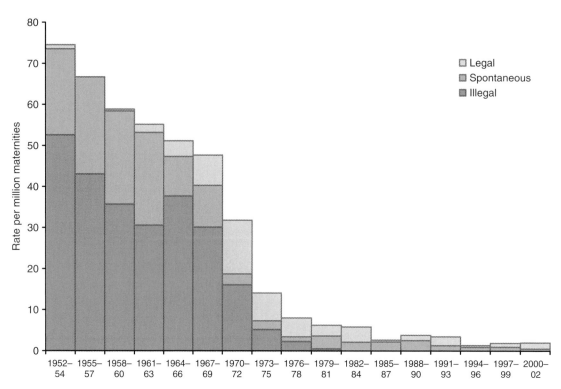

Figure 6.2   Maternal mortality for deaths from miscarriage (embryonic deaths) and terminations of pregnancy; England and Wales 1952–84, United Kingdom 1985–2002

Summary of findings for 2000–02

Fifteen *Direct* deaths attributed to early pregnancy complications are counted in this chapter and shown in Table 6.1. These include 11 deaths from ruptured ectopic pregnancies (seven tubal pregnancies and four cornual pregnancies), one death after miscarriage and three deaths after termination of pregnancy. Two early *Direct* deaths from sepsis are counted and discussed in Chapter 7 Genital tract sepsis and three *Direct* deaths from pulmonary embolism before 24 weeks of completed gestation are counted and discussed in Chapter 2. There are lessons to be learned from the three *Direct* deaths counted in Chapter 9 Anaesthesia, in which general anaesthesia was given for an ectopic pregnancy, an evacuation of retained products of conception or a termination of pregnancy. In addition, one 'unascertained' death which occurred some time after an uncomplicated termination of pregnancy is counted in Chapter 12 Indirect deaths.

These figures are tabulated with those from recent Reports in Table 6.1. Although detailed interpretation of trend is inappropriate because gestational age definitions have changed during this time and because of the fine distinction of whether deaths from miscarriage associated with infection are included in this chapter or in Chapter 7 Sepsis, the table has value in conveying a of lack of progress.

As in previous years, the major challenge is to reduce the number of deaths from ectopic pregnancy and especially those associated with substandard care. In two cases, no information other than autopsy summaries has been made available to the Enquiry. Overall, 66%, ten of the 15 evaluated deaths that are counted in this chapter were assessed as having substandard care. Six of 11 deaths from ectopic pregnancy were

Table 6.1 Numbers of *Direct* deaths in early pregnancy by cause; United Kingdom 1985–2002

	Ectopic pregnancy	Miscarriage	Termination of pregnancy	Total
1985–87	11	1	4	16
1988–90	15	6	3	24
1991–93	9	3	5	17
1994–96	12	2	1	15
1997–99	13	2+5*	2	17+5*
2000–2	11	1+2*	3	15+2*

* There were also five deaths in the triennium 1997–99 and two deaths from sepsis associated with miscarriage or amniocentesis in the triennium 2000–02 counted in **Chapter 7 Sepsis**
Note. Until the 1994–96 Report, early pregnancy deaths were defined as occurring before 20 weeks of pregnancy. In subsequent Reports, 24 weeks has been used as the upper gestational limit. Thus, direct comparisons with data from previous triennia may be inappropriate

associated with substandard care, as were all deaths from miscarriage and termination of pregnancy.

A disproportionate number of women were from ethnic minorities, seven of 11 dying from ectopic pregnancies and two of three dying after termination of pregnancy.

Ectopic pregnancy

Table 6.2 shows that the rate of deaths from ectopic pregnancies has not declined since the last Report and is still an increase on the rates described for 1991–93.

There were 11 deaths from ruptured ectopic pregnancies: seven in the extrauterine tube, and four in the interstitial portion of the tube (cornual pregnancies). Cornual (or interstitial) pregnancies account for 2–4% of ectopic pregnancies and are said to have a mortality rate in the range of 2.0–2.5%.[2] Ultrasound diagnosis is successful in around 70% of cases but there are well-recognised diagnostic difficulties. More conservative methods of treatment, both medical and surgical, have been developed. However, in none of the cases reported here was the diagnosis made before rupture. Haemorrhage can be severe because the pregnancies are often more developed than extrauterine tubal pregnancies and because of the large blood supply to the uterus.

Table 6.2 Deaths from ectopic pregnancies and mortality rates per 1000 estimated pregnancies; England and Wales 1988–1990 and United Kingdom 1991–2002

	Estimated numbers of pregnancies (000s)	Estimated ectopic pregnancies (n)	Ectopic pregnancies per thousand pregnancies		Deaths from ectopic pregnancies (n)	Mortality rate per thousand ectopic pregnancies	
			Rate	95% CI		Rate	95% CI
England and Wales							
1988–90	2,886.9	24,775	8.6	(8.5–8.7)	15	0.6	(0.3–1.0)
United Kingdom							
1991–93	3,137.4	30,160	9.6	(9.5–9.7)	9	0.3	(0.1–0.6)
1994–96	2,911.6	33,550	11.5	(11.4–11.6)	12	0.4	(0.2–0.6)
1997–99	2,873.3	31,946	11.1	(11.0–11.2)	13	0.4	(0.2–0.7)
2000–02	2,739.4	30,100	11.0	(10.9–11.1)	11	0.4	(0.2–0.7)

Source: see Table 21.3

Overall, three of the deaths from ectopic pregnancies occurred suddenly and before any involvement of the clinical services. It is not known if the women had any symptoms before collapse.

Two deaths occurred after substandard care in accident and emergency departments. In one case, a woman with what proved to be an ectopic pregnancy was classed as low priority by a nurse applying the triage system. The woman waited for several hours without seeing a doctor, at which point she collapsed. Another woman was known by the accident and emergency staff to be pregnant but was misdiagnosed as having a urinary tract infection. She was discharged and returned a few hours later, by which time her haemoglobin concentration had dropped from 10 g/dl to 3 g/dl.

These cases reinforce advice in previous Reports that there should be a low threshold for beta-hCG testing in women of reproductive age attending accident and emergency departments with abdominal symptoms. Commercially available dipstick tests for hCG, which are sensitive to values as low as 25 miu/ml, are simple to use, and provide reliable results within 3 minutes. Also, pregnant women with abdominal pain should be reviewed by staff from the obstetrics and gynaecology department.

The previous two Reports have emphasised the problem of women presenting to their general practitioners or accident and emergency departments with atypical symptoms – notably vomiting and diarrhoea – with the diagnosis of ectopic pregnancy not being considered. There was one such case in the current triennium. The woman had nausea and dizziness. The correct diagnosis was not made in primary care.

There was one potentially avoidable death in a woman who had been seen in a specialist service. An ultrasonically empty uterus was interpreted as showing a complete miscarriage. Death occurred 3 weeks later from a ruptured tubal pregnancy. Quantitative beta-hCG testing would almost certainly have established the correct diagnosis.

Early pregnancy deaths: learning points

- Women with ectopic pregnancies may have atypical symptoms suggesting gastrointestinal or urinary tract dysfunction.

- Cornual pregnancies are rare but dangerous types of ectopic pregnancy. Clinicians should be aware of the difficulties with both clinical and ultrasound diagnosis.

Miscarriage

One woman who died after a miscarriage is counted here. She presented in respiratory and renal failure and declined treatment offered in the intensive care unit. There was no sub-standard care.

Termination of pregnancy

There were five deaths that followed termination of pregnancy. Three are counted here. Another death from pulmonary embolism is counted in Chapter 2 Thromboembolism and the other, an anaesthetic death, is counted in Chapter 9 Anaesthesia.

The following vignettes illustrate problems in systems of the provision of termination of pregnancy:

> There were two cases where women, although referred promptly for termination of pregnancy, were not given appointments for more than 5–6 weeks afterwards. National guidelines state that, as a minimum standard, no woman should wait longer than 3 weeks from initial referral to the time of her abortion.[3] In one case, the woman was referred to an NHS hospital for termination early in pregnancy but was not admitted until 16 weeks, when she underwent dilatation and evacuation. Another woman, discussed in Chapter 10 Cardiac disease, was referred for a potentially life-saving termination but did not receive an appointment until after she had died of serious cardiac disease.

> Another woman, although grossly overweight, was referred from an NHS facility to an isolated charitable institution remote from emergency services.

> In the case of a third woman, the report of a routine vaginal swab, taken before the termination, did not reach the relevant clinicians until after the woman had died of group A beta-haemolytic streptococcal septicaemia, secondary to pelvic sepsis, following the termination. The swab grew this same organism. In a further case, investigation of the possible source of infection after a surgical termination was insufficiently rigorous.

In one of these cases there were many major deficiencies in postoperative nursing and medical care. The hospital concerned responded by instituting both internal and external reviews, which has led to many changes in policy.

Other deaths before 24 completed weeks of gestation

In all, 27 women died of *Direct* and 34 of *Indirect* causes of maternal deaths up to and including 24 completed weeks of gestation, of which 15 are counted in this chapter.

Of the 13 other *Direct* deaths occurring before 24 completed weeks of gestation, eight were from thromboembolism and are discussed and counted in Chapter 2, two were from sepsis and counted and discussed in Chapter 7 and three from anaesthesia counted and discussed in Chapter 9.

There were 34 *Indirect* deaths in early pregnancy. Five of these, from cardiac disease, are counted in Chapter 10; three from psychiatric causes are counted in Chapter 11 and one death from cancer is counted in Chapter 13. Twenty-five deaths from *Other Indirect* causes are counted in Chapter 12. Of these, seven had epilepsy, six suffered a cerebral infarct or haemorrhage, three each were diabetic, asthmatic or died of concurrent infections, two had probable autoimmune disease, and in a further two the causes of death remained unascertained.

Seventeen early pregnancy deaths were classified as *Coincidental* and are counted in Chapter 14, representing 50% of the total for this group. Two further deaths from cancer in early pregnancy are counted in Chapter 13.

References

1. Department of Health. Reports on Public Health and Medical Subjects No. 97. Report of Confidential Enquiries into Maternal Deaths in England and Wales. 1952–1954. London: HMSO; 1957.
2. Tulandi T, Al-Jaroudi D. Interstitial pregnancy: results generated from the Society of Reproductive Surgeons registry. *Obstet Gynecol* 2004; 103: 47–50.
3. Royal College of Obstetricians and Gynaecologists. *The Care of Women Requesting Induced Abortion*. National Evidence-based Clinical Guideline No. 7. London: RCOG Press; 2004.

CHAPTER 7
Genital tract sepsis

ANN HARPER on behalf of the Editorial Board

Genital tract sepsis: key recommendations

Service provision

All units should have an antibiotic policy for cases of sepsis; the aim is to control infection without delay and prevent the development of disseminated intravascular coagulation (DIC) and organ failure.

Individual practitioners

When infection develops and the woman is systemically ill, urgent and repeated bacteriological specimens, including blood cultures, should be obtained. Advice from a microbiologist must be sought early to ensure appropriate antibiotic therapy.

When there is strong clinical suspicion of sepsis doctors should commence parenteral broad-spectrum antibiotics immediately, without waiting for microbiology results, even if the presence of diarrhoea suggests gastroenteritis as a possible diagnosis.

Fluid resuscitation and oxygen therapy are also an important part of treatment of the compromised patient.

Education and training

The onset of life-threatening sepsis in pregnancy or the puerperium can be insidious, with rapid clinical deterioration. Vomiting, diarrhoea, abdominal pain, tachycardia, tachypnoea and pyrexia greater than 38°C may all be symptoms and signs of pelvic sepsis. Pyrexia may be absent in some cases of severe sepsis. Education of doctors, midwives and medical students about the risk factors, symptoms, signs, investigation and treatment of sepsis and the recognition of critical illness is recommended.

50 years ago...

Puerperal sepsis (genital tract sepsis) was the leading cause of maternal mortality in the United Kingdom during the 18th, 19th and early part of the 20th centuries.[1] It occurred in epidemics. In 1795, Alexander Gordon described an outbreak of puerperal fever in Aberdeen between 1789 and 1792 and recognised the contagious nature of the disease. In 1847, Ignaz Semmelweiss in Vienna observed that the puerperal sepsis rate was much higher in the wards attended by doctors and medical students compared with those attended by midwives only. After he introduced hand washing in disinfectant for the medical staff after attending autopsies and before carrying out vaginal examinations in the wards, the rate of sepsis in the wards attended by the medical staff decreased greatly. At that time, the cause of the disease was still unknown. Rokitansky, in 1864, first observed organisms in the vaginal discharge of women with puerperal sepsis and in 1865 these were identified as streptococci. Joseph Lister published his work with surgical antisepsis in 1867 and this was gradually introduced into maternity practice.[1]

Despite these advances, it was not until the discovery in 1935 of a dramatically effective treatment, Prontosil® (IG Farben), followed by sulphonamides from 1937 and penicillin from 1945, that mortality from puerperal sepsis began to fall in the United Kingdom.[1] By the early 1950s, when the present series of Confidential Enquiries into Maternal Deaths began, sepsis was well down the list of causes. There were only 42 deaths from puerperal sepsis in the first triennial Report (1952–54), which commented: "At the time of the reports of the Departmental Committee in 1930 and 1932, sepsis was the pre-eminent cause of maternal death, accounting for 37% of the deaths directly due to pregnancy and childbirth in that investigation. In the present series, it accounted for only 3.8%.... Control of infection has made the major contribution to the reduction of maternal mortality. Deaths from other causes have been reduced but not so markedly".[2]

The early Reports had no separate chapter on sepsis. However, as deaths from other *Direct* causes fell, sepsis, in the form of septic abortion, again emerged as a leading cause of maternal mortality (Figure 7.1). The fifth triennial Report (1964–66)[3] was the first to have a chapter devoted to sepsis,. It commented that, if deaths from septic abortion were included "...sepsis would appear as the second commonest cause of maternal deaths, a fact which is not easy to accept". In the fifth Report, 123 (21.2%) of the 579 *Direct* deaths were due to sepsis: 66 (11.4%) due to abortion with sepsis, 28 (4.8%) to puerperal sepsis and 29 (5.0%) to sepsis after surgery. The Abortion Act was passed in 1967. Since then, in the period 1967–2002, there have been only 146 *Direct* deaths

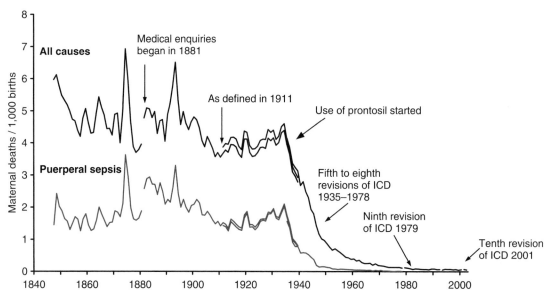

Figure 7.1   Maternal mortality rates from genital tract sepsis and from all causes; England and Wales 1847–2002
Source: General Register Office, OPCS and ONS mortality statistics Birth counts, Tables A10.1.1–A10.1.4

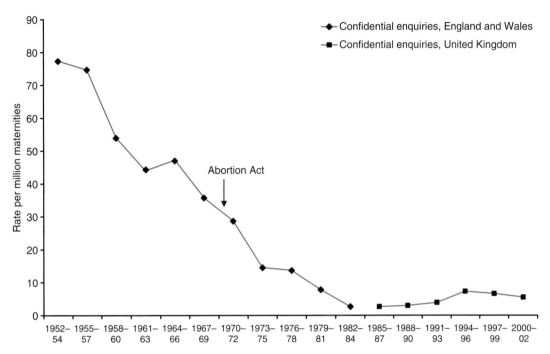

Figure 7.2 Trends in maternal mortality from genital tract sepsis; England and Wales 1952–84, United Kingdom 1985–2002

associated with septic abortion; the majority of these deaths occurred between 1967 and 1972.

In the triennium 1982–84, there were no deaths directly attributable to puerperal sepsis. Unfortunately, deaths from sepsis have risen in subsequent years and there is no room for complacency, as shown in Figure 7.2. In the current triennium there were 13 deaths due to sepsis, accounting for around 12% of all *Direct* maternal deaths. Eleven of these are counted in this chapter and two, due to sepsis following procedures in early pregnancy are counted in Chapter 6 Early pregnancy deaths. The lessons to be learned from these are described in this chapter; most are not new but repeat the recurring themes from previous Reports.

Summary of findings for 2000–02

There were 13 deaths in this triennium directly due to genital tract sepsis. Eleven are counted in this chapter and two more are counted in Chapter 6 Early pregnancy deaths.

The ages of the women ranged from 16 years to 41 years (mean age 30 years). Two were primigravida, seven had already had one or more children and two were of very high parity. Eight babies survived, including one set of twins. There were two miscarriages, one stillbirth and one early neonatal death. Two women died before 24 weeks of gestation, one woman died intrapartum, five women died following vaginal delivery and three women died following caesarean section.

Two women delivered at home but all died in hospital. Five women died within 24 hours of hospital admission and only three women survived for more than 2 days following hospital admission. Some were already gravely ill on arrival at hospital and deteriorated rapidly with little opportunity for altering the course of events. Although a variety of underlying causes and many different organisms were responsible for their sepsis, many presented with abdominal pain, diarrhoea and vomiting; not all had pyrexia. The potential severity of their condition was sometimes unrecognised or underestimated, with resultant delays in referral to hospital, delays in administration of appropriate antibiotic treatment and late involvement of senior medical staff. Awareness of the signs and symptoms of sepsis and recognition of critical illness needs to be raised among staff in maternity units, but also in accident and emergency departments, and among general practitioners, community midwives and health visitors.

The assessors considered that some degree of suboptimal care occurred in 80% of the cases discussed in this chapter, although many of the women were already moribund on admission to hospital. These cases demonstrate that the onset of life-threatening sepsis in pregnancy or the puerperium can be insidious, with extremely rapid clinical deterioration and that rapid referral to consultant care is essential.

The cases discussed in this chapter have been divided into deaths from sepsis in early pregnancy, sepsis before or during labour, puerperal sepsis after vaginal delivery and sepsis after surgery, as shown in Table 7.1. It is important to note that the rates given in Table 7.1 are calculated for all cases in which genital tract sepsis was the *Direct* cause of death, irrespective in which chapter in each Report they were counted, as the allocation of cases by chapter has varied over the years.

Sepsis before delivery

Four cases of genital tract sepsis occurred before delivery, all before 24 weeks of gestation. Two cases of genital tract sepsis in women who had surgical termination of pregnancy are counted in Chapter 6 Early pregnancy deaths but are included in the overall rates described here, for consistency with previous triennia. Two cases are counted in this chapter; one death was due to fulminating septicaemia in a woman with pelvic sepsis and one death followed amniocentesis.

The risk of uterine infection following amniocentesis is estimated to be very low (1/1000)[4] and maternal death is extremely rare. Nevertheless, one case occurred during this triennium and a similar death due to sepsis following amniocentesis was reported in the last triennial Report.[5] Both demonstrate that overwhelming infection can develop in a

Table 7.1 Numbers of *Direct* deaths associated with genital tract sepsis and mortality rate per million maternities; United Kingdom 1985–2002

Triennium	Sepsis in early pregnancy*	Puerperal sepsis	Sepsis after surgical procedures	Sepsis before or during labour	Total	Rate per million maternities	
						Rate	95% CI
1985–87	3	2	2	2	9	4.0	1.8–7.5
1988–90	8	4	5	0	17	7.2	4.2–11.5
1991–93	4	4	5	2	15	6.5	3.6–10.7
1994–96	2**	11	3	1	16	7.3	4.2–11.8
1997–99	6	4***	1	7	18	8.5	5.0–13.4
2000–02	4****	5	3	1	13	6.5	3.5–11.1

   * Early pregnancy includes deaths following miscarriage, ectopic and other causes
  ** In 1994–96, these deaths were included in **Chapter 6 Early pregnancy deaths**
 *** Including two *Late Direct* deaths
**** Including two cases counted in **Chapter 6 Early pregnancy deaths**

matter of hours in previously healthy women. A literature search revealed only one other maternal death related to amniocentesis, probably due to amniotic fluid embolism.[6] The Royal College of Obstetricians and Gynaecologists has recently issued updated guidelines for training and performing amniocentesis, which should be followed in all cases.[7]

Intrapartum deaths

> A woman who died during a perimortem caesarean section had overwhelming sepsis due to group A haemolytic streptococcal septicaemia. She had a short history of diarrhoea, vomiting and abdominal pain and although she was breathless she was apyrexial on admission to hospital. She suffered a cardiac arrest shortly after admission from which she could not be resuscitated.

This case illustrates the deceptive and fulminating nature of streptococcal infection and the challenges facing staff presented with an apyrexial patient who deteriorates so rapidly that there is little time for investigation or treatment. Increasing shortness of breath may predict impending cardiac arrest; regular resuscitation drills may help staff provide rapid and effective resuscitation when such situations arise unexpectedly in clinical practice.

Sepsis after vaginal delivery

Five women died from sepsis after vaginal delivery and are counted in this chapter. Two had had home deliveries. One case also contributes to the general lessons discussed in Chapter 10 Cardiac disease and Chapter 11 Psychiatric causes of death.

Four of the five of these women became ill in the community after discharge home. Attention is drawn to the need for good communication between hospital and community carers and the need for early referral of recently delivered women who feel unwell and have pyrexia. In one case, the woman had declined postnatal visits.

> Two women had risk factors for infection. One woman who had delivered in water with some faecal contamination became unwell with a temperature of 40°C, pain and infection in her buttock and leg. She developed overwhelming sepsis and died, despite intensive medical and surgical treatment. This case highlights the potential dangers of delivering in contaminated water. In another case, community carers were unaware of a history of ragged membranes at delivery and did not immediately suspect sepsis in a recently delivered ill woman.

> A woman with a history of 'panic attacks' developed a persistent tachycardia (130–170 bpm) after delivery and her increasingly bizarre behaviour was repeatedly attributed to a psychiatric cause without further investigation or seeking consultant advice. She was admitted to a psychiatric hospital but quickly transferred to the local general hospital where she died shortly after arrival. Autopsy revealed an infected necrotic uterus and several different organisms (*Streptococcus* groups B and D, *Staphylococcus aureus*, *Bacteroides*, *Escherichia coli*, Gram positive rods) were identified in the uterus, blood and gastrointestinal tract. There was also marked left ventricular hypertrophy, which probably accounted for some of her symptoms and was possibly due to peripartum cardiomyopathy, although histological examination was not done to confirm this diagnosis.

Sepsis: Learning points for diagnosis and management in the community

- Sepsis should be considered in recently delivered women who feel unwell and have pyrexia.

- Sepsis can be insidious in onset and have a fulminating course. The severity of illness should not be underestimated; early referral to hospital may be life saving.

- The risk of sepsis is increased after prolonged rupture of membranes, emergency caesarean section and if products of conception are retained after miscarriage, termination of pregnancy or delivery.

- Delivery in water carries a risk of infection for mother and baby due to faecal contamination of the perineum and genital tract.

- Any problems noted during the hospital stay should be reported directly to the community carers (GP, midwives and health visitors) at the time of the woman's discharge so that appropriate follow up visits may be arranged and the significance of developing symptoms recognised. This is particularly important in early postpartum discharge from hospital, which is now an increasingly common practice.

Sepsis after surgery

Three deaths in women who had a caesarean section and died from genital tract sepsis are counted in this chapter. Two were already ill from sepsis before the emergency caesarean section. Both had chorioamnionitis and developed coagulopathy; one died suddenly a few hours after delivery, the other after a protracted illness in intensive care. The severity of the illness may have been initially underestimated. Starting intravenous antibiotics immediately, involving consultants sooner, continuity of care with a lead consultant and considering ICU admission earlier might have made a difference, although all were extremely ill.

Comments

The most common pathogen identified among the 11 cases counted in this chapter was the beta-haemolytic *Streptococcus*: Lancefield groups A (3), B (2) and D (1). *S. aureus* (1) and coagulase-negative *Staphylococcus* (1); *E. coli* (2); mixed anaerobes/bacteroides (2) and *Fusobacterium necrophorum* (1) were also identified. More than one organism was identified in three women. No pathogen was identified in one obviously septic patient despite repeated investigation; in two others, results were unavailable or tests were not performed. One case of genital tract sepsis following surgical termination of pregnancy, counted in Chapter 6 Early pregnancy deaths, was due to group A beta-haemolytic streptococcal infection; in the other case, results were unavailable or tests were not done.

One women who died had a fulminating and overwhelming genital tract sepsis due to an unusual organism, *F. necrophorum*. This is an anaerobic Gram negative bacillus is usually sensitive to penicillin. Death from is rare and usually follows oropharyngeal infection, although death from *F. necrophorum* genital infection has been reported.

Sepsis learning points: investigating sepsis

Although the number of maternal deaths *Directly* due to genital tract sepsis has decreased from previous triennia, these cases of genital tract sepsis and the cases of overwhelming sepsis counted in other chapters indicate that infection remains a significant cause of maternal death in the United Kingdom.

If sepsis is suspected, vaginal swabs and urine culture should be taken, wound swabs taken, if appropriate, and throat and rectal swabs considered. Blood cultures should always be taken. Blood should also be taken for haemoglobin, white cell count, platelets, C-reactive protein, coagulation screen, group and hold, urea and electrolytes, and liver function tests.

In the event of maternal death due to suspected sepsis where the source of infection and the organisms responsible have not been identified during life, swabs from all possible sites of infection and tissue samples for histology of suspect organs (with informed consent from next-of-kin) should be taken at autopsy.

In many situations, infection may be so rapid and overwhelming that death is unavoidable despite the best efforts of all concerned. Previous Reports have emphasised the often-insidious onset, rapid spread and fulminating course of genital tract sepsis, particularly where it is due to streptococcal infection. This is seen in many of the present cases where the women had a short duration of illness and in some cases were moribund by the time they presented to primary care or hospital.

The importance of prompt aggressive treatment of suspected sepsis with adequate intravenous doses of appropriate broad-spectrum antibiotics must be emphasised, as early intervention may prevent the situation becoming irreversible. In some of the cases reported, there was delay in starting appropriate antibiotic treatment due to imprecise prescribing by medical staff. Doctors prescribing antibiotics and other drugs should ensure that midwives have clear written instructions. Treatment should be started immediately without waiting for results and sensitivities of microbiological investigations, as they may not be available for days. A combination of co-amoxiclav and metronidazole could be used initially. The choice of drug will be influenced by local antibiotic policy and the advice of a consultant microbiologist should be sought. If the woman is already extremely ill, deteriorates or does not improve within 24 hours of treatment, then additional or alternative intravenous antibiotics such as piperacillin/tazobactam or gentamicin and clindamycin should be used. Microbiological specimens should be repeated and urgent results requested.

There is an increased risk of infection in some clinical situations. Previous Reports have highlighted the importance of continuing close surveillance and assessment of antenatal patients with prolonged rupture of membranes for signs and symptoms of sepsis, avoiding vaginal examinations in these women unless essential, when careful aseptic technique should be observed, and the evidence-based use of routine prophylactic antibiotics for caesarean section. In the postpartum woman with possible sepsis, any history of ragged membranes or possibly incomplete delivery of the placenta should be sought, and the woman examined for the presence of uterine tenderness or enlargement. If retained products of conception are suspected, vaginal swabs and an ultrasound scan

to confirm that the uterine cavity is empty should be done before discharging the woman from hospital. Any relevant information about the woman's hospital stay should be communicated to her GP and community midwife or health visitor at the time of discharge from hospital.

There is evidence from the cases reported that when faced with extremely ill patients, junior doctors sometimes failed to seek timely advice from consultants, perhaps due to a lack of awareness of the possibility of serious infection and its signs and symptoms. In the past, obstetricians were very aware of sepsis and its consequences, but life-threatening sepsis is now rare and many doctors have never seen a case. As general practitioners, junior hospital doctors and nurses or midwives usually have the first contact with these women and it is important to raise their awareness of the possibility of sepsis and their skills in the recognition of developing critical illness. Pregnant women who present to accident and emergency units should be seen and assessed promptly by an experienced doctor. Improved education of 'front-line' staff, emphasising the importance of appropriate timely investigation and treatment and early communication with and involvement of consultants, may help to avoid some future maternal deaths due to sepsis. Obstetricians should seek advice from other specialists, such as anaesthetists, haematologists and microbiologists, at an early stage. All staff should regularly update and practice their resuscitation skills. In pregnant women, correction of aortocaval compression by placing the woman on her left side or using a wedge is important during resuscitation. Maternity units should develop their own guidelines for the management of women with suspected sepsis.

Vomiting, diarrhoea and abdominal pain are all symptoms of underlying genital tract sepsis but are often attributed to gastroenteritis. There may be a rash. Discoloration or mottling of the skin may indicate cellulitis. Significant pyrexia should always be

Signs of critical illness[8]

Physiological
- Signs of sympathetic activation: tachycardia, hypertension, pallor, clamminess and peripheral shutdown.
- Signs of systemic inflammation: fever or hypothermia, tachycardia and increased respiratory rate.
- Signs of organ hypoperfusion: cold peripheries, hypoxemia, confusion, hypotension and oliguria.

Biochemical
- Metabolic acidosis.
- High or low white cell count.
- Low platelet count.
- Raised urea and creatinine concentrations.
- Raised C reactive protein concentration.

investigated and treated but is not always present in cases of severe septicaemia. Elevated C-reactive protein, raised white cell count or neutropenia are important signs that should be investigated. Vital signs should be monitored and fluid balance recorded. Blood gases should be checked at an early stage to detect metabolic acidosis. Persistent tachycardia, peripheral vascular shutdown, oliguria, metabolic acidosis, increased respiratory rate and reduced oxygen saturation indicate critical illness that needs urgent management. Younger women may maintain their blood pressure and conceal serious illness for a long time and appear deceptively well, alert and talking before sudden cardiovascular decompensation occurs.

In some of the cases reported, delays in treatment caused by physical separation of facilities did not facilitate the situation, e.g. transfer to theatre delayed because it was on a different floor, making a lift journey necessary, or transfer to an intensive care unit on a different site, making an ambulance journey necessary. Ideally, there should be an operating theatre on the same floor as the delivery suite and intensive care facilities in the same building as the maternity unit.

Acknowledgements
This chapter has been read and commented on by Professor W Thompson MD FRCOG, Dr CH Webb, BDS MB FRCPath FFPRCPI, Consultant Microbiologist, and Dr JG Barr, PhD CBiol FIBiol FRCPath, Consultant Microbiologist.

References

1. Drife J. Infection and maternal mortality. In: MacLean AB, Regan L, Carrington D, editors. *Infection and Pregnancy*. London: RCOG Press; 2001. p. 355–64.
2. History and Method. In: Ministry of Health. *Report on Confidential Enquiries into Maternal Deaths in England and Wales,1952–54*. Reports on Public Health and Medical Subjects No. 97. London: HMSO; 1957. p. 1–5.
3. Puerperal sepsis. In: Ministry of Health. *Report on Confidential Enquiries into Maternal Deaths in England and Wales, 1964–66*. Reports on Public Health and Medical Subjects No. 119. London: HMSO; 1969. p. 89–91.
4. Wilson RD. The role of invasive fetal testing in prenatal diagnosis of inheritable diseases. In: Harman CR, editor. *Invasive Fetal Testing and Treatment*. Oxford: Blackwell Scientific; 1995. p. 1–19.
5. Thompson W. Genital tract sepsis. In: Lewis G, Drife J, editors. *Why Mothers Die 1997–1999. The Fifth Report of the Confidential Enquiries into Maternal Deaths in the United Kingdom*. London: RCOG Press; 200. p. 121–9.
6. Bell JA, Pearn JH, Wilson BH, Ansford AJ. Prenatal cytogenetic diagnosis – a current audit. A review of 2000 cases of prenatal cytogenetic diagnoses after amniocentesis, and comparisons with early experience. *Med J Aust* 1987;146:12–15.
7. Royal College of Obstetricians and Gynaecologists. *Amniocentesis*. Guideline No. 8A. London: RCOG; 2004.
8. Cooper N. Acute care: recognising critical illness. *Student BMJ* 2004:12;12–13.

CHAPTER 8
Other *Direct* deaths

JAMES O DRIFE on behalf of the Editorial Board

Genital tract trauma: key recommendation

A consultant facing the prospect of carrying out hysterectomy for genital tract trauma should have support available from another consultant.

Bowel perforation: key recommendations

Women who have undergone caesarean section must be looked after by midwives appropriately trained in postoperative care.

Medical staff must check a woman's progress after caesarean section, as they would after any surgical procedure. This is particularly important during holiday periods and at times of staff changeover.

Fifty years ago. . .

The brevity of this chapter, with its single death from genital tract trauma, is a powerful illustration of how things have changed over 50 years. In 1952–54, the Enquiry's first Report listed 23 deaths after "delivery complicated by disproportion or malposition of the fetus", 63 deaths after "delivery complicated by prolonged labour of other origin", 55 after "delivery with other trauma", and 66 after "delivery with other complications of childbirth". These deaths were not discussed in detail.

The 1955–57 Report included a chapter on "uterine rupture". It discussed 33 deaths, five of which occurred after previous caesarean section and two after manual removal of the placenta. Most of the 33 cases were associated with obstructed labour or intrauterine manipulations. The eight cases of spontaneous rupture all occurred in multiparous women: "two were having their eleventh babies, and one each their tenth, ninth, eighth, sixth, fifth and fourth babies. Both the women having their eleventh and tenth babies had been allowed to make arrangements for their confinement to take place at home, surely a most unwise procedure".

A chapter on uterine rupture was included for 30 years, from 1955–57 to 1982–84. The early ones emphasised the risks of older, highly parous women being confined at home or in a maternity home. The 1964–66 Report, which included 30 cases, commented that "ruptured uterus due to obstructed labour or traumatic delivery ought not to occur under proper supervision, and yet it is far more common than rupture of a uterine scar". By this time, the Report was also commenting on "the importance of oxytocic drugs as a factor in causing rupture".

The 1967–69 Report included 19 deaths (nine traumatic, eight spontaneous and two scar ruptures) and commented that the symptoms may be masked by epidural block. The next Report criticised "failure to examine the uterine cavity or delay in performing laparotomy when uterine rupture is suspected because of bleeding or shock". This lesson is still applicable today.

In 1973–75 the total fell to 11 deaths. High parity was no longer a factor but concerns were still being expressed over the use of oxytocic drugs. In 1979–81, with only four deaths, delays in performing caesarean section were criticised. The total continued at a low level until 1991–93, when a chapter on "genital tract trauma" appeared for the last time. The later Reports commented that some deaths were due to junior doctors having to perform procedures without adequate supervision.

A chapter "Other *Direct* Deaths" has been included since 1985–87, with no major trends developing over these 20 years. Deaths from liver disease have occurred at the rate of one or two a year. Bowel injury after caesarean section has been reported from time to time and it remains to be seen whether or not the increase in this complication in the present Report is a worrying new trend.

Summary of findings for 2000–02

Eight deaths are counted in this chapter, compared with seven in 1997–99 and in 1994–96 (Figure 8.1). The causes are the same as in the last Report. Acute fatty liver caused two deaths in late pregnancy and one after delivery. Genital tract trauma caused one death. The management of trauma requires urgent and skilled intervention and hospitals need to have a surgical team readily available. Bowel perforation caused four *Direct* deaths and one *Late* death, compared with one in 1997–99 and none in 1994–96. All five deaths from bowel perforation occurred after caesarean section and all involved

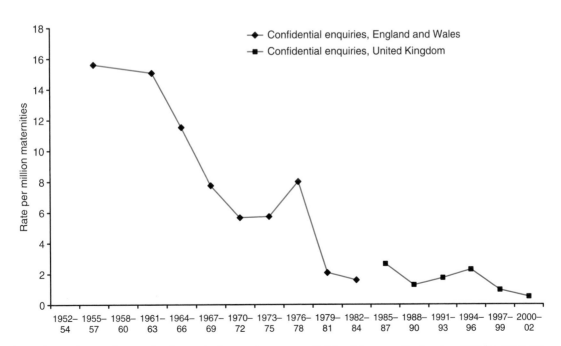

Figure 8.1 Maternal mortality from uterine rupture or genital tract trauma; England and Wales 1955–84, United Kingdom 1985–2002

substandard care. Signs of peritonism are difficult to detect in the puerperium and there is inadequate awareness that ileus after caesarean section may be fatal. Lessons about such rare complications can be learned only by aggregating experience in Reports like this.

Acute fatty liver

There were three deaths from this cause, compared with four in 1997–99 and two in 1994–96. One of the deaths occurred about 3 weeks after delivery but no other details are available. The other two occurred in late pregnancy and in each of these cases the woman presented with epigastric pain followed by deteriorating liver function tests. In both cases, delivery was by caesarean section and the woman was admitted to an intensive care unit. In one case, liver rupture occurred and the woman received a portocaval shunt before dying of fulminant liver failure.

Acute fatty liver is an unpredictable complication with a high mortality and is very difficult to prevent or treat. In one of the cases in this triennium, the anaesthetic care was considered substandard because, although a specialist registrar provided good care, a consultant anaesthetist did not attend the caesarean section or help in the early postoperative assessment. It is unlikely, however, that this would have affected the outcome.

Genital tract trauma

Genital tract trauma accounted for one death, compared with two in 1997–99 and five in 1994–96. In this case, a woman who had an induction of labour with prostaglandins had a precipitate labour and a forceps delivery. She collapsed within a few hours of delivery. At laparotomy, a uterine tear was found and hysterectomy was carried out. She died after several days in the intensive care unit.

Such cases require urgent, skilled intervention and hospitals need to have this readily available. Cases are now rare and a UK consultant obstetrician is likely to have limited experience of dealing with life-threatening haemorrhage from genital tract trauma. The consultant should not hesitate to call a colleague.

Bowel perforation

Four *Direct* deaths and one *Late* death were due to bowel perforation. This compares to one death in 1997–99 and none in 1994–96. All five deaths followed caesarean section. The rising caesarean section rate may be a factor in the increasing number of deaths from this cause. The other feature common to all cases was delay in making the diagnosis and, in most cases, there was substandard postoperative care.

In all four *Direct* deaths, abdominal distension occurred a few days after caesarean section. Three of these deaths were due to Ogilvie's syndrome and the other was due to perforation of the sigmoid colon. Ogilvie's syndrome involves bowel pseudo-obstruction with distension leading ultimately to bowel perforation[1] and is not associated with any bowel perforation occurring at the time of operation. In one of the three cases in this triennium, death occurred without bowel perforation, probably due to biochemically induced arrhythmia.

In one case, the woman had been discharged home and was not readmitted to hospital despite marked intestinal dilatation, which must have been evident before death but which was noted only at autopsy. Nowadays, midwives may have no general nursing training and, with a caesarean section rate of around 20%, attention must be paid to education of midwives in postoperative management.

The other three *Direct* deaths had strikingly similar case histories. When abdominal distension occurred, the women were reviewed by junior doctors from the obstetric and general surgical teams and the initial diagnosis was paralytic ileus. There was delay in diagnosing bowel perforation and further delay in carrying out laparotomy and bowel resection. In one case, the woman initially refused laparotomy. In each case death occurred weeks later in the intensive care unit.

Recurrent features of substandard care were lack of continuity during postoperative care and lack of consultant input. For example, a woman who initially refused laparotomy should have had the chance to discuss her management with a consultant.

The one *Late* death is counted in Chapter 15. In this case, a woman had suffered dehiscence of a low transverse incision after caesarean section. It was re-sutured and healed well. Some months later she developed diarrhoea, vomiting and abdominal pain, which continued for several days until she was admitted to hospital, where she suffered cardiac arrest. Autopsy revealed small bowel volvulus, with bowel adherent to the abdominal scar.

This is a very rare complication and it is not surprising that the GP failed to diagnose it. Trainees are now taught not to suture the parietal peritoneum at caesarean section: it is not yet known whether there has been a change in the incidence of wound dehiscence, which is very unusual in a low transverse incision.

Other Direct deaths: learning points

- The management of genital tract trauma requires urgent and skilled intervention. A surgical team needs to be readily available. More than one consultant may be needed.

- Ileus after caesarean section may be fatal. Bowel perforation may not be easy to recognise. Signs of peritonism are difficult to detect in the puerperium and young women can tolerate peritonitis until it is well advanced.

References

1. Ogilvie H. Large intestinal colic due to sympathetic deprivation. A new clinical syndrome. *BMJ* 1948; ii: 671–3.

CHAPTER 9

Anaesthesia

GRISELDA M COOPER and JOHN H McCLURE
on behalf of the Editorial Board

Anaesthesia: key recommendations

Service provision

Dedicated obstetric anaesthesia services should be available in all consultant obstetric units. These services should be capable of taking responsibility for epidural analgesia, anaesthesia, recovery from anaesthesia and management of mothers requiring high dependency care.

Isolated consultant obstetric units present major difficulties in terms of immediate availability of additional skilled anaesthetic backup and assistance from other specialties, including critical care. When presented with problem cases requiring special skills or investigations, obstetric anaesthetists should not hesitate to call on the assistance of anaesthetic colleagues in other subspecialties, as well as colleagues in other disciplines.

Anaesthesia training must ensure competence in airway management, especially the recognition and management of oesophageal intubation.

Obese pregnant women (body mass index, BMI, greater than 35) are at greater risk from anaesthesia and should be referred to the anaesthetist early.

Adequate advance notice of high-risk cases must be given to the obstetric anaesthetic service. The notice must be sufficient to allow consultation with the woman, specialist advice, investigation and assembly of resources needed for the safe management of high-risk women.

Women who are needle phobic are at greater risk from anaesthesia and an anaesthetic consultation in the antenatal period should be arranged to establish a management plan.

Supportive counselling of anaesthetic personnel involved in a maternal death is essential. It should be remembered that such an event represents a tragedy not only for the mother's family but also for the anaesthetist involved, who commonly assumes full responsibility for the death.

Individual practitioners

Invasive monitoring via appropriate routes should be used, particularly when the cardiovascular system is compromised by haemorrhage or disease. Invasive central venous and arterial pressure measurement can provide vital information about the cardiovascular system. Samples for arterial blood gas estimation should be taken early and any metabolic acidosis should be taken seriously.

Care of women at high risk of, or with, major haemorrhage must involve a consultant obstetric anaesthetist at the earliest possible time.

Intensive care beds may not be available in an emergency. Early consultant to consultant referral is recommended to facilitate the creation of a bed and to help with the early institution of intensive therapy while awaiting bed availability.

Women with suspected raised intracranial pressure require a full neurological assessment to help determine the optimal mode of delivery and type of anaesthesia or analgesia if required.

Fifty years ago...

The preface of the first Report of the Confidential Enquiries 50 years ago drew attention to the fact that anaesthesia was a major primary or associated factor in maternal death. Anaesthetic deaths were not separately classified in the early Reports but 49 deaths were ascribed to anaesthesia in the first triennial Report (1952–54) and at least 20 more were identified where anaesthesia was contributory.

The dramatic reduction in the number of maternal deaths due to anaesthesia has been one of the notable success stories of these Reports. There were between 30 and 50 deaths in each triennium ascribed directly to anaesthesia until 1981. In the 1982–84 triennium, this figure was 19 deaths and the same total number of deaths due to anaesthesia was reported during the years 1985 to 1996 spanning four triennia or twelve years. Because of the small numbers of deaths now reported it is too early to say whether the increase in deaths due to anaesthesia in this triennium is real cause for concern.

The numbers of deaths due to anaesthesia should not be examined in isolation from the numbers of general and regional anaesthetic procedures given. Epidural analgesia services started in the late 1960s and 24% of women received epidural analgesia in labour in 2000. It is notable how few deaths have occurred as a result of regional anaesthesia since the late 1960s. There were no *Direct* deaths attributed to regional anaesthesia in this triennium.

The number of anaesthetics given during pregnancy and the postpartum period are not known with certainty, but the numbers for caesarean sections can be estimated from the caesarean section rate and the numbers of maternities. Although the Reports from 1955 until 1963 did not specify the numbers of deaths where anaesthesia was given for caesarean section, a large number of general anaesthetics were given for delivery by forceps during this time.

Caesarean section data for the triennia 1964–66, 1982–84 and this one, and the number of anaesthetic deaths for each, are summarised in Table 9.1. This shows that anaesthesia (spinal, epidural and general) for caesarean section is more than 30 times safer now than it was in the 1960s, when the majority of caesarean sections were performed under general anaesthesia.

Table 9.1 The estimated numbers of caesarean section (CS) operations performed, the caesarean section rate expressed as a percentage of maternities, the numbers of *Direct* anaesthetic maternal deaths and the rate of maternal deaths from anaesthesia given for caesarean section; England and Wales 1964–84, United Kingdom 1982–84 and 2000–02

Triennium	Maternities (n)	Caesarean section (n)	Caesarean section (%)	*Direct* Deaths due to anaesthesia	*Direct* deaths due to anaesthesia for CS	Rate of *Direct* deaths due to anaesthesia per 100,000 CS*
1964–66	2,600,000	88,000	3.4	50	32	36
1982–84	1,884,000	190,000	10.1	19	11	6
2000–02**	1,997,000	425,000	21.0	7	4	1

* This figure excludes other causes of death at or after caesarean section
** Caesarean section data for the UK (2000–02) are grossed from Hospital Episode Statistics for England

The predominant cause of anaesthetic death used to be related to airway management, either through failure to oxygenate the mother while trying to achieve tracheal intubation or because of aspiration of gastric contents resulting in either immediate asphyxiation or later respiratory failure from adult respiratory distress syndrome. It is obvious from reading the older Reports that practice was very different from now. Examples that illustrate this include: "In five, and possibly six, cases the anaesthetic was administered by the single-handed obstetrician" (1955–57).[2] "Anaesthesia (spinal anaesthesia for caesarean section) initially appeared satisfactory but respiratory difficulties occurred before the operation was completed. By this time the anaesthetist was busy elsewhere and not immediately available." (1961–63)[3]

These illustrations speak for themselves, although it is worth noting that abolishing operator-anaesthetists in dentistry did not occur until 1983. It is now unthinkable that the anaesthetist would not be present throughout the procedure.

The problem of acid aspiration was tackled by a series of changes. The technique of rapid-sequence induction involving preoxygenation, cricoid pressure, use of succinyl choline and avoidance of mask ventilation before tracheal intubation, was developed in a piecemeal fashion, as documented in the first five Reports.

The widely adopted policy of limiting oral intake during labour has ensured that relatively few women are anaesthetised with a genuinely full stomach. Perhaps the most effective measure has been the widespread administration of drugs to prevent acid secretion from the stomach to women anticipated to need anaesthesia. In the UK, in 98% of cases, this is achieved with H_2 blockers coupled with a drug such as sodium citrate to neutralise any gastric acid already present.[1]

The requirement for tracheal intubation for caesarean section in order to reduce aspiration risk had become accepted by the 1960s. Unfortunately, this led to a marked increase in deaths from failed intubation and failed oxygenation and other airway problems; 16 deaths from these causes were recorded in the 1976–78 Report, eight in 1979–81 and ten in 1982–84. This had become unusual in recent Reports, presumably as a result of better training and assistance, use of failed intubation drills and monitoring such as capnography and oximetry throughout induction, maintenance and recovery from anaesthesia. It is a concern that unrecognised oesophageal intubation has re-emerged as a cause of death from anaesthesia in this Report.

One of the key ways of avoiding airway management problems has been the increased use of regional anaesthesia. In the year 2000, 91% of elective and 77% of emergency caesarean sections were performed under regional block.[1] Assuming an 80% frequency of use of regional anaesthesia for caesarean section in the 2000–02 triennium, it is possible to estimate the risk of death due to general anaesthesia for caesarean section as one death per 20,000. Unfortunately, this estimated risk does not seem to have altered from the 1982–84 triennium. When general anaesthesia is required, there is some concern now over the lack of experience attained by some anaesthetists and their confidence in its delivery.

Successive Reports have highlighted the lack of consultant involvement. At a time when specialist input was sparse, the recommendation from the 1964–66 Report recognised that "patients with obstetric emergencies are gravely at risk and require knowledge and skill of an experienced anaesthetist who must be readily available". Rationalisation of maternity services has reduced the frequency of trainees working in isolation and the training of anaesthetists new to the discipline of obstetric anaesthesia has improved considerably. There has been a concerted effort to improve consultant anaesthetist staffing of obstetric services but the trainee anaesthetist is still sometimes isolated from senior backup out of hours.

Summary of findings for 2000–02

The central assessors in anaesthesia reviewed the cases of all the women who died of either a *Direct* or *Indirect* cause and identified as having received an anaesthetic for this triennium, 120 of the 161 *Direct* and *Indirect* deaths.

In this triennium, six deaths are ascribed as being directly due to the conduct of anaesthesia. One other *Late* death is ascribed to anaesthesia, although death occurred several years after the anaesthetic event, which occurred in the previous triennium for 1997–99. Lessons from this death are included in this chapter, although it is not counted here for statistical purposes. The numbers of maternal deaths and death rates for this and the preceding triennia are shown in Table 9.1 and Figure 9.1.

In addition to these six *Direct* anaesthetic deaths, there were 20 deaths in which perioperative/anaesthesia management contributed to the death. These deaths have

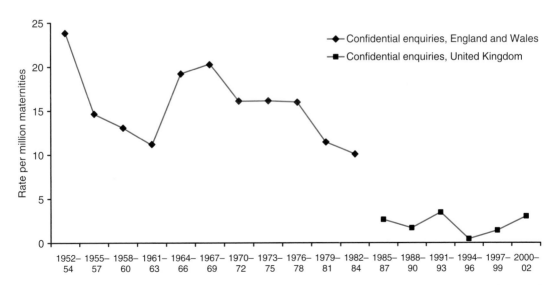

Figure 9.1   Maternal death rates from anaesthesia for all obstetric or maternity procedures; England and Wales 1952–1984, United Kingdom 1985–2002

been assigned to the core chapters but anaesthesia services were regarded as substandard.

In most cases the standard of record keeping was good but some records were very poor. Reviewing the records of some deaths showed that the anaesthesia service does not always meet the declared standards of the relevant Departments of Health and professional bodies. These units were often isolated from anaesthetic backup and other medical specialties and in particular critical care services. The workload and challenges presented to the obstetric anaesthetist are increasing in number, complexity and severity. In several of the cases, including those where anaesthesia was contributory, earlier consultant anaesthetic involvement was warranted and was either not sought or was not as prompt as was indicated.

It was a matter of consensus judgment assigning a death as being a direct result of anaesthesia and whether substandard care contributed to the mother's death. Key points of the cases illustrated here result from the central assessors' judgment.

In reviewing the cases, especially where anaesthesia was the cause of death, the profound effect of the maternal death on the anaesthetist was clear. Good record keeping is crucial in these situations. The need for proper support for the anaesthetist(s) involved in a maternal death is vital although the best source of support will vary between individuals. The Joint Committee on Good Practice is setting up a counselling service and can be contacted through the Royal College of Anaesthetists or the Association of Anaesthetists of Great Britain and Ireland.

Deaths due to anaesthesia

There were six *Direct* deaths (plus one *Late Direct* death) due to anaesthesia, representing a regrettable increase from the three deaths directly attributable to anaesthesia in the 1997–99 Report. All the deaths in this triennium were associated with general anaesthesia.

Misplaced tracheal tubes

In this triennium, there were two deaths and one *Direct Late* death that resulted from oesophageal intubation during anaesthesia. In two of the cases, anaesthesia was being given for urgent caesarean section and in one it was for a presumed ruptured ectopic pregnancy. In all cases, SHO-grade trainees, without immediate senior backup, administered the anaesthetics.

The need for proper checking of anaesthetic machines before use is highlighted, as it transpired in one of these cases that the fresh gas flow from the common gas outlet had been disconnected during a previous case. It is recommended that a separate oxygen supply is used when patients receiving regional anaesthesia are given oxygen supplementation and that the anaesthetic breathing system is not disconnected. One of the reasons for caesarean section being performed under general anaesthesia is because of urgency of delivery but guidelines published in 2004 and not available during this triennium suggest that the monitoring equipment, breathing system and ventilator should be checked before each new patient.[4] There also needs to be comprehensive check of equipment and emergency drugs at each change of shift.

In one case, a death from anaesthesia occurred due to inadequate supervision. The anaesthetist, who was new to the country and the hospital, had not undergone any assessment of competence and gave general anaesthesia without direct supervision or immediate backup being available. The woman sustained irreversible brain damage.

At the time of this anaesthetic being given it was not common practice for anaesthetists new to a hospital to have to perform basic competency tests formally.[5] The need for a formal test of competency of all new anaesthetic trainees is emphasised by this case.

It is noteworthy that, in all the cases, auscultation of the lung fields gave false reassurance that the tracheal tube was correctly placed. Only in one of the cases was capnography use, and in that case the tubing to the capnograph became blocked with gastric contents. The Royal College of Anaesthetists issued a statement in 1998 that "No trainee anaesthetist should be put into the position of having to intubate the trachea without a capnograph being available. If a capnograph is not available, either the patient or the equipment should be moved".[6] In the year 2000, it was further clarified that anaesthetists should not be required to deliver anaesthesia without using monitoring equipment which complies with the recommended minimum monitoring standard current at that time. When intubating the trachea during induction of anaesthesia or managing an intubated patient during anaesthesia, a capnograph must be used as part of the monitoring procedure.[7]

The isolation of relatively inexperienced trainee anaesthetists (SHO grade) was considered to be a factor in all of these cases. It was not possible to receive urgent experienced help that might have been able to recognise and correct the misplaced tracheal tubes. Even with experienced anaesthetists, when unexpected difficulties occur the ready availability of a second pair of hands may be life saving. It is clear that previous recommendations of "a failed intubation drill" were not implemented and each patient's oxygenation was not maintained while allowing spontaneous respiration to return and awaiting more senior help. In all these cases, there appeared to be a major reluctance on behalf of the anaesthetist to consider the possibility that the oesophagus had been intubated in error. Anaesthesia training must concentrate on airway management skills, especially the recognition and management of oesophageal intubation. The small numbers of general anaesthetics given in obstetrics mean that some of this training will have to be delivered in other clinical areas; the use of simulators may be explored usefully.

In those having caesarean section, general anaesthesia was the patient's choice. One of these women did not speak English. It may have been possible to explain the option of regional anaesthesia through a translator.

In addition to the cases above, where the relative isolation of the trainees was a relevant factor, there are two further cases where the proximity of additional early help may have averted maternal death.

Isolated sites

Two women had general anaesthetics in isolated sites where the delay in being able to obtain help was a contributory factor in the death. Both women suffered hypoventilation which was inadequately managed. One woman was undergoing caesarean section and the other mid trimester termination of pregnancy. One of the women was obese (BMI 40) and one of the women was needle phobic. In one of the cases, a capnograph was not used, contrary to recommendations.[8] In one of the cases the cardiac arrest was inadequately managed, the administration of any drugs being delayed until help arrived. In another case, amniotic fluid embolism was thought to be a possible cause of death on clinical grounds but this was specifically excluded by autopsy including detailed histology.

It is relevant to note that on sites remote from general hospitals, the Department of Health standard[9] is that non-consultant career grade staff with NHS appointments should be working under the line responsibility of a named consultant anaesthetist. They should also be proficient in advanced cardiac life support. It also recommends that only anaesthetists holding a higher qualification should give general anaesthetics for terminations of pregnancy.

Aspiration of gastric contents

An obese woman (BMI greater than 35) died after aspiration of gastric contents following failure to intubate the trachea after induction of general anaesthesia for caesarean section, having declined a regional block because of needle phobia. The assessors were unable to determine whether the woman had received antacid prophylaxis.

Aspiration of gastric contents remains a clear risk during induction of general anaesthesia and this risk is higher when there is difficulty experienced intubating the trachea. Obesity is a major factor in causing difficulty with tracheal intubation and obesity and late pregnancy predispose to hiatus hernia, which make regurgitation of gastric contents more likely to occur.

Anaphylaxis

A woman presented with bleeding due to an incomplete miscarriage. An SHO induced anaesthesia with propofol and succinyl choline was given to facilitate tracheal intubation. She developed the classic signs of acute anaphylaxis and cardiac arrest rapidly ensued

The diagnosis was confirmed by a raised mast cell tryptase in a sample of blood taken shortly after the collapse. This is a helpful investigation in a case of suspected anaphylaxis.

Deaths to which anaesthesia contributed

In addition to the six *Direct* anaesthetic deaths detailed above, there were 20 deaths in which perioperative anaesthesia management contributed. These deaths are counted in the relevant chapters, as shown in Table 9.2, and are discussed here in the broad categories of perioperative care where anaesthesia services were regarded as substandard or where there are lessons for anaesthesia services.

These deaths highlight examples of the following aspects of care with some deaths falling into several categories:

- lack of multidisciplinary cooperation

- lack of appreciation of the severity of the illness

- lack of perioperative care

- the management of haemorrhage.

Table 9.2 *Direct* and *Indirect* causes of death in which perioperative anaesthetic management contributed counted in other chapters; United Kingdom 2000–02

Chapter	Cause of death	Deaths associated with anaesthesia (*n*)
2	Thromboembolism	1
3	Eclampsia and pre-eclampsia	2
4	Haemorrhage	5
5	Amniotic fluid embolism	2
7	Sepsis	1
8	*Other Direct*	2
10	Cardiac	3
12	*Other Indirect*	4
Total		20

Lack of multidisciplinary cooperation

There were three deaths in which there were failings in multidisciplinary working. In two women, cardiac arrest occurred but the resuscitation teams failed to find the patients in good time. In another case resuscitation was confused and ineffective. This failure and inability to provide basic and advanced life support on hospital wards is substandard. It is recommended that cardiac arrest drills are practised routinely in all maternity units and all medical and midwifery staff maintain their resuscitation skills.

All team members need to be aware of the vital contributions that can be made by anaesthetists and intensive care specialists when adequate warning of women with serious illness is given and the harm that can result when it is not. Obstetric anaesthetists must also remember that they have colleagues with different, but invaluable, skills provided that the anaesthetist calls on their help in good time. It is evident that intensive care consultants should be part of the multidisciplinary team planning the care of those pregnant women with serious co-existing disease. Beds in an intensive care unit are always at a premium but consultant to consultant referral can facilitate the creation of a bed in an emergency in a seriously ill woman.

Lack of appreciation of the severity of illness

There were nine deaths in which a common theme emerged where trainee obstetric and anaesthetic staff sought help from a senior anaesthetist or other senior specialist too late, owing to failure to realise the severity of illness. The major learning points from these cases are:

- Not all headaches are due to spinal anaesthesia

  A postdural puncture headache is not associated with severe difficulty with communication. Neurological symptoms and signs may indicate serious intracranial or spinal pathology and a neurological opinion needs to be sought urgently.

- Pre-eclampsia with haemolysis, elevated liver enzymes and low platelets (HELLP syndrome) accompanied by intrauterine death from placental abruption can be anticipated to result in severe haemorrhage.

  When this occurs further assistance should be sought early, invasive monitoring used and arterial blood gases measured.

- Overwhelming sepsis can be rapidly fatal and requires urgent intensive therapy, which may be started in the maternity unit while waiting for an intensive care unit bed to become available.

  For example, in one case, the attention of the obstetric staff was directed towards the management of an intrauterine death without fully appreciating the serious condition of the mother, who was systemically unwell but apyrexial. She died shortly after admission from disseminated streptococcal sepsis, although this outcome could probably have not been prevented.

- Fetal compromise may be due to severe maternal disease.

  An underweight woman with an undelivered premature baby was referred from another hospital because of the need for neonatal intensive care for her baby. A consultant anaesthetist commendably noticed cyanosis and delayed caesarean section. A cardiologist diagnosed Eisenmenger's syndrome and she died 1 week after delivery.

- Coexisting disease should be properly assessed in good time and managed by a multidisciplinary team.

  There were several cases where the woman could have been anticipated to have needed preoperative anaesthetic assessment and management. Clinical records should be clearly flagged to alert staff of women with serious medical conditions.

Perioperative care
There were five deaths in which poor perioperative care was a contributing factor and the lessons to be learned from these can be summarised as:

- Good blood pressure control in proteinuric hypertension is required to avoid cerebral haemorrhage.

  Inadequate treatment of blood pressure was evident in one case while awaiting the availability of a neonatal cot. Liaison with neonatologists needs to stress where delivery is urgent for the mother's health.

- Unexpected readings from a monitor should not be dismissed.

  In one case, a woman said to be behaving strangely had a general anaesthetic for an urgent caesarean section. A locum anaesthetist considered that the woman's low oxygen saturation was due to a malfunctioning probe because of nail polish or poor peripheral circulation. She suffered a cardiac arrest after surgery and amniotic fluid embolus was confirmed at autopsy.

- Proper monitoring should alert staff to the existence of concealed haemorrhage

  An anaesthetist was called to see a woman as it was thought that she had a retained placenta. The anaesthetist found the woman bleeding heavily from the vagina and laparotomy later revealed a uterine tear. There appeared to be some reluctance on the part of the obstetric staff to consider the possibility that she was also bleeding intra-abdominally. Ultrasound guidance for the placement of a central venous line may have helped with her resuscitation.[10]

- Consultant anaesthetic attendance must be forthcoming for sick women.

In several cases the consultant anaesthetist, although aware of major problems in the anaesthetic management or high-dependency care of acutely ill women, did not attend.

The management of haemorrhage

Major haemorrhage is still one of the most common causes of *Direct* maternal death. In looking at the deaths due to haemorrhage, multifactorial causation is clear. Pathological process, poor obstetric management and care, poor inter-specialty communication and inadequate anaesthetic response all appear in various combinations. Anaesthetists are trained to recognise and treat major haemorrhage that they encounter in many areas of their professional practice. Obstetric haemorrhage is often sudden and massive and accompanied by a coagulopathy, which is sometimes difficult to manage. Excellent anaesthetic care was provided in many of the cases, sometimes involving large volumes of blood replacement. However, responsibility for substandard care in five of the 17 deaths from haemorrhage, described in Chapter 4 Haemorrhage, rests in part with the anaesthetic services. In addition, there were two deaths in women who declined to receive blood products and lessons may also be learned from their anaesthetic management. From these deaths the following factors were relevant:

- In young fit women the severity of haemorrhage may not be recognized until the cardiovascular system decompensates suddenly.

  Tachycardia will usually indicate hypovolaemia and blood pressure may not fall until the circulating blood volume is very low. However, some patients may not exhibit the normal tachycardic response to haemorrhage, such as women with pregnancy-induced hypertension treated with beta-adrenergic blockers.

- Care of women who suffer a major haemorrhage or are at high risk of major haemorrhage must involve consultant obstetric anaesthetists at the earliest possible time.

  Help from several anaesthetists may be required for optimal management of massive blood loss.

- Blood and a device to rapidly infuse warmed blood must be immediately available in all cases at high risk of major haemorrhage.

  Blood is regularly removed from blood bank refrigerators by blood transfusion technicians and therefore a check that the blood is actually available is essential.

- Isolated maternity units distant from blood transfusion services and the intensive care unit present a particular risk when major haemorrhage occurs.

- Central venous and direct arterial pressure monitoring should be used when the cardiovascular system is compromised by haemorrhage or disease.

  When difficulty is encountered, ultrasound guidance for the insertion of a central venous catheter is recommended.[10]

- Surgical compression with packs and aortic compression may allow time to restore the circulating volume while waiting for more senior surgical and anaesthetic help.

  The anaesthetist may need to request this from the obstetrician. The anaesthetist should be aware that surgical manoeuvres that may be considered include the B-Lynch suture, uterine or internal iliac artery ligation, or hysterectomy.[11]

The placement of bilateral iliac artery balloon catheters under portable image intensifier control may also help to control haemorrhage in an emergency. Arterial embolisation is also an option but may be more difficult to deliver where haemorrhage has occurred without warning or if the woman's condition does not permit safe transfer to the radiology department.[11]

- Postoperative care frequently needs to be provided in an intensive care or high-dependency unit.

  Stabilisation of cardiovascular parameters prior to transfer is necessary and improvement of a metabolic acidosis can be a helpful indication of success. Hands-on help from an intensivist, such as providing appropriate inotropic support, in theatre before transferring the patient may be life saving.

- A plan of management for women at high risk of placenta accreta, such as those with an anterior placenta praevia after a previous caesarean section, should be evident.

  These women require particular preparation, as they are at very high risk of major haemorrhage.[12] The placement of bilateral iliac artery balloon catheters immediately prior to caesarean section should be considered in high-risk elective cases.

- The use of a 'cell saver' is something that could be considered for a woman having a caesarean section who declines homologous blood transfusion on religious grounds.[13]

The management of haemorrhage is a shared responsibility of midwifery, obstetric, anaesthetic and blood transfusion personnel. Anaesthetists should be ready to suggest that the obstetrician summons help in the face of major haemorrhage regardless of the obstetrician's grade or experience. Good communication is vital and regular practice of emergency drills is crucial, particularly in units with a high turnover of staff.

Acknowledgements
This chapter has been seen and discussed with the National and Regional Assessors in Anaesthesia.

References

1. Royal College of Obstetricians and Gynaecologists. Clinical Effectiveness Support Unit. *The National Sentinel Caesarean Section Audit Report.* London: RCOG Press; 2001.
2. Ministry of Health. *Report on Confidential Enquiries into Maternal Deaths in England and Wales 1955–1957.* London: HMSO; 1960.
3. Ministry of Health. *Report on Confidential Enquiries into Maternal Deaths in England and Wales 1961–1963.* London: HMSO; 1966.
4. Association of Anaesthetists of Great Britain and Ireland. *Checking Anaesthetic Equipment 3.* London: Association of Anaesthetists; 2004.
5. Royal College of Anaesthetists. *The CCST in Anaesthesia.* 2nd ed. London: RCA; 2003.
6. Royal College of Anaesthetists. *Guidance for Trainers.* London: RCA; 1999. p. 8.
7. Royal College of Anaesthetists. *Guidance for Trainers.* London; RCA; 2000. p. 13.

8. Association of Anaesthetists of Great Britain and Ireland. *Recommendations for Standards of Monitoring During Anaesthesia and Recovery.* London: Association of Anaesthetists; 2000.

9. Department of Health. *Procedures for the Approval of Independent Sector Places for the Termination of Pregnancy.* London: Department of Health; 1999.

10. National Institute for Clinical Excellence. *Ultrasound Locating Devices for Placing Central Venous Catheters.* Guideline number 49. London: NICE; 2002.

11. Hong T-M, Tseng H-S, Lee R-C, Wang J-H, Chang C-Y. Uterine artery embolisation: an effective treatment for intractable obstetric haemorrhage. *Clin Radiol* 2004;59:96–101

12. Royal College of Obstetricians and Gynaecologists. *Placenta Praevia: Diagnosis and Management.* Guideline No. 27. London: RCOG; 2001.

13. Catling SJ, Freites O, Krishnan S, Gibbs R. Clinical experience with cell salvage in obstetrics; 4 cases from one UK centre. *Int J Obstet Anesth* 2002;11:128–34.

Section

3

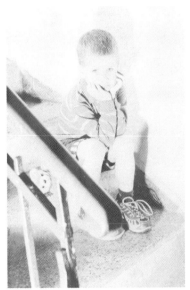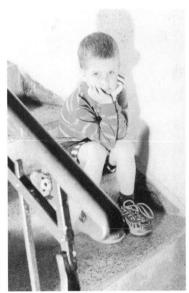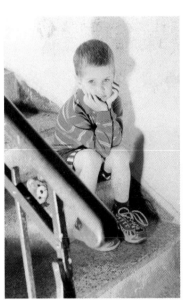

Indirect deaths

CHAPTER 10
Cardiac disease

MICHAEL de SWIET and CATHERINE NELSON-PIERCY
on behalf of the Editorial Board

Cardiac disease: recommendations

Service provision

Women requesting or requiring assisted conception are often at higher risk of obstetric complications, partly because of their increased age and associated other medical conditions. Women with known cardiac disease should receive thorough prepregnancy counselling.

Family members must not be relied upon to act as interpreters. This is particularly important in women with heart disease. The desire of family members for the woman to have a child may stop them passing on details of a past medical history or potential symptoms of heart disease to healthcare staff. It may also prevent them telling the pregnant woman the true risk of her continuing her pregnancy.

Cardiac arrests are rare in maternity units but they can and do happen and their management is often suboptimal. All medical and nursing staff should be trained to a nationally recognised level (basic, intermediate, advanced life support; BLS, ILS or ALS) as appropriate. Emergency drills for maternal resuscitation should be regularly practised in clinical areas in all maternity units. These drills should include the identification of the equipment required and appropriate methods for ensuring that cardiac arrest teams arrive promptly. Specialised courses such as Advanced Life Support in Obstetrics (ALSO) and Managing Obstetric Emergencies and Trauma (MOET) provide additional training for obstetric and midwifery staff.

Termination of pregnancy services should be readily available and accessible for women with medical conditions precluding safe pregnancy.

Guidelines and protocols

Individual obstetric units should develop protocols for the management of pregnant women who are extremely ill for non-obstetric reasons. This must involve liaison with other hospital services, such as cardiology, and with emergency services and accident and emergency departments regarding the most appropriate site (accident and emergency, local delivery suite or another hospital) to ensure women receive speedy resuscitation.

Individual practitioners

Isolated systolic hypertension should not be ignored. Severe systolic hypertension can damage the heart and should be treated with antihypertensive therapy.

Increased age, obesity and hypertension are risk factors for heart disease that should be noted at booking.

If a woman dies from a genetic or inheritable condition (such as Marfan's syndrome) or potentially inheritable disease such as sudden adult death syndrome (SADS), her family members should be counselled and offered screening.

50 years ago...

Fifty years ago the maternal mortality rate from cardiac disease was two and a half times the rate in the current triennium, as shown in Figure 10.1. In the first Report, for 1952–54, 121 women died from cardiac causes compared with 44 reported cases for this triennium. Of the 11 women whose deaths were assessed for the first Report, 84% had rheumatic heart disease, of whom the vast majority had mitral stenosis. Perhaps it is not therefore surprising that 25% of all these maternal cardiac deaths occurred in labour. In this current Report there were no deaths from rheumatic heart disease and there have only been six such deaths in the last 20 years. Despite this marked difference in the pattern of cardiac disease, two of the four recommendations made in that first confidential Enquiry remain as pertinent today:

- "All patients known or suspected to be suffering from heart disease should be referred for their care in pregnancy and confinement to a hospital where they can receive the necessary supervision."

- "The need for efficient and conscientious antenatal care and the use of an infallible system of immediate check-up of all non-attenders is also emphasised."

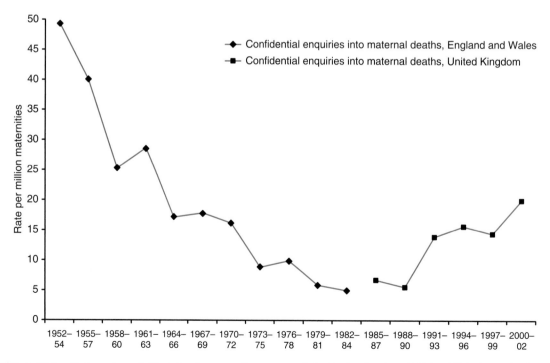

Figure 10.1 Maternal mortality rates from cardiac causes of death; England and Wales 1952–84, United Kingdom 1985–2002

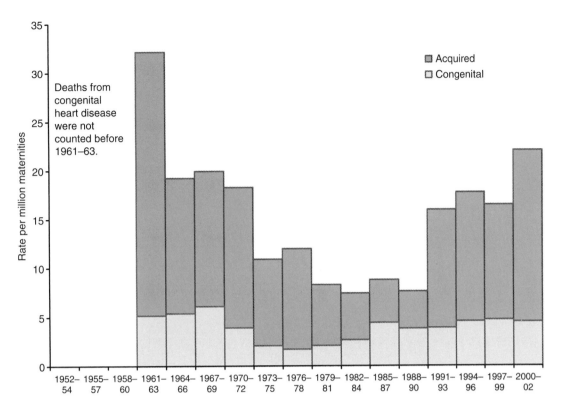

Figure 10.2 Maternal mortality rates for congenital and acquired cardiac disease; England and Wales 1961–1984, United Kingdom 1985–2002

The message continued in the 1958–60 Report: "no effort should be spared by all concerned to convince any pregnant woman who is suffering from heart disease that hospital care and responsibility is her chief safeguard".

In the 1961–63 Report deaths from congenital heart disease were included for the first time, as shown in Figure 10.2. The striking fact is that the mortality rate from congenital heart disease is almost the same today as it was 40 years ago.

Unsurprisingly, there have been between one and seven deaths from Eisenmenger's syndrome and pulmonary vascular disease in each Enquiry since 1961–63, reflecting the 30–50% maternal mortality associated with pulmonary hypertension and the lack of clinical advance in treating women with this condition. The conclusions of the 1982–84 Enquiry are also relevant today in light of some of the deaths from congenital heart disease in this Report: "The surgical correction of a congenital lesion is often of necessity incomplete and any such lesion, corrected or not, leaves the patient at risk . . . Small blood losses are not well tolerated and equally it is easy to produce right heart failure with minor degrees of circulatory overload following transfusion".

Enquiries from 1966 onwards repeatedly highlighted the fact that women over 34 years of age were at increased risk of death from acquired heart disease. This also is true today, although it is surprising that, despite the increased prevalence of ischaemic heart disease and associated risk factors, particularly smoking, in women, deaths from ischaemic heart disease have not increased more. It may be that increasing rates of obesity and hypertension in the general population, combined with the trend of increasing maternal age, are contributing to the increase in maternal deaths from acquired heart disease, particularly from causes such as peripartum cardiomyopathy, where obesity, increased age and hypertension are all established risk factors. However, acquired causes such as coronary artery and aortic dissection are very much pregnancy specific and there are currently no data relating these to the above demographic factors. Increases in attributable deaths from these causes are therefore more likely to represent more accurate ascertainment of cause of death.

Summary of findings for 2000–02

There were a total of 44 deaths from heart disease related to pregnancy reported to the Enquiry in 2000–02. This compares with 35 deaths in 1997–99, as shown in Table 10.1. Cardiac disease is now the second most common cause of maternal death after psychiatric causes and more common than the most frequent *Direct* cause of maternal death, thromboembolism. This gives a maternal mortality rate of 2.2/100,000 maternities for this triennium.

The lessons from 15 further deaths from cardiac disease counted elsewhere in this Report contribute to the learning points and key messages contained within this chapter. There was one death from sepsis where cardiomyopathy may have been a contributing feature and one from epilepsy where myocardial fibrosis may have contributed. These are counted in Chapter 7 Sepsis and Chapter 12 *Other Indirect*, respectively. Thirteen *Late* deaths from cardiac disease are counted in Chapter 15.

The assessors considered that some degree of substandard care was present in 40%, 18 of the 44 cases. A similar proportion was found for the *Late* deaths.

The cardiac causes of maternal death can be broadly divided into congenital and acquired. Pulmonary hypertension is the major cause of deaths from congenital heart disease and cardiomyopathy (predominantly peripartum), myocardial infarction, aneurysm or dissection of the thoracic aorta or its branches are the leading causes of deaths from acquired cardiac disease. Put together, any one of these four causes is responsible for about as many deaths as all other conditions put together. Table 10.2 also shows the numbers of deaths by major cause for this triennium and as a total for 1991–2002.

Congenital heart disease

Twenty percent of the women who died from cardiac disease and whose deaths were reported to the Enquiry during this triennium died from congenital heart disease. Of these nine deaths four were associated with pulmonary vascular disease.

Table 10.1   Maternal deaths from congenital and acquired cardiac disease; United Kingdom 1985–2002

| | Congenital | | Acquired | | | | |
| | | | Ischaemic | | Other | | |
Triennium	(n)	(%)	(n)	(%)	(n)	(%)	Total cases (n)
1985–87	10	44	9	39	4	17	23
1988–90	9	50	5	25	4	25	18
1991–93	9	24	8	22	20	54	37
1994–96	10	26	6	21	23	53	39
1997–99	10	29	5	15	20	56	35
2000–02	9	20	8	18	27	62	44

Table 10.2 Causes of maternal deaths from heart disease; United Kingdom 1991–2002

Cause of death	2000–02	Totals 1991–2002
Cardiomyopathy and myocarditis	8	34
Aneurysm of thoracic aorta and its branches	7	28
Myocardial infarction	8	27
Pulmonary hypertension	4	22
All other heart disease	17	39
Valve disease including endocarditis	4	12
Other congenital	2	9
Sudden adult death syndrome	4	6
Myocardial fibrosis	3	4
Other Acquired	4	8
All cardiac deaths and totals for 1991–2002	44	150*

* This total of 150 is less than the total of 155 given in Table 10.1 because the precise cardiac causes of death of five cases could not be determined

The key lessons to be learned from the management of women with congenital heart disease can be drawn from the following representative vignettes:

> A woman with a tetralogy of Fallot, corrected as a child, developed symptoms and signs of right heart failure in the third trimester of her pregnancy. She was treated with diuretics and labour was induced. After delivery she had a postpartum haemorrhage (PPH) which required a blood transfusion; she developed atrial flutter and right heart failure from which she eventually died.

In this case, echocardiograms performed prior to her pregnancy had shown right ventricular dilatation and impaired function suggesting that the cardiac defect had only been partially corrected or that she had re-stenosed her pulmonary valve. It is unclear whether she received appropriate prepregnancy advice or counselling Undoubtedly, the anaemia that followed her PPH and the transfusion to correct this contributed to her right heart failure.

This case, together with others discussed in this chapter, highlights the importance of ensuring that all women with significant congenital heart disease are closely monitored by a cardiologist with expertise in the care of adult congenital heart disease in pregnancy during and after pregnancy. Their care should be provided in close conjunction with a consultant obstetrician preferably at a joint clinic.

> Another woman had a ventricular septal defect (VSD) repaired as a child, as she had developed slight right ventricular hypertrophy and pulmonary hypertension. As a teenager her pulmonary artery pressure was reported as normal and an echocardiogram was also reported as normal only months before she became pregnant. During her antenatal period a cardiologist, who did not note anything unusual, reviewed her and she had a normal vaginal delivery. Shortly afterwards she collapsed with cyanosis and died.

At autopsy, the successful VSD repair was noted but there were features of very marked right ventricular hypertrophy. Her pulmonary blood vessels showed well established and advanced pulmonary hypertension with medial hypertrophy, atheroma and numerous angiomatoid and plexiform lesions. A specialist cardiac histopathologist agreed with the findings and commented that pregnancy could itself have accelerated her pulmonary hypertension, possibly in association with haemodynamic or thrombotic changes.[1,2] It was stated that it was impossible to know for how long the changes had been present but postulated that some histological changes would have developed by the time she had her original surgery.

This case, although unusual, provides other learning points for the management of women with potential pulmonary vascular disease, predominantly those at risk for Eisenmenger's syndrome, primary pulmonary hypertension and those with antiphospholipid syndrome. Echocardiographic studies in women at risk, which show normal or near normal pulmonary artery pressures must be repeated through pregnancy. Prepregnancy counselling for women living with, or at risk of developing, significant pulmonary hypertension therefore needs to include a discussion concerning their increased risk of death or severe morbidity.

> Another woman had a history of VSD in childhood, which was thought to have closed spontaneously. Her GP had noted a murmur but thought it was physiological. Her pregnancy and delivery were uneventful but she saw her GP a few days after delivery with tachycardia, cyanosis and increasing breathlessness. She was immediately admitted to a regional cardiac centre where primary pulmonary hypertension was diagnosed. An echocardiogram showed no evidence of a VSD. Despite excellent treatment she suffered a cardiac arrest from which she could not be resuscitated. The diagnosis was confirmed at autopsy where a residual small VSD was also noted.

This woman's case is typical of the course of pulmonary hypertension, primary or secondary, after delivery, i.e. a relentless deterioration despite supportive therapy. Although the very small VSD was not detected by the echocardiogram it was not considered to have contributed to her pulmonary vascular disease. However, in the light of the previous vignette, it is possible that her pulmonary vascular disease did indeed arise because of her initial cardiac defect.

> A woman with severe social problems booked late. She had been so severely breathless in a previous pregnancy that she could not speak but this had not been investigated. During this pregnancy she was referred to a tertiary obstetric centre because of fetal growth restriction, for which she required a caesarean section. She was first noted to be cyanosed by the anaesthetist. Her cyanosis was probably the cause of the fetal growth restriction. She was markedly polycythaemic so her cyanosis would not have been a new feature and should have been identified earlier. Indeed her high haemoglobin concentration (16 g/dl) should, in itself, have warned her healthcare professionals that she had a significant medical problem. Subsequent investigations revealed Eisenmenger's syndrome due to an atrial septal defect with pulmonary hypertension (pulmonary pressures being at systemic level) and she died some days later from pulmonary artery dissection.

Her management, once her condition had been diagnosed, was exemplary. However, although the diagnosis of pulmonary hypertension is often difficult, there was probably undue delay in noticing that she was cyanosed, possibly because of her skin colour. There was also a delay in investigating her high haemoglobin concentration, an abnormal finding in pregnancy and in failing to diagnose her condition in a previous pregnancy despite her being obviously very unwell.

This account is characteristic of maternal death from Eisenmenger's syndrome, a condition that carries a maternal mortality rate of about 40% per pregnancy. The mother often dies after delivery and there is currently no agreed management plan or intervention that will reduce this risk. As a consequence these women, too, should always be offered prepregnancy counselling. It also appears quite common for women who die from Eisenmenger's syndrome or pulmonary vascular disease to come from a minority ethnic group; this is an area that requires further study.

> A woman with an aortic valve replacement was seen at a combined obstetric/adult congenital heart disease clinic in the second trimester of her pregnancy. She was advised to continue warfarin anticoagulation because of concern about a previous possible valve thrombosis which led to a myocardial infarction. Her pregnancy remained uneventful until she collapsed at home near term. Resuscitation, including a postmortem caesarean section, was unsuccessful.

Her autopsy showed marked cardiomegaly, presumably from long standing aortic valve disease, and a very recent extension of the previous myocardial infarction. There was no valve thrombosis and her coronary arteries were normal with no thrombosis. No details are available of the adequacy of her anticoagulation. Her infarct was either caused by another coronary embolus, which broke up during resuscitation, or due to her cardiomegaly and the increased demands of pregnancy. This case emphasises the difficulty of managing pregnant women with artificial heart valves.

Learning points: congenital heart disease

- Eisenmenger's syndrome still carries a 40% chance of maternal death during or after pregnancy. There is no known effective management or treatment except heart/lung transplantation.

- Prepregnancy counselling for women living with, or at risk of developing, significant pulmonary hypertension needs to include a discussion concerning the increased risk of death or severe morbidity.

- All pregnant and recently delivered women with congenital heart disease should be supervised by a consultant cardiologist or physician with an interest and expertise in the care of adult congenital heart disease in pregnancy both during and after pregnancy. Their care should be provided in close conjunction with a consultant obstetrician, preferably at a joint clinic.

- Echocardiographic studies in women at risk of developing pulmonary hypertension from their congenital heart disease which show normal or near normal pulmonary artery pressures must be repeated through pregnancy.

Delay in obtaining termination of pregnancy

Chapter 6 Early pregnancy deaths has already highlighted the issues relating to the availability of a termination of pregnancy as a matter of urgency in cases where the woman's life is at risk. One woman, whose death is counted in this chapter, had a life-threatening cardiac disease and decided to terminate the pregnancy after counselling. She died while waiting for an outpatient appointment that had been significantly delayed because an administrator rejected the referral letter as the woman was 'out of area'. This case highlights the need for protocols for the management of women such as these and strengthened communications between primary care, medicine and community gynaecology services regarding requests for urgent terminations of pregnancy when the woman's life is at risk. Regardless of which gynaecology unit holds 'the contract' for terminations or where the woman lives, termination should be readily obtainable for women with significant medical problems precluding safe pregnancy.

Acquired heart disease

Ischaemic heart disease

Three women died of ischaemic heart disease and a further five of myocardial infarction due to coronary artery dissection, a recognised complication of pregnancy. All three women who died from ischaemic heart disease died before delivery, two in the third trimester. All had identifiable risk factors; all were parous, two were smokers and two had a family history of heart disease.

Of the five deaths from coronary artery dissection, four occurred in the first month after delivery and one in mid-pregnancy. Although rare in general, coronary artery dissection is a not uncommon cause of coronary artery occlusion in pregnancy. In one series of 25 cases, 21 were in women and eight occurred after delivery.[3] Dissection and rupture of all blood vessels are more common in pregnancy. The vessels that are particularly vulnerable include the aorta, as demonstrated later in this chapter, and the adrenal, splenic and coronary arteries.

The following vignette shows a recurrent concern about the standard of care provided for some of the women whose deaths are counted in this chapter:

> A woman who rarely attended for antenatal care had known hypertension in each of her previous pregnancies and a family history of ischaemic heart disease. During her last pregnancy she had sustained systolic hypertension (170–180 mm/Hg) but no action was taken, perhaps because her diastolic blood pressure was about 75 mm/Hg. Just before term she collapsed and died. The autopsy showed severe coronary atheroma without actual infarction and "massive" left ventricular hypertrophy, presumably due to long-standing hypertension.

Her systolic hypertension should not have been ignored and warranted specialist referral. There should also have been better arrangements for the follow-up of a woman known to be at high risk of cardiac complications who failed to attend for regular antenatal care.

Learning points: cardiac disease, coronary artery dissection

- Coronary artery dissection is a common (63%) cause of death from myocardial infarction in pregnancy.

- There should be a low threshold for angiography when myocardial infarction occurs in pregnancy or the puerperium since demonstration of dissection allows the possibility of intervention.

Aortic aneurysm and dissection

Despite the fact that dissecting aortic aneurysm is rare in pregnancy, 28 women have died from this cause over the last ten years; 19% of all cardiac deaths. As a cause of maternal death it is equal to myocardial infarction, cardiomyopathy or pulmonary vascular disease.

Seven women died from a dissecting aneurysm of the aorta during this triennium. For example:

> An obese woman, who was well during her pregnancy, developed crushing chest pain radiating to her back near term. She was started on low-molecular-weight heparin in case she had suffered a pulmonary embolism but this was discontinued when standard investigations were normal. No diagnosis was made and she was sent home some days later. When reviewed in the antenatal clinic she seemed better but she died shortly afterwards from a ruptured aortic aneurysm, which had dissected into the pericardium.

Patients with severe crushing chest pain requiring opiate analgesia should not be sent home without a diagnosis. The appropriate investigation, which was not undertaken, would have been a CT chest scan or MRI, despite the extra radiation exposure to the fetus from the former.

> Another woman, who died of aortic dissection due to undiagnosed aortic coarctation soon after delivery, also received substandard care. She had severe systolic hypertension during pregnancy that was neither appropriately treated nor investigated. Once again, the presence of high systolic readings of up to 190 mm/Hg was accepted because of the presence of relatively normal diastolic readings.

There was a *Late* death counted in Chapter 15 in a woman with Ehlers Danlos type IV (vascular) syndrome who died from aortic rupture at the level of the coeliac axis. Ehlers Danlos type IV is known to predispose to large-vessel rupture.

Learning points: dissecting aortic aneurysm

- Staff should remain vigilant about the possibility of dissection as a cause of chest or interscapular pain in pregnancy, particularly if the woman is hypertensive. Dissecting aneurysms can be successfully treated surgically, although this is a very high-risk procedure.

- Aortic dissection should always be considered in pregnant women with atypical chest pain and features of pulmonary embolus who do not get better with treatment. Other diagnostic features include pulse deficits and signs of aortic regurgitation.

- Clinicians should communicate suspected aortic dissection as the indication for CT/MRI/echocardiography to the radiologist/technician.

- At autopsy histology of the aorta should be performed and may show cystic medial degeneration, a finding of normal pregnancy and not necessarily due to any connective tissue disease. Nevertheless, if this is found, Marfan's syndrome needs to be excluded and the family screened.

Other acquired cardiac disease

Cardiomyopathy

Eight women died from cardiomyopathy. Four deaths were due to peripartum cardiomyopathy and one each from probable dilated cardiomyopathy, hypertrophic obstructive cardiomyopathy and probable left ventricular failure of undiagnosed aetiology. One further death was probably due to cardiomyopathy.

Three of the four women who died from peripartum cardiomyopathy had pregnancies complicated by hypertension, two were multiparous and two were obese. All presented postpartum, three within 1–2 days after delivery. The following vignettes show the importance of early diagnosis:

> An older woman who developed moderate hypertension and intermittent proteinuria later in pregnancy delivered following the early spontaneous rupture of membranes despite ritodrine treatment. Shortly afterwards, she became acutely unwell with breathlessness and echocardiography showed that she had a dilated, possible peripartum cardiomyopathy. Her sudden death shortly after treatment with heparin and diuretics was ascribed to pulmonary embolus. No autopsy was performed.

The ritodrine treatment for premature labour may have contributed to her heart failure, even though it was stopped 24 hours before she became overtly symptomatic. Her cardiomyopathy may have also been longstanding and therefore not peripartum, since she had mild breathlessness and palpitations even before pregnancy. Her age must have been a factor in her death, both with regard to possible pulmonary embolism and cardiomyopathy.

> Another woman had a VSD repaired some years ago. She was investigated for supraventricular tachycardia (SVT) during pregnancy and admitted after delivery with a stroke, pulmonary oedema and poor left ventricular function with an ejection fraction of less than 20%. There was also thrombus in her left ventricle. She collapsed and died shortly after admission to an intensive care unit. An autopsy confirmed cardiomyopathy and identified a small, non-contributory pulmonary embolus despite heparin prophylaxis.

Antenatal presentation with SVT and a reduced ejection fraction (30–35%) is suggestive of cardiomyopathy. Repeat echocardiograms should be performed after any episodes of SVT have been treated and may show continuing impaired left-ventricle function despite lack of symptoms. If dilated cardiomyopathy is considered, this suggests prophylactic anticoagulation and more active investigation after delivery. However, it is debatable whether more aggressive therapy would have affected the outcome in the above case.

Learning point: cardiac disease, cardiomyopathy

- Peripartum cardiomyopathy is more common in older, obese, multiparous women with hypertension in pregnancy and should be suspected when tachycardia, tachypnoea, dyspnoea or pulmonary oedema develop in the context of these risk factors in the last months of pregnancy or within the first 6 months following delivery.

Myocardial fibrosis

Three women died from myocardial fibrosis, a condition notoriously difficult to predict and diagnose:

> One woman collapsed while using an exercise machine but none of the attendant staff were familiar with cardiopulmonary resuscitation and no resuscitation was performed until the ambulance team arrived. On arrival at hospital she could not be resuscitated.

At autopsy, idiopathic myocardial fibrosis was confirmed by a specialist cardiac pathologist, who recommended offering screening to her family members, as in all cases of SADS.

Two pregnant women with known sickle cell disease had myocardial fibrosis. One died of epilepsy and is counted in Chapter 12; the other had chest pains in pregnancy and collapsed while in hospital undergoing treatment for a sickle cell crisis. Chest pain in women with sickle cell disease may be due to sickle bony crisis, pulmonary infection or pulmonary infarction. In the latter case, her chest pain may have represented symptomatic myocardial fibrosis.

Hypertensive heart disease

Two extremely obese women died from hypertensive heart disease. Both had characteristics of social exclusion and the following vignette describes the key learning points in relation to the planning and provision of care for women known to be at higher risk of medical complications:

> A woman with pre-existing hypertension and morbid obesity (BMI greater than 40) was booked for shared rather than hospital care. She repeatedly failed to attend for antenatal care and was not followed up. She was also known to be non-compliant with her antihypertensive medication. At term, she collapsed and died, despite a perimortem caesarean section performed in the accident and emergency department.

At autopsy, a severely enlarged heart was found without evidence of infarction. The cause of death was given as hypertensive heart disease; however, no histology was performed and it was not possible to exclude a phaeochromocytoma or the possible contribution of pre-eclampsia or hypertension.

Some of the difficulties encountered in this case relate to the fragmentation of care between community midwives from different hospitals and a lack of communication with the GP. However, there was also no continuity of care, even within the hospital where she was booked.

Sudden adult death syndrome

SADS is defined as sudden death in an adult for which no cause can be found. Three mothers died of SADS during this triennium and the symptoms are suggestive of SADS as the cause of death in a fourth case.

This condition is identified for the first time in this Report because of increasing awareness of it as a separate syndrome and one for which genetic screening may be possible. These cases are counted in this chapter because, historically, this is the chapter where most cases of unexplained death tended to be counted. It is not clear whether pregnancy is a risk factor for SADS but, on the assumption that it is, these cases have been counted as *Indirect* rather than *Coincidental*. The classification of SADS within acquired rather than congenital heart disease is arbitrary. However, in whatever way it is classified, there is a need to counsel family members of the possibility of a genetic component for this condition.

The following vignette is a typical example of the characteristics of a death from SADS:

> Following a normal pregnancy a young mother collapsed, by chance near a healthcare facility, a few weeks after delivery. She could not be resuscitated. A very detailed autopsy only revealed pulmonary oedema and a careful examination of the heart by a national expert showed no abnormality. The cause of death was given as SADS.

Sudden deaths in the young, including women of childbearing age, usually have an attributable cause such as cardiomyopathy, myocarditis or congenital coronary artery anomalies, but this is not necessarily so. In England, there are about 200 sudden truly unexplained deaths per year[4] and in this triennium about one per year occurred in association with pregnancy. Those relatives left behind find the uncertainty particularly unsettling and this distress is compounded by the death of a young mother.

A recent Australian study[5] has shown that in one-third of those cases of women aged less than 35 years referred to a forensic medicine department, the cause of sudden death could not be established at autopsy and was presumed to be due to primary arrhythmogenic disorders. In a UK study of 32 SADS cases,[6] 109 first-degree relatives were studied. Twenty-two percent of the families had evidence of potential heritable heart disease. The majority had a condition, such as long QT syndrome, that would lead to dysrhythmia but hypertrophic cardiomyopathy was also identified.

At present, it is uncertain how best to offer counselling and screening for occult heart disease to the surviving relatives. The very least that family members deserve is a careful autopsy (not something that can be taken for granted from the data of the Confidential Enquiries) and a thorough exploration of the woman's and her family's past medical histories, preferably by an interested cardiologist. A standard 12-lead electrocardiograph will diagnose some but by no means all of those at risk from long QT syndrome. An echocardiograph would go a long way to screen for cardiomyopathy.

Bacterial endocarditis

> A young obese woman died from group B streptococcus endocarditis a week following a normal vaginal delivery. Although she had had some dental treatment 6 weeks previously, group B streptococcus was isolated from a high vaginal swab following spontaneous rupture of membranes in this pregnancy and on the placenta and baby in an earlier pregnancy. The pathologist thought that the genital tract was therefore the most likely source of the organism.

The GP is to be commended for making the correct diagnosis, although the symptomatology was non-specific and there was no previous known heart disease. This case raises important issues regarding the timing of surgery in bacterial endocarditis. Although the woman was referred to a tertiary centre for consideration of valve replacement, this was understandably postponed, awaiting better control of her septicaemia. In the event, although treated with antibiotics to which the organism was fully sensitive, she developed worsening aortic regurgitation with left ventricular dysfunction and died.

This case is extremely unusual both because the bacterial endocarditis occurred on a normal (non-bicuspid) aortic valve and because group B streptococcus does not normally cause bacterial endocarditis. Antibiotic prophylaxis to prevent neonatal morbidity in maternal group B streptococcus colonisation was not given because the result of the high vaginal swab was not available when she was in labour. The clinicians involved have now changed their protocol to include any previous proven group B streptococcus colonisation. It is not known whether such prophylaxis would have prevented the maternal disease.

Late deaths and those counted in other chapters

There were seven *Late* deaths due to cardiomyopathy reported to this Enquiry. An additional death from sepsis in which cardiomyopathy may have been an additional factor is counted in Chapter 7 Sepsis. These deaths were all associated with the known risk factors of multiparity, obesity, increased age and hypertension for peripartum cardiomyopathy.

There were two reported *Late* deaths from ischaemic heart disease, one from pulmonary hypertension, one from congenital heart disease; two others were probably cardiac in origin.

The following vignette raises the issue of post-delivery care for women with known cardiac disease:

> A woman was known to have left bundle branch block and had a family history of ischaemic heart disease. During her pregnancy she was seen by a general physician rather than at the local joint cardiac/obstetric clinic. She was not referred for multidisciplinary care and was managed entirely in the community. She presented in labour with angina, which was treated with a nitrate inhaler. The medical team was contacted and recommended low-molecular-weight heparin treatment and further investigation but she was discharged 2 days later with no cardiology follow up. She died from ischaemic heart disease some months after delivery.

Left bundle branch block must always be considered indicative of heart disease. This woman was at high risk because of her known heart disease and also because she was older. Women with risk factors such as these should be encouraged to have obstetric-led consultant care managed jointly with a cardiologist. While it is not possible to say with certainty whether different treatment might have altered the outcome in any of the cases discussed in this chapter, maternal and neonatal outcomes in cases such as these may be different if a cardiologist is involved in the woman's continuing care after delivery.

References

1. Brach Prever S, Sheppard MN, Somerville J. Fatal outcome in pregnancy in Eisenmenger's syndrome. *Cardiol Young* 1997;7:238–40.

2. Daliento I, Somerville I, Presbitero P, Menti I, Bach-Prever S, Rizzoli G, *et al.* Eisenmenger syndrome. Factors relating to deterioration and death. *Eur Heart J* 1998;19:1845–5.

3. Silver M, Gotleib AI, Schoen FR, editors. Cardiac Pathology. 3rd ed. Edinburgh: Churchill Livingstone; 2001.

4. Lee A, Ackerman MJ. Sudden unexplained death: evaluation of those left behind *Lancet* 2003;362:1429–31.

5. Doolan A, Langlois N, Semsarian C. Causes of sudden death in young Australians. *Med J Aust* 2004;180:110–12.

6. Behr E, Wood DA, Wright M, Syrris P, Sheppard MN, Casey A, *et al.* Cardiological assessment of first-degree relatives in sudden arrhythmic death syndrome *Lancet* 2003;362:1457–59.

CHAPTER 11
Deaths from psychiatric causes

Introduction

For this Report, the concept of psychiatric death has been broadened to include not only deaths from suicide but also includes deaths from substance misuse, physical illness, accidents and other misfortunes which, in the opinion of the assessors, would not have occurred in the absence of a psychiatric disorder. However, as the characteristics of the deaths and lessons to be learned from these different groups of women are dissimilar, the Editorial Board took the decision to split this chapter into two parts:

- **11A**, which relates to lessons to be drawn from maternal deaths from suicide and other psychiatric causes; and the second, new section,

- **11B**, on lessons to be learned from deaths associated with drug and/or alcohol misuse.

This distinction has also been made because the problems and needs of women with substance misuse were distinctively different to those of women with psychiatric illness and because neither group was best served by including them under one generic title, 'Psychiatric disorder'.

For statistical purposes, the actual numbers of deaths from all psychiatric causes will continue to be counted under one overall category for psychiatric causes of death.

Although a psychiatrist has been a member of the Enquiry Board and a central assessor for the last three triennia, CEMACH will be introducing a network of Regional Psychiatric Assessors for 2003–2005, to reflect the importance of the lessons to be learned from these deaths.

CHAPTER 11A

Deaths from suicide and other psychiatric causes

MARGARET OATES on behalf of the Editorial Board

Psychiatric deaths from suicide or attributed to physical causes: key recommendations

Service provision

Guidelines for the management of women who are at risk of a relapse or recurrence of a serious mental illness following delivery should be in place in every Trust providing maternity services.

A specialist perinatal mental health team with the knowledge, skills and experience to provide care for women at risk of or suffering from serious postpartum mental illness should be available to every woman.

Women who require psychiatric admission following childbirth should be admitted to a specialist mother and baby unit, together with their infant. In areas where this service is not available then admission to the nearest unit should take place.

Sufficient regional psychiatric mother-and-baby units should be developed to meet the needs of the population.

Individual practitioners

Systematic enquiries about previous psychiatric history, its severity, care received and clinical presentation should be routinely made at the antenatal booking visit.

General practitioners should ensure that all relevant information concerning a woman's current or previous psychiatric history is included in referral letters to the booking clinic.

The term 'postnatal depression' or 'PND' should not be used as a generic term for all types of psychiatric disorder. Details of previous illness should be sought and recorded in line with the recommendations above.

Women who have a past history of serious psychiatric disorder, postpartum or non-postpartum, should be assessed by a psychiatrist in the antenatal period. A management plan regarding the high risk of recurrence following delivery should be agreed with the woman, her maternity team and GP and placed in her handheld records.

Women who have suffered from serious mental illness either following childbirth or at others times should be counselled about the possible recurrence of that illness following further pregnancies.

Education and training

The Royal Colleges of Psychiatry, Obstetrics and Gynaecology, General Practice and Midwives should ensure that perinatal psychiatry is included in their curricula and requirements for continuing professional development.

Local training must be put into place before routine screening for serious mental illness is implemented.

Obstetricians and midwives should be aware of the laws and issues that relate to child protection and when and to whom to refer if concerned.

Introduction

Perinatal psychiatric disorder

Psychiatric disorder associated with childbirth is common, both new episodes specifically related to childbirth and recurrences of pre-existing conditions. Ten percent of new mothers are likely to develop a depressive illness,[1] of whom between one-third and one-half will be suffering from a severe depressive illness.[2] Two percent of delivered women will see a psychiatrist during the first year after delivery. Four per thousand will be admitted to a psychiatric hospital, of which two per thousand will suffer from a puerperal psychosis.

The majority of women who develop postnatal mental health problems will suffer from mild depressive illnesses, often with accompanying anxiety. Such illnesses are equally prevalent in pregnancy. However, there is little evidence that mild depression is any more common during pregnancy or the postpartum period than at other times.[1]

In contrast, the risk of developing a severe mental illness, either a severe depressive illness or a puerperal psychosis, is substantially elevated, particularly in the first 3 months postpartum. The relative risk of suffering from a severe depressive illness following childbirth is 5, of seeing a psychiatrist 7 and of being admitted with a psychosis in the first three months following childbirth 324. The relative risk of suffering from a new onset serious psychiatric disorder in pregnancy is lower than at other times.[4] However, it should not be forgotten that the prevalence of all psychiatric disorders including substance misuse, schizophrenia and obsessional compulsive disorders is the same at conception as in the nonpregnant female population.

While psychosocial factors are undoubtedly in the ascendancy as etiological factors in the mild to moderate postnatal depressive illnesses,[4] it has been thought that biological factors (genetic and neuroendocrine) are the most important etiological factors in the severe postpartum onset conditions. It is known that a family history of bipolar disorder increases the risk of a woman developing such an illness after childbirth.[5] Women who have had a previous episode of non-postpartum serious mental illness are at an increased risk of developing a postpartum-onset illness, a risk estimated at between 1 in 2 and 1 in 36 and women who have had a previous manic episode either postpartum or non-postpartum are at particularly elevated risk of recurrence following childbirth, a risk estimated at 1 in 2.[6] The last Report[7] revealed that one-half of the women who died from suicide had a previous history of serious mental illness, one-quarter related to their last childbirth.

Specialist perinatal psychiatric services

The serious mental illnesses following childbirth tend to have an early and rapid onset, with the illness often developing very quickly over a period of 24–48 hours. Fifty percent of these illnesses have presented by day 7 and 90% by 3 months postpartum.[4] This, together with the distinctive symptoms[8] and the special needs of women and their infants at this time has led to national and international acceptance of the need for special services for perinatal psychiatric disorder.[9] It is also generally recommended in the United Kingdom that, if such women require admission to hospital, they should be admitted together with their infant to a specialised mother-and-baby unit. The finding of the last Report that none of the women who died as a consequence of severe postnatal mental illness had been admitted to a mother-and-baby unit underpins the importance of this Health Service strategy.

Maternal suicide

Despite the frequency of maternal psychiatric disorder in general and the increased risk of serious postnatal psychiatric disorder in particular, suicide is a rare event during pregnancy and the postpartum period. Until recently it had been thought that pregnancy and the postpartum period exerted 'a protective effect' on suicide and that the maternal suicide rate was lower than would be expected.[10,11] The last Report found that overall maternal suicide was more common than previously thought and was in fact the leading cause of maternal death. Four times as many suicides occurred following delivery than in pregnancy itself.

As shown in Chapter 20, the rate of suicides in women who have given birth up to 1 year after delivery is less than that for the nonpregnant population of the same age. This 'protective effect of pregnancy' is even more striking among pregnant women, who have the lowest suicide rate of all.

Risk of recurrence

Of great importance to the findings of this Enquiry is the risk of recurrence posed by childbirth to women who have a past history of severe mental illness, postpartum or at other times. The recommendations made in the last two Reports that women should be asked in the antenatal clinic about a previous history of psychiatric illness is strengthened in this Report, which once again emphasises not only the identification of risk but also its psychiatric management.

Fifty years ago...

Over the last 50 years, suicides have been reported to the Confidential Enquiries into Maternal Deaths. However, it is only in the last three Enquiries covering the triennia 1993–96, 1997–99 and this current Enquiry for 2000–02 that they have been separately analysed and described. The concept of psychiatric death has been broadened to include not only suicide but also deaths from substance misuse, physical illness, accidents and other misfortunes which would not have occurred in the absence of a psychiatric disorder. It is also only in the last three triennia that a psychiatrist has been a member of the Enquiry and a central assessor.

Suicide research over the last 40 years has consistently shown that suicide rates based on coroners' verdicts alone are underestimated. The record-linkage study by the Office for National Statistics (ONS) conducted at the end of the last Report and repeated for this, clearly demonstrated that around half of all maternal suicides had not been reported to this Enquiry. This is because these women died once they had lost contact with maternal health services, whose professionals are well used to reporting all cases of maternal death of which they are aware. To date, psychiatrists, community mental health nurses, general practitioners and others have not been sufficiently aware of the need to report such cases, and some women will have died out of contact with any services at all. Such under-reporting is likely always to have been true, making it difficult to compare the rates of suicide in the current Enquiries (and other psychiatric causes of deaths) with those over the last 50 years. Maternal suicide and postnatal mental illness have not been seen in the past as the direct consequence of the effects of childbirth. While the reporting of early suicide may be improving, those occurring after 42 days, particularly later in the postpartum year, are still under reported. Advice to pathologists, coroners and regional assessors will hopefully improve this situation in future Enquiries.

The previous Report for 1997–99

Chapter 11 in the previous Report described 42 psychiatric deaths; 68% of those deaths were due to suicide, which was the leading cause of *Indirect* death and the second leading cause of maternal death overall. However, when the additional cases discovered by the ONS linkage study were added, suicide emerged as the leading cause of maternal death. Other important findings to emerge from the 1997–99 Report were that the great majority of women who committed suicide died violently, very few dying from an overdose of prescribed medication. This, together with the fact that the majority of suicides were over 30 years of age and from comfortable social circumstances, suggested that the profile of women at risk of suicide at this time might be different to that of other women and men. A further important finding was that half of the suicides had a previous psychiatric history. Had their risk of recurrence been recognised and managed then the outcome might have been different. These findings informed the recommendations of the previous Report and included the recommendations that all women should be asked about a previous history of serious mental illness at booking and that management plans should be put in place for those women at high risk of recurrence following delivery. These and other recommendations have now been widely implemented in maternity Trusts throughout the United Kingdom[12] and have been incorporated into the NICE guidelines for antenatal care,[13] the Scottish National Maternity Framework (National Service Framework),[14] the Women's Mental Health Strategy,[15] and the Children and Maternity National Service Framework for England.[16]

An important cause of maternal death revealed in the last Report was overdosing of illicit drugs, mainly heroin. Those women suffering from substance misuse who committed suicide by other methods were counted as suicides. However, for most of the 'accidental' overdoses it is difficult to know whether the overdose was intentional. It was clear from the last Report that many of these women had difficulties engaging with Substance Misuse Services and that few of those services were well integrated with maternity care. In this Report, the deaths from substance misuse that occurred in pregnancy and in the first 42 days following delivery are counted in this chapter. All the deaths from substance misuse including the *Late* deaths are described in further detail in Chapter 11B.

Summary of the findings for 2000–02

As in the previous Report, the number of cases of suicide and other deaths associated with psychiatric causes were under-reported to the Enquiry. By using the numbers of cases of suicide actually reported to the Enquiry it appears to be the second leading cause of maternal death after cardiac disease. However, as shown in Figure 11.1, the ONS record linkage study, described more fully in Chapter 1, has identified additional deaths in England and Wales not reported to the Enquiry shows that suicide was in fact the leading cause of *Indirect* or *Late Indirect* maternal death over the whole year following delivery. Figure 11A.1 shows the number of deaths due to drugs and substance misuse, violence, accidents and misadventure that were also unreported. It is likely that a number of these also include cases of suicide.

Suicide is the leading cause of maternal death

As in the last Report, the majority of women who committed suicide after childbirth but within 1 year after delivery were not known to the Enquiry. This is mainly because they were out of contact with the maternity services by the time they died and their deaths were not coded as due to maternal causes on the death certificate. The ONS record linkage study identified around 50 women in England and Wales who were known to have died of suicide or whose deaths were recorded under an open verdict. Only 18 suicides were known to the Enquiry, including cases from Scotland and

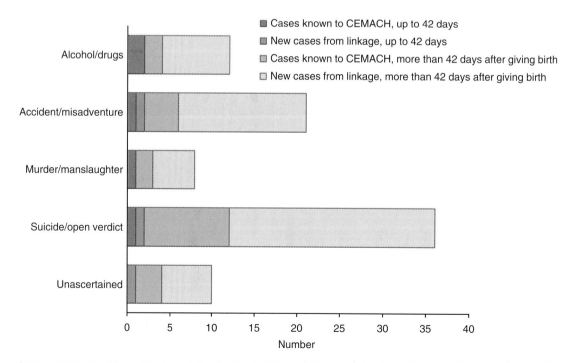

Figure 11A.1   Number of maternal deaths idenitifdied by ONS record linkage from psychiatric, accidental, violent of unascertained causes; England and Wales 2000–02

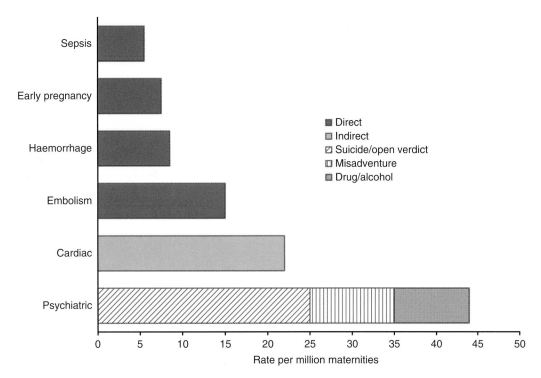

Figure 11A.2 Deaths per million maternities from leading causes of death as identified by ONS Linkage study for England and Wales; 2000–02

Northern Ireland. Further, another 14 women had verdicts of deaths due to accidental causes or misadventure and another ten died from drugs and/or alcohol and in both categories some of these too would have probably been self-inflicted. Figure 11A.1 shows the additional cases identified for England and Wales and Figure 11A.2 shows the overall UK maternal mortality rate if these deaths are included. It is important to note that many women who died as a result of puerperal psychosis did so after the first 6 weeks following delivery had elapsed, the timeframe usually taken to define a maternal death. Although these cases are classed as *Late Indirect* deaths they are still counted in the overall maternal mortality rate from suicide.

In this, as in previous Reports, the majority of the women died by their own hand, mostly suicide but a significant number from self-administered recreational drugs. As in previous Reports, there were a smaller number of women who died from other causes. However, all these deaths were caused, or significantly contributed to, by a psychiatric illness.

There were 60 deaths reported to this Enquiry which had psychiatric aspects and which are described in this Chapter. Details for four cases, two suicides and two to physical causes are incomplete and they are excluded from many of the tables in this chapter. However, only the 16 deaths, from suicide or recreational drugs overdose that occurred during pregnancy or in the first 42 days following delivery are counted in this chapter to accord with the international definitions of maternal deaths described on page 9 of this Report. A further 18 suicides and four illicit drug overdoses took place after 42 days, *Late* deaths, and are counted in Chapter 15. Eighteen women died from physical causes attributable to psychiatric disorder and are counted in the relevant chapters. There were three deaths: a death in a house fire, a murder and a road traffic accident, which have been counted as *Coincidental* deaths in Chapter 14. The details of how these deaths

Table 11A.1 Chapters in which maternal deaths reported to this Enquiry caused by or linked with psychiatric illness are counted; United Kingdom 2000–02

	Chapter 11 *Indirect*	Chapter 15 *Late*	Other chapters	Total
Suicide	10	18		28*
Drug overdose**	6	5		11
Other physical cause of death		3	15	18*
Other**			3	3
Total	16	26	18	60

* Two cases in each section have very few details and are excluded from the majority of the tables in this Chapter
** One death from alcoholism
*** Road traffic accident, murder or house fires in which psychiatric conditions may have played a part

have been classified are shown in Table 11A.1. The timing of the deaths in relation to pregnancy are shown in Table 11A.2.

Causes of death

There were 28 reported suicides. Further details were not available for two cases. Five of these occurred in pregnancy, including a woman who died in a road traffic accident, which did not have a coroner's suicide verdict but was probably intentional. Five women who committed suicide died within 42 days after delivery and there were 18 *Late* reported deaths from suicide. There were 11 deaths from an overdose of illicit drugs, four in pregnancy, two early after delivery and five *Late* deaths. Eighteen women died from physical causes, directly or indirectly related to a psychiatric condition, mainly in the immediate postpartum period. Three other deaths counted in Chapter 14 Coincidental deaths, probably had an underlying psychiatric component.

Deaths from physical illness

The three deaths in pregnancy included a woman who died of meningitis who was an intravenous drug user and a woman who died from HELLP syndrome who was an intravenous heroin user and homeless and whose psychosocial problems interfered with the earlier identification and management of her medical syndrome. A woman from an ethnic minority also died from infection. Her behavioural disturbance, probably due to a toxic confusional state, again interfered with her initial diagnosis and management.

Table 11A.2 Timing of reported maternal deaths associated with psychiatric causes; United Kingdom 2000–02

Cause	During pregnancy	Up to 42 days after delivery	Late (42 days to one year after delivery)	Total
Suicide	5	5	18	28*
Illicit drugs overdose	4	2	5	11
Physical illness	3	12	3	18*
Other	2	1	0	3
Total	14	20	26	60

* no further details available for two of these cases

Table 11A.3 Maternal deaths from physical illness associated with psychiatric disorders; United Kingdom 2000–02

Cause	During pregnancy	Within 42 days of delivery	Late	Total
Thromboembolism:				
Cerebral thrombosis		2		2
Pulmonary embolus		1		1
Central nervous system:				
Cerebral haemorrhage		1	1	2
Wernickes encephalopathy		1		1
Acute hydrocephalus			1	1
Infection:				
Meningitis	1			1
Uterine sepsis		1		1
Not known	1	1		2
Obstetric haemorrhage		2		2
Others	1	3	1	5*
Total	3	12	3	18

* details not available for 2 of these cases

Many of the lessons to be learned from the 12 deaths from physical causes in which psychiatric causes played a part are described in the relevant chapters. Some are briefly mentioned here and the major lessons to be learned from these cases are discussed later in this chapter (Table 11A.3).

In the immediate postpartum period, two women's deaths were due to cerebral thromboembolism and their symptoms, in one case attributed to hysteria, had led to them receiving inappropriate psychiatric care prior to the correct diagnosis. Another woman's symptoms of meningitis were ascribed to depression. This probably delayed their treatment.

Of the *Direct* deaths, one woman who died from sepsis a few days following delivery had a severe tachycardia, which was mistaken for panic attacks. Two women died from postpartum haemorrhage. They had both concealed their pregnancies and had unassisted deliveries. In one case there was clear evidence to suggest a major personality disorder and in the other the circumstances of the concealment and unassisted delivery strongly suggest psychological problems.

There were three other early postpartum deaths. One woman, a chronic alcoholic, died from a ruptured pancreatic cyst shortly after delivery. A second, with a long history of major psychosocial problems, was thought to have psychogenic vomiting and died from the consequences of a ruptured oesophagus. In the third, a woman with a long history of emotional and behavioural disturbance died from a ruptured adenoma after having been transferred to a psychiatric unit with a presumed diagnosis of puerperal psychosis. It is possible that her psychiatric medication contributed to her respiratory arrest.

There were three *Late* deaths from physical causes, two of which are discussed in the section on drug and alcohol misuse. The final woman who died had a sudden unexplained cardiac death, which may have been due to her antidepressant medication.

Table 11A.4 Timing of deaths from or associated with psychiatric causes reported to this Enquiry during pregnancy or in 6-week intervals up to following delivery; United Kingdom 2000–02

| | Timing | | | | | | | |
| | Pregnancy (completed weeks of gestation) | | | Up to 42 days after delivery (weeks) | Late (weeks after delivery) | | | |
Cause of death	< 28	28–33	34–40	0–6	7–12	13–25	> 26	Total (n)
Suicide	1	0	4	5	5	7	6*	28
Drugs	3	1	0	2	0	3	2	11
Physical Illness	0	1	2	12*	2	1	0	18
Other	1	1	0	1	0	0	0	3
Total	5	3	6	20	7	11	8	60

* further details not available for two cases

Timing of psychiatric deaths from suicide, overdose or other causes

The known epidemiology of perinatal psychiatric disorders suggests that psychiatric disorder presenting in the last trimester of pregnancy is both unusual and predictive of problems following delivery. It is also known that the majority of serious mental illnesses have presented by 90 days following delivery. For this reason, together with the fact that deaths from psychiatric causes may occur some weeks after the early onset of the illness, the psychiatric deaths were analysed in 6-week periods relating to childbirth. Four out of five suicides in pregnancy occurred between 34 and 40 weeks of gestation. Details are shown in Table 11A.4. Twelve of the 26 reported suicides therefore occurred between the last trimester of pregnancy and the first 3 months following delivery. In two more, the timing was not known to the assessors.

The timings of death of the women who died from an overdose of drugs are also shown in Table 11A.4, as are those for women who died of other causes. There were no deaths from physical causes beyond 18 weeks post-delivery. All the *Coincidental* deaths occurred during or shortly after delivery.

Overall therefore, almost more than 50% (34 out of 60, according to the Reports to this Enquiry) of all maternal deaths from psychiatric causes occurred either in the 3 months before or the 3 months after childbirth.

Method of suicide

As in the last Confidential Enquiry, the method of suicide was predominantly violent. In two women the method of death was not disclosed on the death certificate and further information not available.

Of the suicides where the method of death was known only nine women died from an overdose of prescribed medication. Seventeen women died violently, eight from hanging, four from jumping, one each from a cut throat, self-immolation and drowning; two were from intentional road traffic accidents. Two-thirds of the suicides assessed for this triennium were violent. Table 11A.5 shows the percentage of deaths from suicide by method for 1997–2002.

Table 11A.5 Chosen method of suicide; United Kingdom 1997–2002

Method of suicide	1997–99 (n)	2000–02 (n)	Total (n)	(%)
Hanging	10	8	18	35
Jumping from a height	5	4	9	17
Cut throat	4	1	5	10
Intentional road traffic accident*	1	2	3	6
Self-immolation	1	1	2	4
Drowning	1	1	2	4
Gunshot	1	0	1	2
Total violent deaths	23	17	40	77
Overdose of prescribed drugs	3	9	12	23
Total	26	26**	52	100

* Open verdict but the details of the cases led the opinion of the Assessors to classify these as suicides
** Details missing for two further cases

Age at death

In the last Report it was noted that the women who committed suicide tended to be older than for those dying of other causes of maternal death with over half the women being aged 30 years more. For this triennium, 42% of the women who committed suicide were 30 years or older as shown in Table 11.6. The details are missing for two cases.

Social characteristics

Unlike the women who died from drug- or alcohol-related deaths, the social circumstances of the women who committed suicide were favourable, and there was no social class gradient or link to deprivation as seen for many other causes of maternal death. The majority of the women came from comfortable backgrounds, were in stable relationships and had partners who were in employment. Many had completed higher education and several had higher professional qualifications. As in the last Report, a number were healthcare professionals.

Ethnicity

Four of the women who committed suicide were from ethnic minority groups, two being Indian. None of the suicides was African or Caribbean, although three women from these groups died of physical causes. Fifty-three of the total number of 60 women who died from psychiatric deaths were White.

Table 11A.6 Age at death from psychiatric causes; United Kingdom 2000–02

Age (years)	Suicide (n)	Illicit drugs (n)	Physical illness (n)	Other (n)	Total (n)
18 & under	1	1	0	1	3
19–24	3	3	2	0	8
25–29	11	3	7	0	21
30–34	6	2	4	2	14
35+	5	2	5	0	12
Total	26*	11	18	3	58*

* Excluding two suicides for which very few details were available

Table 11A.7 Psychiatric diagnosis and underlying causes of death; United Kingdom 2000–02

Diagnosis	Suicide (n)	Illicit drugs O/D (n)	Physical illness (n)	Other (n)	Total (n)
Organic state	0	0	5	0	5
Psychosis	9	0	1	1	11
Severe depressive illness	5	0	0	0	5
Anxiety/depression adjustment	5	0	2	0	7
Alcohol dependent	2 (1*)	0	3 (1*)	1	6
Drug dependent	2 (1*)	9 (3*)	5	0	16
Personality disorder	1	0	1	1	3
Unascertainable	2	0	1	0	3
Total	26**	9	18**	3	56

* Co-morbidity anxiety and depression
** Detail not available in two cases

Diagnosis of psychiatric disorder

In all but three cases, there was sufficient information to make a probable or definite psychiatric diagnosis. In nine of the 18 women whose deaths were due to physical causes the probable psychiatric diagnosis immediately prior to deaths were of an acute confusional state. However, their symptoms were attributed to a functional psychiatric disorder and this may have delayed appropriate diagnosis and treatment. Details of the psychiatric diagnosis and cause of death are given in Table 11A.7.

In all, there were 11 cases of psychosis, nine of the 26 women who committed suicide, one who died from physical causes and a woman who was murdered. Five other women who committed suicide were suffering from a severe depressive illness. Therefore, more than 50%, 14 of 26, women who died from suicide were suffering from a serious mental illness during the index maternity.

There were seven cases of mixed anxiety and depression or adjustment reaction, five who committed suicide and two who died from a physical illness.

Six women were alcohol-dependent, of whom two committed suicide, one of whom had co-morbid anxiety and depression. A further three women with chronic alcoholism died from physical illness, and the other woman died in pregnancy in a house fire.

Details of the women who died from drug- or alcohol-related deaths are given in Chapter 11B but two heroin addicts committed suicide by hanging.

Three women had personality disorders. One woman with an explosive personality disorder and co-morbid alcohol misuse committed suicide, and another profoundly personality disordered woman, with a history of at least 12 concealed pregnancies and unassisted deliveries, died of a postpartum haemorrhage. A young girl with conduct disorder and personality difficulties died when pregnant in a road traffic accident in a car driven by her young disordered boyfriend.

Although over half of the suicides were seriously ill, there was a wide range of psychiatric disorders in the deaths overall.

Substance misuse (see Chapter 11B)

There were 22 deaths in women who misused alcohol or illicit drugs, six in alcohol misusers and 16 in drug misusers. Eleven died of overdoses and five hanged themselves.

Three women died from the physical consequences of chronic alcoholism. Apart from the suicides and deaths due to alcohol the remainder were either accidental overdoses or deaths from physical consequences of drug misuse. Another nine women who died from other causes were known to be substance misusers.

Current level of contact with services

In the previous Report, 68% of all women who died from psychiatric causes and 86% of those who committed suicide were receiving some form of psychiatric treatment during the index maternity, and over half were in contact with psychiatric services. In this triennium, ten women had been admitted to a psychiatric hospital in the index maternity, six of whom subsequently committed suicide and three of whom died from physical illness. Only one woman had received inpatient care in a specialist mother and baby unit.

A further 13 women had been in contact with a community mental health team or a psychiatrist during the index maternity: eight suicides, two who died from physical causes, one woman who was murdered and a girl who died a road traffic accident.

Five women were being treated by their general practitioner for depression, four of whom committed suicide and one who died of a drug overdose and who was being managed by her general practitioner for co-morbid anxiety and depression.

Overall out of the 60 psychiatric deaths from all causes, 37 were receiving treatment for their condition during the index maternity, 23 of these by psychiatric services, ten as inpatients. Twenty of the 26 women who committed suicide were receiving treatment, 15 by psychiatric services. Seven of these women had been admitted for psychiatric care during the index maternity (Table 11A.8).

Previous psychiatric history

In the last Report half of the women who died from suicide had had a psychiatric history prior to the index maternity, of which half had followed a previous childbirth. These findings are consistent with this Report. In this triennium, 17 of the 26 suicides had a prior psychiatric history. Six of these had been treated as an inpatient, three with a previous puerperal psychosis. Seven had been managed as psychiatric outpatients or by the community mental health team, including one woman with a previous history of severe postnatal depression. A further two women were being managed by their

Table 11A.8 Highest level of current psychiatric care, by cause of death, provided during the index pregnancy; United Kingdom 2000–02

Level of care	Suicide	Illicit O/D drugs	Physical illness	Other	Total
Inpatient	7	0	3	0	10
Outpatient	8	0	2	3	13
Substance misuse services	1	6	2	0	9
GP only	4	1	0	0	5
None	6	2	11	0	19
Total	26*	9	18*	3	56

O/D = overdose; * details for not available for 2 cases

Table 11A.9 Previous contact with psychiatric services past history of psychiatric disorder all causes; United Kingdom 2000–02

	Cause of death				
Type of care	Suicide	Illicit drugs overdose	Physical illness	Other	Total
Inpatient	6(3*)	0	0	1	7
Outpatient	7 (1*)	0	3	2	12
Substance misuse services	2	5	4	0	11
GP only	2 (1*)	0	2	0	4
None	9	4	9	0	22
Total	26	9	18	3	56**

* = postnatal illness   ** details not available for four cases

general practitioners, including one with a history of postnatal depression. Two substance misusers who committed suicide had been seen previously by the substance misuse services.

Half of the 18 women who died from physical illness had been previously treated for a psychiatric disorder, mainly by community mental health teams or their general practitioners for anxiety and depression (Table 11A.9).

The woman who was murdered had previously been an inpatient for schizophrenia, the road traffic accident victim had been treated by the child and adolescent services for conduct disorder and the woman who died in a house fire by the community mental health services.

Overall, therefore, 34 out of 56 psychiatric deaths had a prior psychiatric history, 19 out of the 56 a previous history of serious psychiatric disorder, treated by psychiatric services and a further 11 women previously treated by substance misuses services. In this triennium only five women had a previous psychiatric history of postpartum illness.

Risk identification and management

Thirty-four of the women who died from psychiatric causes had a previous history of a psychiatric disorder treated by psychiatric services, substance misuse services or their general practitioner. Of these, 17 had their history identified during the index pregnancy and 17 did not. Of the 17 suicides 'at risk', in seven cases the risk was antenatally identified by either or both maternity and psychiatric services but in ten cases it was not identified. For women dying from other causes including accidental overdoses of illicit drugs, ten were identified antenatally but ten were not. Overall, therefore, in half of the cases 'at risk', risk factors were not identified during the index pregnancy.

Further, of the 34 women with a previous history of treated psychiatric disorder, in only ten cases was an adequate psychiatric management plan put into place in the antenatal period. Of the 17 suicides with a previous history only four had an adequate management plan and of the 17 deaths from other causes with a previous history only six had an adequate management plan, as shown in Table 11A.10.

Contact with specialist services

Of the 60 deaths, only one woman, who died from suicide in pregnancy, was cared for by specialist perinatal mental health services and only one woman, a *Late* suicide, was

Table 11A.10 Appropriate management of risk in women with a known previous psychiatric history; United Kingdom 2000–02

| Cause of care | Management of risk | | | | Total (n) |
| | Plan in place | | No plan | | |
	(n)	(%)	(n)	(%)	
Suicide	4	24	13	76	17
Other	6	55	11	65	17
Total	10	42	24	71	34

admitted to a mother and baby unit. However, this latter woman was admitted many miles from her home and discharged herself after only a few hours. None of the women who had been in contact with psychiatric services after a previous childbirth had been treated by specialist services during the current pregnancy.

Communication between professionals and services

Despite the fact that two thirds of the women who died from psychiatric causes were receiving some form of psychiatric treatment during the index maternity, and the fact that almost two thirds of the women had a previous psychiatric history, there was very little evidence of communication between the specialties of general practice, psychiatry and obstetrics. With two notable exceptions, there appears to have been an absence of communication in the following areas:

- GPs did not reveal previous psychiatric history or current psychiatric involvement to obstetricians on referral.

- Psychiatric services seemed to be unaware in many cases that their patient was pregnant and, if they were aware, did not communicate their management plans or concerns to the obstetricians.

- Obstetricians and midwives did not appear to communicate with psychiatric services.

The children

Twenty-five women who died of psychiatric causes had no living children prior to the index maternity. Thirty-one women had one or two older children and only three women had more than two older children including a woman who died from a haemorrhage after a concealed pregnancy and unassisted delivery. She had at least 12 children. Half the women who died from suicide had older children but only five had a previous history of postnatal mental illness.

Infanticide and filicide

There were four cases, all suicides, where the woman died and killed her infant; three suicide/infanticides and one death of the infant was followed by suicide some weeks later. In two cases, an older child was killed at the same time. To these cases can be added four suicides that occurred in pregnancy, near term, therefore killing a viable infant.

Comparison with the findings of the last Report

The overall numbers of maternal deaths due to psychiatric causes and the numbers of suicides in particular were broadly similar to the 1997–99 Enquiry. Also the same were the findings that the majority of women were older, White, had a previous history of psychiatric disorder, and that in the majority of cases the risk of recurrence was neither identified nor managed in the index pregnancy. Sadly, the predominantly violent method of suicide was also found in the current Enquiries.

However, there were some differences. There were relatively fewer women in the current Enquiries with a previous history of puerperal psychosis and postnatal depression. While over half of the suicides were seriously mentally ill, there was a wider range of psychiatric diagnoses in deaths from all causes than previously. The proportion of women who died from the consequences of illicit drug misuse seems to have increased. There were fewer early deaths and there seemed to be an increase in the number of women who died from physical illness as a consequence of their psychiatric disorder. On this occasion, unlike the two previous Enquiries, four women died together with their infants or older children.

Emergent themes

Suicide profile

Although there were fewer earlier deaths after childbirth than in the last Report, 57% of the women who died from suicide and whose deaths were assessed by this Enquiry died within 3 months of childbirth and 78% within 6 months. This highlights the need to be particularly vigilant about the mental health of women in late pregnancy and the first 3 months postpartum. The following points summarise the findings in this Report.

Of the women who committed suicide:

- 87% were White
- 83% were over the age of 25 years
- 46% were over the age of 30 years
- 55% had previous children
- 54% were seriously ill, either suffering from a postpartum psychosis or a very severe depressive illness
- 50% had a previous history of serious illness, of whom half had been admitted to a psychiatric unit
- 50% were in contact with psychiatric services during their index maternity, 75% of whom were receiving some form of treatment
- Only one woman with significant postpartum mental illness had been admitted to a specialist mother and baby unit
- 65% of the suicides died violently, half from hanging or jumping from a height, clearly reflecting the profound disturbance of their mental state and intention to die
- Only 35% died from an overdose of prescribed medication.

These illnesses were therefore neither hidden nor undetected.

However, in this Report, only five women had a previous history of postpartum mental illness, despite the fact that over 50% of the women who killed themselves had had a previous child.

Learning point: profile of women who commit suicide due to perinatal mental illness

The most common profile of women at risk of suicide in late pregnancy and following delivery is of a White older woman in her second or subsequent pregnancy, married and living in comfortable circumstances. She is likely to have a previous history of mental illness and contact with psychiatric services, is probably currently being treated and whose baby is under 3 months old. She is likely to die violently. This highlights the importance of alerting psychiatric services to the fact that risk factors for maternal suicide may be different to those for other women and men.

Risk detection and management

Sixty percent of all maternal psychiatric deaths and 77% of suicides had a previous history of treated psychiatric disorder and were therefore 'at risk' of a recurrence of that disorder following childbirth. For 57% of the women who committed suicide, this previous psychiatric history was of serious mental illness and had been managed by the psychiatric services. Despite this, 50% of the maternal deaths overall and 60% of suicides had not had these risk factors identified during the index pregnancy either by maternity or psychiatric services. A higher percentage, 70% of all those at risk and 76% of the suicides at risk, had no psychiatric management plan for the peripartum period. For some women, therefore, even though their risk had been identified, no further action had been taken.

This finding underlines the importance of the recommendation made in the last Confidential Enquiry that routine inquiry should be made about previous psychiatric history during pregnancy and that management psychiatric plans should be put in place for those at risk of a recurrence of their condition following delivery.

In 50% of all cases and 60% of suicides where the risk was not identified during the index pregnancy, the GP records would have contained the relevant information. In some cases, it is evident that the GP did not inform the obstetrician or midwifes of the previous psychiatric history. In other cases, including once more a previous history of puerperal psychosis recorded as 'PND', the midwife did not seek further information.

The following vignette demonstrates the importance of GPs sharing their knowledge of a woman's previous history and how this information might have altered the significance of the events that followed:

> A professional woman died from violent means, together with baby and another child. At the booking clinic she revealed a family history of mental illness but denied any personal psychiatric history. Her GP records contained the evidence that she had taken several previous overdoses and had been

treated previously by a psychiatrist but this was not shared with her maternity care providers. There were no concerns about her mental health until the very end of pregnancy when she called her GP saying that she was unable to leave the house. She was diagnosed with agoraphobia and was referred to the community mental health team. She declined psychological intervention on the unusual grounds that the resultant anxiety would harm the baby. This was accepted and no arrangements were made for her to be seen again. Following her death, the family revealed that the woman had wished them to conceal her previous history and that she was developing a paranoid psychosis.

Both her previous psychiatric history and family history were risk factors for the development of her fatal psychiatric illness. If more information had been available, the community mental health team might have perceived her presentation late in pregnancy as an additional risk factor and visited her following delivery.

The central role of the GP and the information contained in their records to assist in the accurate identification of risk cannot be overemphasised.

The following vignette gives an example of a case, even when the history of previous serious mental illness and its treatment had been accurately noted at the Booking Clinic by the midwife, in the risk seems to have been under-estimated by others and no proactive plans put into place:

> A professional woman killed herself and her baby by self-immolation some weeks following delivery. She had a history of bipolar illness with several previous inpatient admissions. Despite this, she had been well for many years and functioning at a very high level. At booking, the midwife accurately recorded her previous psychiatric history but the fact that she had been well for many years seems to have diminished the risk of a recurrence in the view of others. No proactive management plan was put into place. The early signs of a developing depressive psychosis were misattributed before her death.

This woman, as with others with a previous history of bipolar disorder, was at a one in two risk of a postpartum recurrence. A proactive management plan of supportive vigilant monitoring in the early weeks following delivery and perhaps prophylactic medication might have altered the outcome.

A further case illustrates the theme that risk identification in the absence of risk management is of little use:

> An older parous woman killed herself a few days following delivery by jumping from a height. She had a substantial psychiatric history, which included a number of previous puerperal psychoses. Following the birth of a previous child she survived a serious suicide attempt. She had been chronically mentally unwell and physically disabled since that time. Her substantial risk of relapse was correctly identified by all involved. However, no plan was put into place for her peripartum management. She first tried to kill herself by jumping a few days after delivery and, shortly afterwards, succeeded.

In view of her previous psychiatric history and life-threatening suicide attempt, this woman should have received intensive psychiatric care and close observation throughout the peripartum period. Neither of this woman's earlier puerperal psychoses had been treated in a mother and baby unit.

Misattribution of symptoms to functional psychiatric disorder

A worrying new theme emerging from this Enquiry is that 32% of psychiatric deaths were due to physical illness, 18 of the 56 psychiatric deaths. In 50% of these, nine cases, either physical symptoms or behavioural disturbance were mistakenly attributed to functional psychiatric disorder rather than to serious and ultimately fatal physical illness. In all of these cases, the presumed psychiatric diagnosis led to a delay in making the correct diagnosis. One case serves as a reminder to exercise caution in attributing atypical neurological signs to hysteria, particularly in a woman with no previous psychiatric history. It also underlines the importance of involving obstetricians and midwives in the care of a pregnant woman who is admitted to a non-maternity facility. In three cases, the women were admitted initially to a psychiatric hospital, which may also have delayed the onset of effective treatment.

The following case demonstrates the difficulty of distinguishing clinically the symptoms of anxiety from tachycardia of physical origin:

> A woman died within days of delivering her second child from sepsis and cardiac arrhythmia. At postmortem, she was discovered to have a gangrenous uterus and gross cardiac dilatation. Towards the end of her pregnancy, she complained of palpitations and had a tachycardia recorded at between 140 bpm and 170 bpm. She revealed a previous history of anxiety and depression treated many years ago by her GP and a diagnosis of recurrent panic attacks was made. Following delivery, her complaints continued and again a diagnosis was made of panic attacks and a selective serotonin reuptake inhibitor antidepressant was started. Her complaints continued and she was referred to the community mental health team. On the day of her death she became acutely disturbed and doubly incontinent. She was admitted to a psychiatric hospital. Shortly afterwards, she was transferred to an intensive care unit where she died.

This case is a reminder that a tachycardia of over 110 bpm and double incontinence are unlikely to be due to a functional psychiatric disorder. It is probable that the attribution of this woman's symptoms to an anxiety state delayed appropriate diagnosis and treatment.

Clinicians should be reminded that serious physical illness can coexist with mental illness. Great caution should be exercised before attributing unusual physical symptoms to psychiatric causes. The possibility that new emotional and behavioural changes in later pregnancy and the early postpartum period may be due to an acute confusional state with serious underlying pathology should not be overlooked.

Suicide and Infanticide

The majority of suicides did not involve the death of a living child. There were four exceptions to this. In addition, four suicides occurred in the last few weeks of pregnancy and a viable infant died. This could be seen, psychologically, as indistinguishable from infanticide.

As in the last Enquiry, there was little information about the infants and children of the women who died, despite the evidence that social services had been involved with previous children or with the index pregnancy in a number of cases. However an exception was a very full social services report on a woman who died from a postpartum haemorrhage. She had given birth to at least 12 children previously with at least three infant deaths and one stillbirth. In most other cases it could be surmised that the infant and older children were alive and well.

There were four previous described cases in which women died and killed their infant and, in two cases, older children. The first was a suicide/infanticide in a woman with a prior history of bipolar disorder. The second was an early death of a woman who committed suicide by jumping together with her infant and older child. Both of these have already been described. The third case was of a woman who was depressed with a previous history who killed herself just before delivery by cutting her throat having first killed her existing child. The last, a woman who had had an unassisted delivery, killed herself by taking an overdose of psychotropic medication during court proceedings for having been charged, together with her partner, with wilful neglect causing the death of their infant.

Most cases of infanticide due to serious maternal mental illness will be associated with either a significant suicide attempt or a successful suicide. In late pregnancy and the early weeks postpartum, maternal suicide risk should therefore be also regarded as a risk for infanticide. However, implementing child protection procedures alone is not only unlikely to protect the mother and infant but may increase the risk by increasing guilt and the fear that the child may be removed. The most effective way of protecting both the mother and the infant's life is early risk identification and rapid and effective treatment.

Child protection issues

Some of these women had no prior indications for the involvement of social services and were devoted mothers. Their acute psychiatric disorder posed the only, fatal risk to their children. However, in two further cases, knowledge of and correct use of child protection procedures might have influenced the outcome. One was the woman who killed herself after she and her husband had been charged with causing death by wilful neglect. In this case, there were multiple risk factors for child abuse present prior to the death of the child that could have been identified during pregnancy. In one further case a woman killed herself during court proceedings after her child had been removed into the care of the local authority for non-accidental injury to her child at the hands of her husband. This child had presented previously with a lacerated lip, which was probably the first episode of non-accidental injury. If it had been acted upon at that time, then perhaps the second episode, which resulted in the infant being severely brain damaged, might have been prevented. In the case of the schizophrenic woman who was murdered, her preterm infant was safely in special care baby unit. However, in the light of her lifestyle and severe chronic illness, childcare social services should perhaps have been involved.

Clinical isolation and communication

From the evidence available to the Enquiry, it seems that, although the majority of women who died were receiving psychiatric treatment during the index maternity and that the majority had a previous history of prior treatment, this information was not elicited at antenatal clinic nor was the information provided by general practitioners or psychiatric services. Communication between these services also appears not to have occurred during the immediate postpartum period. The fact that psychiatric services are often geographically isolated from maternity units and have separate management and patient information systems no doubt increases the problem. This theme can be seen to run through all the other emergent issues and made a significant contribution to the deaths of many of these women.

When different Trusts and professions are involved in the care of a pregnant or postpartum woman and where there has been a history in the past of such involvement, it is essential that obstetric and psychiatric services communicate with each other and that the pivotal role of the general practitioner is recognised.

Conclusion

More than 25% of the women who died from *Direct, Indirect* or *Late Indirect* causes had some form of psychiatric disorder associated with their death. Excluding the women who died from physical causes initially wrongly attributed to psychiatric disorders, 42 actually died as a result of their mental health problems, although a majority died in the *Late* postnatal period.

The introduction to this chapter shows that the deaths from suicide reported to this Enquiry are the second leading reported cause of maternal death, but the number of unreported cases identified by subsequent record linkage reveals psychiatric causes to be the leading cause of maternal death overall.

Nevertheless, maternal suicide is rare, particularly in pregnancy. Although the fact that suicide is the leading cause of maternal death overall and has led to the key recommendations made in this Report, the results of the survey discussed in Chapter 20 show pregnancy itself to have a protective effect on suicide until at least 1 year after delivery.

In the absence of full information from psychiatric sources and the absence of a control group, it is not possible to know the frequency of the risk factors found in this study in women with severe psychiatric morbidity but who did not die. The findings of this study of deaths from psychiatric causes are therefore not only important for suicide prevention but also important in improving the care of equivalently ill women.

Psychiatric deaths: key learning points

- Although the number of cases reported to this Enquiry suggests that death from mental illness is the second leading cause of maternal mortality, the ONS linkage study has shown that a large number of deaths were not reported; if these were included then deaths from psychiatric causes would be the leading cause of maternal morality.

- Women who have had a past episode of severe mental illness following delivery have a one in two to one in three chance of recurrence.

- 50% of the women were seriously mentally ill but a wide range of psychiatric disorders was found.

- The risk of recurrence was neither identified nor managed.

- GPs, obstetricians, midwives and psychiatrists are not sharing information or psychiatric management plans.

- Women requiring specialist inpatient care after delivery are still not being admitted to specialist mother and baby units.

- The suicide profile of childbearing women is different in many respects to that of other women and men.

- Psychiatric disorder is a risk to the physical health of women. Serious physical illness can present with psychological symptoms, result from or complicate mental illness. In many causes a psychiatric diagnosis delayed the treatment of a fatal physical illness.

Acknowledgements

This chapter has been seen and discussed with Dr Alan Lee, Consultant Psychiatrist, University Hospital, Nottingham, and Emeritus Professor TJ Fahy, National University of Ireland, Galway.

References

1. O'Hara MW, Swain AM. Rates and risk of post partum depression – a meta-analysis. *Int Rev Psychiatry* 1996; 8: 37–54.
2. Cox J, Murray D, Chapman G. A controlled study of the onset prevalence and duration of postnatal depression. *Br J Psychiatry* 1993; 163: 27–41.
3. Oates M. Psychiatric Services for women following childbirth. *Int Rev Psychiatry* 1996; 8: 87–98.
4. Kendell RE, Chalmers KC, Platz C. Epidemiology of puerperal psychoses. *Br J Psychiatry* 1987; 150: 662–73.
5. Dean C, Williams, RJ Brockington IF. Is puerperal psychosis the same as bipolar manic-depressive disorder? A family study. *Psychol Med* 1989; 19; 637–47.
6. Wieck A, Kumar R, Hirst AD, Marks MN, Campbell IC, Checkley SA. Increased sensitivity of dopamine receptors and recurrence of affective psychosis after childbirth. *Br J Psychiatry* 1991; 303: 613–16.
7. Lewis G, Drife J, editors. *Why Mothers Die 1997–1999. The Fifth Report of the Confidential Enquiries into Maternal Deaths in the United Kingdom.* London: RCOG Press; 2001.
8. Dean C, Kendell RE. The symptomatology of puerperal illness. *Br J of Psychiatry* 1981; 139: 128–33.
9. Royal College of Psychiatrists. *Perinatal Mental Health Services. Recommendations for Provision of Services for Childbearing Women.* CR88. London: Royal College of Psychiatrists; 2001.
10. Apleby L. Suicidal behaviour in childbearing women. *Int Rev Psychiatry* 1996; 8: 107–15.
11. Hawton K, Sex and suicide: gender differences in suicidal behaviour. *Br J Psychiatry* 2000; 177: 484–5.

12. Clinical Negligence Scheme for Trusts. *Clinical Risk Management Standards for Maternity Services.* London: NHS Litigation Authority; 2002.

13. National Collaborating Centre for Women's and Children's Health. *Antenatal Care. Clinical Guideline.* London: RCOG Press; 2002.

14. Scottish Executive. *Framework for Maternity Services in Scotland.* Edinburgh: NHS Scotland; 2001.

15. Department of Health. *Women's Mental Health: Into the Mainstream 2002.* Strategic Development of Mental Health Care for Women. London: DoH; 2001.

16. Department of Health, Department for Education and Skills. *National Service Framework for Children, Young People and Maternity Services.* London: DoH; 2004 [www.doh.gov.uk].

CHAPTER 11B

Drug and/or alcohol related deaths

MARY HEPBURN on behalf of the Editorial Board

Key recommendations: drug and/or alcohol related deaths

Service delivery

Pregnant women with significant problem drug and/or alcohol use may have other social problems and their care should reflect this. They should not be managed in isolation but by maternity services that are part of a wider multi-agency network, which should include both addiction and social services.

Women with problems with substance misuse, and their babies, also require close multi-disciplinary follow-up in the postnatal period.

The management of pregnant women who are substance misusing should be according to best practice guidelines. National guidelines for Scotland were published in 2003[1] and suggested guidelines for England and Wales in 1997.[2]

Individual practitioners

Staff providing antenatal care for pregnant women should ask sensitively, but routinely, about all substance use, prescribed and non prescribed, legal and illegal, including tobacco and alcohol.

Information on social problems, including substance misuse, that could affect medical or social outcomes of pregnancy should be provided in all referral letters.

Women with problem drug and/or alcohol use have potentially high-risk pregnancies and an obstetrician should supervise their management. However, most of their care can be usually be delivered by midwives.

Education

All maternity and primary care staff require training so that they have the knowledge and skills to identify substance misuse, assess its severity and refer women to specialist services.

Staff in specialist services, including obstetricians, midwives, health visitors, social and addiction workers, require ongoing training and all staff, mainstream and specialist, need support in caring for such women.

Obstetricians and midwives should be aware of the laws and issues that relate to child protection and when, and to whom, to refer if concerned.

Introduction

Such is the growing impact of problem drug and alcohol use on the outcome of pregnancies for mother, child and the wider family, that this separate section has been included in this Report for the first time. The aim of this section is to give a brief summary of the main issues and to summarise the general lessons and recommendations that can be drawn from the management of the women who died, from whatever cause, who were known to use drug and or alcohol inappropriately.

The prevalence and patterns of problem use

The huge increase in problem drug use that has occurred nationally and internationally since the 1980s has been disproportionately large among women of childbearing age. The effects of substance abuse on the mother include poorer overall health, addiction and occasionally death by either an intentional or unintentional overdose. Consequently, there has been a large increase in the numbers of pregnant drug-using women. No such change appears to have occurred in numbers of pregnant women with problem alcohol use. The possible effects on the baby are given in Box 11B.1, which has been taken from the 2003 Scottish guidelines for working with families and children affected by problem drug misuse.[1]

There is a general under-identification of women with problem substance abuse in maternity services. This may reflect inadequate history taking or a reluctance to disclose the information. Problem drug use is usually illegal and is socially unacceptable and therefore women may not wish to admit to an activity that could lead to loss of custody of their child or children. Alcohol is socially acceptable but levels of consumption are often underestimated by pregnant women, not recognised as problematic or may be hidden. Nevertheless, there is increasing awareness of the need to provide specialised services for such women and specialist care is increasingly provided to varying degrees in many maternity units throughout the UK.

Box 11B.1   The effects of substance misuse on the baby during and after pregnancy[1]

Substance misuse during pregnancy increases the risk of:

- having a premature or low weight baby
- the baby suffering symptoms of withdrawal from drugs used by mother during pregnancy
- the death of the baby before or shortly after birth
- sudden infant death syndrome
- physical and neurological damage to the baby before birth, particularly if violence accompanies parental use of drugs or alcohol
- pregnant women drinking to excess risk delivering babies with fetal alcohol syndrome.

Some pregnant women who misuse substances do not seek antenatal services until late in pregnancy or when in labour. They may not realise they are pregnant because of the effects of some substance use on the menstrual cycle. Their substance misuse and associated lifestyle may make other more urgent demands on their time. They may fear that their drug use or drinking will be detected through routine urine or blood tests, or that if they tell staff they will be treated differently, or that child protection agencies will be contacted automatically. They may feel guilty about their drug or alcohol use and want, or feel they ought, to stop but are worried they will not succeed. They may be worried that their baby will be damaged or display withdrawal symptoms after birth. Many of these problems can be overcome by provision of accessible antenatal services that tackle these worries honestly and sympathetically.

Problem drug use is closely associated with socio-economic deprivation.[1] Alcohol consumption occurs throughout all groups of society but problem alcohol use may also be exacerbated by deprivation. Problem drug and alcohol use both cause significant morbidity and mortality aggravated by coexisting social problems and both can lead to additional social problems. Associated problems may include smoking, a poor diet, homelessness and a chaotic lifestyle that can prevent adequate access to services and consequently compromise childcare.

A multi-agency approach

Since the mid 1980s, informal guidelines have existed for the management of drug-using families. The current guidelines were drawn up in collaboration with all relevant professional bodies, both healthcare and non-healthcare and, like earlier versions, address the issue of problem drug and/or alcohol use during pregnancy. The most recent suggested guidelines for England and Wales were published in 1997,[2] while those applicable to Scotland were published in 2003.[1] All the guidelines recognise the impact of drug and alcohol use and their associated social problems on the health and social outcomes of pregnancy and emphasise the importance of integrated multi-agency management.

Women with significant problem drug and/or alcohol use may have other social problems and their care should reflect this. Pregnant women with substance misuse problems should not be managed in isolation but by maternity services that are part of a wider multi-agency network, which should include both addiction and social services. The multidisciplinary service should be led by a healthcare professional with a special interest in the area.

If, during pregnancy or at booking, it emerges that a woman may have a problem with drugs or alcohol, she should be encouraged to attend addiction services, or specialist maternity services where available, and her healthcare professional should offer to make the referral. Antenatal services should arrange a multidisciplinary assessment of the extent of the woman's substance use – including type of drugs, level, frequency, pattern, method of administration – and consider any potential risks to her unborn child from current or previous drug use. If the woman does not already have a social worker, her obstetrician, midwife or general practitioner should ask for her consent to liaise with the local service to enable an appropriate assessment of her social circumstances.

The related medical and social problems associated with substance abuse also increase the likelihood that these women will have a high-risk pregnancy. They should have an assessment by an obstetrician and a joint care plan agreed and the obstetrician should continue to supervise those pregnancies considered to be at medium or high risk. For the majority of women, care can be mainly midwifery-led if they so choose, and they should have access to the same range and quality of services as all other women throughout their pregnancy and childbirth.

Whatever the local arrangements for delivery of maternity care, a multidisciplinary approach is essential, with local protocols drawn up to ensure effective collaboration between agencies and services. Such protocols should prescribe the arrangements for assessment and care.

Summary of findings for 2000–02

During this triennium, 31 women whose deaths were reported to the Enquiry were known to have problem drug and/or alcohol use, although, for some, this may not have directly led to their deaths. This is three times as many as the 11 women identified in the last Report. Part of the rise for this triennium may be due to increased case ascertainment. Additionally, ten cases were discovered through the ONS record linkage study for England and Wales, described in Chapter 1, although many of these deaths took place some months after delivery. The cases are counted in the chapter that best reflects the underlying causes of death. Many of these are counted in Chapter 11 Deaths from psychiatric disorders, or in Chapter 15 *Late* deaths, but others who died from other *Direct* or other *Indirect* causes are counted elsewhere in this Report.

Of the 31 women in this triennium who were know to have problem substance misuse, insufficient information was available to enable a full assessment to be made in nine cases. The discussion in this chapter is therefore restricted to the 22 cases, for which full details were available. Twelve of these deaths were associated with drug use, six with alcohol use and four with combined drug and alcohol use.

The women who died

All but four of the 22 women who died were aged 25 years or older and half were in stable relationships. All but two had existing children, although in two cases no information on parity was provided. Only one pregnancy appeared to have been actively planned and two women had opted for a termination of pregnancy. All but four of the women had features of marked social exclusion.

The timing of death

Of the 22 cases, six women died during pregnancy, six died early in the postpartum period and ten were *Late* deaths, occurring more than 42 days after delivery. While many of the deaths that occurred after pregnancy, especially the *Late* deaths, were considered *Coincidental*, it appeared very likely that the birth of the baby added to the pressures experienced by the women and may have contributed indirectly to their deaths. However, in many of these cases, no or minimal information was provided, suggesting that the services did not recognise the possibility of any link. In almost all cases, including those women who received a lot of specialist support during pregnancy, it was apparent that little support was provided in the postnatal period. In some cases this demonstrated a lack of awareness of the difficulties experienced by the women but in others it may have reflected the lack of resources and consequently the lack of sufficient community support available for such disadvantaged women.

The causes of death

Eleven women died from drug overdose and five hanged themselves. Six women died from medical conditions and, in four of these cases, there were additional complications due to their drug or alcohol use. While death by hanging was clearly intentional it is less clear whether overdoses were suicide. However, in some cases where death by overdose was deemed to be accidental, circumstances suggest that the death may have been intentional or at least there was a lack of concern about living:

> A woman with multiple deprivation factors had already had at least one previous child adopted. A child protection case conference was held during her next pregnancy and the decision was taken to remove the child to statutory care at delivery. Shortly after this, she died from an overdose.

> Another woman with a combined drug and alcohol problem had a stillbirth at term. She was provided with some short-term postnatal support in the community but this ended abruptly. Shortly afterwards, on a particularly significant day for her, she looked after the children of a close relative. She was found dead a few days after the children had left her care. Death was due to drug overdose.

Identification of substance misuse

Fifteen of the 22 women were known by maternity services to have a drug and/or alcohol problem. The problem was sometimes identified because the woman had specifically reported it and asked for advice and help and sometimes because the information was provided to the maternity services.

In the seven cases where it was not known that the women had a problem, it was recorded in the notes that the women had 'no special needs' but it is not clear whether they were proactively asked about substance misuse. The absence or paucity of information provided in a number of the reports suggests that there may be a lack of recognition of the need for, and importance of, such a routine enquiry. However, it is also possible that the women chose not to disclose this information.

In two cases, despite a long history of substance misuse known to the general practitioner, the information was not provided to maternity services until long after the booking visit. For a further woman, information was only provided when the midwife contacted the general practitioner because of an abnormal blood result. Another woman changed to a different general practitioner, who noticed her intoxication and notified the midwife and for one, not registered with a general practitioner, her pregnancy and substance misuse were only picked up when she attended the accident and emergency department with a drug-related problem. In four cases it is not clear whether maternity services were aware of the problem (but in two of these the general practitioner definitely was aware) while in a further two cases both the general practitioners and maternity services were unaware of the problem. Four women changed general practitioners during pregnancy.

Coexisting mental health problems

Mental illness can be a cause or effect of substance misuse and a number of these women had mental health problems. Many had depression before, during and/or after pregnancy and at the time of their deaths seven women were receiving antidepressant therapy. Two of these women were also drinking heavily, two were also using illicit drugs and three women were also receiving prescribed substitute medication for their drug problem. Two were prescribed methadone and one was prescribed dihydrocodeine.

All of the seven women on antidepressant therapy died from a drug overdose, a recognised risk in such cases, and dual therapy with medication for drug use and mental illness is recognised as a particular risk factor associated with drug deaths in general. Where women were on prescribed substitute medication, it was not clear whether this was dispensed daily under supervision according to recognised good practice.

Experience of violence or abuse is a risk factor for mental illness and for substance misuse and for seven of the women there was reference to experience of violence at some time in their lives. Among these women there was minimal overlap with those receiving antidepressant therapy.

A number of women who were clearly mentally unwell or had psychological problems were not referred for psychiatric assessment or support. For such women, there may be a lack of appropriate services to meet their needs and this was evident in the group of women who died during this triennium. Some were referred for psychiatric assessment and then deemed not to need psychiatric care but there were others whose psychiatric problems appear to have been disregarded by the maternity services. Most of these women received very little support from services particularly after delivery and most did not have effective support systems within family and friends networks. Consequently, many of these women who died were very isolated.

Other stressful factors

Bereavement or loss was a common factor and was documented in ten cases. One woman had had at least six miscarriages, her current pregnancy also ending in miscarriage, while two women had experienced the death of one of their children. In one case the pregnancy had ended in a stillbirth while another woman whose earlier child had died was informed just prior to her death that the child she was carrying would be taken into care at delivery. A further five women had had all or some of their previous children removed from their care and in two cases these children had been adopted. One woman's partner had been killed and the close relative of another woman was terminally ill during her pregnancy and died shortly before she did.

The services they received

The majority of women appeared to have been managed within mainstream services. In many reports to this Enquiry the women's addiction problems seemed to be viewed only in terms of the impact on their obstetric care, with little acknowledgement of the other medical, psychological or social effects of the addiction on the women, their babies and their social or other circumstances. A few of the women attending mainstream services appeared to have been referred to addiction services and, in such cases, it was sometimes recorded that they attended or defaulted but in others there was no further comment.

There also seemed to be little recognition that pregnancies complicated by problem drug and /or alcohol use are potentially at high risk and consequently that management provided in the main by midwives (as it should be) ought to be supervised by an obstetrician. The management, in many cases, was not according to established guidelines and this may indicate that the care providers were not familiar with the guidelines.

For three women it was recorded that a specialist midwife contributed to their care, with inputs that ranged from providing regular support to a one-off consultation. These women also attended addiction and social services but did so in parallel, with no inter-agency liaison. As with a further three women who received good multidisciplinary care services during pregnancy, there was little ongoing postnatal support.

While the women who were managed within integrated services all received good antenatal care, some women attending mainstream services were also clearly looked after by committed and caring staff. However, the absence of integrated services may have compromised care, with women falling through the gaps between services. Moreover, the lack of multi-agency collaboration clearly left many staff feeling isolated, with obvious distress when these women died.

Child protection issues

While in some cases the clinical and social information provided for the cases of the women who died was often inadequate, there was even less information about referral to social services because of concerns about the baby, even when there had been previous child protection issues. According to all published guidelines, a multidisciplinary planning meeting should be held at 32 weeks of gestation. If there are child protection concerns these should be separately addressed and a child protection case conference held if appropriate.

On the whole, the women who died had significant addiction problems and many had associated chaotic lifestyles, so child protection issues could have been anticipated in many cases. For seven women, death occurred before 32 weeks of gestation, although, in one of these cases, because of her history, a child protection case conference was held the day prior to her death. In only one other case was it recorded that a case conference was held and in the remainder there was no reference at all to formal or informal social services procedures. While the lack of information about referral and procedural management does not necessarily mean that such issues were not addressed, it may imply that those providing information did not recognise their relevance or importance.

The management of substance misuse during the pregnancies

Only four women were documented to be in contact with addiction services at the time of antenatal booking. Most drug-using women were polydrug users. Only half of the ten women using opioids were recorded to be receiving prescribed methadone during pregnancy and dispensing arrangements were not noted. One woman who was on a reducing dose of prescribed dihydrocodeine also continued to use several other drugs. Another was on a reducing dose of prescribed methadone with continued reduction postnatally. She had regular urine screens carried out, which all showed the presence of benzodiazepines and other opioids but, despite this, reduction of her methadone dose continued. Urine screening has a limited role in the management of drug use in pregnancy and the postpartum period. However, in the presence of evidence that the woman was not coping with withdrawal, her continued reduction in dosage was inappropriate. While many women can manage to achieve major reductions in their dose of methadone during pregnancy, in the interests of the baby, they often find it difficult to maintain stability at these lower levels after delivery, especially with the dual stresses of caring for a baby and fear of loss of custody of the child. It is therefore common for women to require an increase in methadone dosage postnatally.[3]

The management of substance misuse in pregnancy should be undertaken by a specialist in addiction medicine and according to best practice guidelines.[1,2] Methadone has, for many years, been prescribed as an opioid substitute, including during pregnancy, and its medical and social benefits, when prescribed as a constituent of addiction treatment, have been demonstrated.[4] Consequently, methadone has been and remains the opioid substitute of choice during pregnancy. Buprenorphine has recently been introduced as a prescribed opioid substitute and there are therefore insufficient data to compare use of buprenorphine and methadone in pregnancy.

Reproductive choices and the planning of pregnancies

Only one of the pregnancies discussed in this chapter appears to have been definitely planned and there was no indication that any of the women had received prepregnancy counselling about the effects of drugs and alcohol on their reproductive health or about reproductive choices. Even where women were already in contact with specialist addiction services there was no evidence that contraception had been discussed. After delivery, most women were discharged without adequate contraception.

Experience has shown that drug and alcohol using women are keen to receive appropriate nondirective reproductive health care information to enable them to regain some control of their lives, to plan and space their pregnancies and to improve their health prior to conception. However directional counselling for drug and/or alcohol using women is unsuccessful and will also alienate or discourage women, including those who are planning to become pregnant, from attending services.

These women often have chaotic lifestyles that compromise access to services so frequently their first contact with reproductive health care is with the maternity services. Contraception should be discussed during pregnancy and after birth and, if requested, should be commenced prior to postnatal discharge. Long-acting reversible methods, particularly progestogen intrauterine devices and implants, are proving popular and appropriate for such women using the integrated Reproductive Health Services in Glasgow.

Ideally, contraception for drug and/or alcohol using women (and indeed all women with severe social problems that lead to an inability to access a number of services) should either be provided by the same service that provides maternity care or by services operating in such close collaboration that they are perceived by the women as a single service. This allows not only the provision of contraception but also the earlier identification of the next pregnancies and, since the women are already under the care of the relevant maternity service or perceive themselves to be so, there is less opportunity for the women to be lost between services.

Drug and/or alcohol use in pregnancy: learning points

- Pregnant women with drug and/or alcohol problems, and their babies, are at higher risk of maternal and perinatal morbidity and mortality.

- There are guidelines for England and Wales[2] and Scotland[1] on the multi-agency management of drug using families. Both sets of guidelines address the management of pregnant women affected by substance misuse.

- Pregnant women with significant problem drug and/or alcohol use may have other social problems and their care should reflect this. They should not be managed in isolation but by maternity services that are part of a wider multi-agency network, which should include both addiction and social services.

- In order to provide the best possible care, a full social history should be taken from all women at booking that includes the use of prescribed or illicit drugs, alcohol and tobacco.

- Women using opioids should be prescribed appropriate substitution therapy during pregnancy.

- Polydrug using women should not undergo detoxification from opioid substitution while they are unstable and continue to use other drugs.

- Substance misuse is often associated with past and/or current experience of violence and/or abuse and with psychiatric problems or psychological problems which, while not constituting mental illness, cause major morbidity and contribute to death.

- Management of women with substance misuse and mental illness co-morbidity requires especially close supervision during pregnancy.

Acknowledgements

Extracts from *Getting our Priorities Right,* produced by the Scottish Executive, are published with their kind permission.

References

1. Scottish Executive. *Getting our Priorities Right: Policy and Practice Guidelines for Working with Children and Families Affected by Problem Drug Use.* Edinburgh: Scottish Executive; 2003.
2. Hogg C, Chadwick T and Dale-Perera A (LGDF/SCODA). *Drug Using Parents: Policy Guidelines for Inter-agency Working (England and Wales).* London: LGA Publications; 1997.
3. Hepburn M. Drugs of addiction. In: Cockburn F, editor. *Advances in Perinatal Medicine.* Carnforth: Parthenon Publishing; 1997. p. 120–4.
4. Perlmutter J. Heroin addiction and pregnancy. *Obstet Gynecol Surv* 1974; 29: 439–46.

CHAPTER 12

Other Indirect deaths

MICHAEL de SWIET on behalf of the Editorial Board

Indirect deaths: key recommendations

See also the general recommendations in Chapter 13 Deaths from cancer.

Service provision

All pregnant women with medical conditions requiring treatment and care by other specialists should have an integrated care plan developed and agreed between all specialties involved. For some more common medical conditions, such as diabetes and epilepsy, joint clinics should be provided.

Regular communication between specialties is crucial and this should be monitored and ensured by the woman's lead maternity care provider, who will usually be her midwife.

Isolated maternity units without intensive care, advanced imaging and cardiology on site cannot look after sick women properly. There may even be a problem if hospitals are all on one site but an ambulance needs to be called for patients to be transported from one department to another. These facts must be taken into consideration, in terms of general healthcare planning and where to refer individual women with potential problems in pregnancy.

Pregnant women with complications must be seen early in pregnancy by consultant obstetricians. If the complications are outside the experience of the local obstetrician they should be referred to tertiary centres for a further opinion. This would not necessarily entail delivery at the tertiary centre.

Women admitted with medical or surgical complications outside the experience of their obstetrician should be managed jointly with consultant physicians or surgeons. This may necessitate moving them to a medical or surgical ward however great the pressure on these beds.

Sick pregnant women should be anaesthetised by consultant anaesthetists.

Individual practitioners

Pregnant women who are seriously ill from conditions not immediately related to pregnancy require exceptional care and routine referral patterns are not good enough for them.

Clear, relevant and complete information must be passed from the general practitioner to the antenatal care team, at booking, accurately detailing any past medical history including previous malignancies, abnormal cervical smears, operations and any relevant family history.

When a woman says that she is or has been treated by an oncologist or any other consultant, such as a respiratory or cardiac physician, for an ongoing condition, these consultants should be contacted and up-to-date records made available. It should not be left to the woman to give her complete medical history or act as a go-between.

Pregnant women undergoing intercurrent treatment or investigation for medical or surgical conditions should be reviewed by a consultant obstetrician even though they may appear to be obstetrically well.

Women with persistent chest symptoms must be referred for specialist review. Chest X-rays should not be withheld because a woman is pregnant.

Introduction

Indirect maternal deaths are defined as deaths resulting from previously existing disease or disease which develops during pregnancy and which were not due to direct obstetric causes, but which were aggravated by physiological effects of pregnancy. Section One of this Report describes the definitions and categories of maternal deaths in more detail.

Examples of *Indirect* deaths include deaths from epilepsy, diabetes, cerebral haemorrhage and HIV infection. Cardiac causes of death are also classified as *Indirect* but, such is their importance, they have their own chapter in this Report. The international definitions of maternal death exclude deaths from suicide due to perinatal mental illness and those from hormone-dependant malignancies, both of which the UK Assessors consider to be linked to the woman's pregnancy. These causes of death also have their own separate chapters in this Report. The remaining deaths due to *Indirect* causes are counted and discussed in this chapter and are classified as *Other Indirect*. However, all these other causes of death also contribute to the overall *Indirect* mortality rate calculated for this Report.

Fifty years ago...

Death rates from associated causes, which include those now classified as either *Indirect* or *Coincidental* fell during the 1950s and 1960s. Because of better ascertainment, *Indirect* deaths rates are now higher than *Direct* death rates, as Figure 12.1 and Table 12.1 show. A more detailed description of time trends for *Indirect* deaths can be found in Chapter 22.

Table 12.1 shows the more recent changes in the number and rate of *Direct* and *Indirect* deaths for the United Kingdom since 1985. The *Direct* mortality rate has remained virtually static and it is the increase in *Indirect* mortality that has caused the overall increase in maternal mortality since 1993. The *Indirect* mortality rate for deaths reported to this Enquiry has been higher than the maternal death rates for deaths from *Direct* causes for the past two triennia. However, some of this increase may be attributable to increased reporting of these cases.

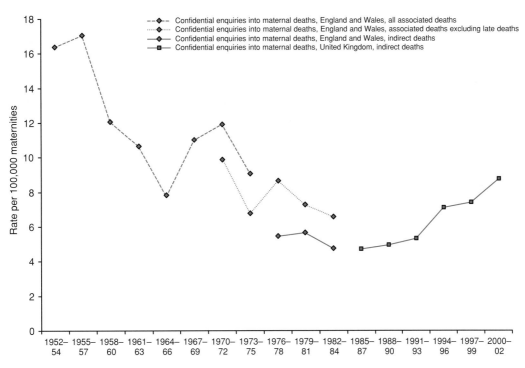

Figure 12.1 Maternal mortality rates for associated and *Indirect* deaths, per million maternities; England and Wales 1952–84, United Kingdom 1985–02

Part of the recent increase in *Indirect* mortality relates to an increase in cardiac mortality, as described in Chapter 10. This in turn is partly related to changes in the way that deaths have been classified as due to cardiac causes. *Indirect* deaths from suicide and cancer are now counted and discussed in Chapter 11 and Chapter 13, respectively. Some of these deaths and, in particular, deaths from suicide, are likely to have been under-reported in the early years. Since 1987, deaths from cancer, heart disease and suicide have all been rising but so too have deaths from all *Other Indirect* causes. As already indicated, the change in the definition of cardiac deaths as described in Chapter 10 would account for some of the rise in this category but such factors would not account for the rises in other causes of *Indirect* deaths, which are most likely due to better case ascertainment, particularly since the Office for National Statistics (ONS) has been able to identify more deaths from underlying causes coding, as discussed in Chapter 1. Nevertheless, the importance of all *Indirect* deaths as the major cause of maternal mortality which are often associated with substandard care should not be underestimated.

Table 12.1 *Direct* and *Indirect* deaths notified to the Enquiry and maternal mortality rates per 100 000 maternities; United Kingdom 1985–02

Type of death	Triennium											
	1985–87		1988–90		1991–93		1994–96		1997–99		2000–02	
	(n)	*Rate*	*(n)*	*Rate*	*(n)*	*Rate*	*(n)*	*Rate*	*(n)*	*Rate*	*(n)*	*Rate*
Direct	139	*6.1*	145	*6.1*	128	*5.5*	134	*6.1*	106	*5.0*	106	*5.3*
Indirect (all)	84	*3.7*	93	*3.9*	100	*4.3*	134	*6.1*	136	*6.4*	155	*7.8*
Direct and *Indirect* total	223	*9.8*	238	*10.1**	228	*9.8**	268	*12.2*	242	*11.4*	261	*13.1*
Total maternities	2,268,766		2,360,309		2,315,204		2,197,640		2,123,614		1,997,472	

* Figures do not add up because of rounding

Summary of cases for 2000–02

Table 12.1 shows that in 2000–02 there was a total of 90 *Other Indirect* deaths compared with 75 deaths in 1997–99(Table 12.2). In some cases very few details were available to the assessors. Note that *Indirect* deaths from heart disease are counted in Chapter 10, those due to cancer are counted in Chapter 13 and those due to psychiatric causes are counted in Chapter 11. In addition, there were 18 deaths mentioned in this chapter but counted elsewhere.

Diseases of the central nervous system

Intracranial haemorrhage

There were 21 cases of intracranial haemorrhage, 17 due to subarachnoid haemorrhage and four to intracerebral haemorrhage.

Subarachnoid haemorrhage
The ages of the women with subarachnoid haemorrhage varied between 19 years and 39 years and were evenly distributed, with a mean of 32 years. In three cases the timing of bleeding in relation to stage of pregnancy was unknown. Four of the bleeds occurred antenatally, two in the first trimester and two in the third. No case occurred in labour; ten occurred after delivery at between 5 days and 4 weeks. Therefore, labour is unlikely to be a risk factor for subarachnoid haemorrhage. Seven of the bleeds were from aneurysm. In the other cases the source of bleeding is unknown. There were no cases of substandard care.

Table 12.2   Causes of *Other Indirect* deaths; United Kingdom 1997–02

Cause	1997–99	2000–02
Diseases of the central nervous system	34	40
Subarachnoid haemorrhage	11	17
Intracerebral haemorrhage	5	3
Cerebral thrombosis	5	4
Epilepsy	9	13
Other (see text for further details)	4	3
Infectious diseases	13	14
HIV	1	4
Other (see text for further details)	12	10
Diseases of the respiratory system	9	10
Asthma	5	5
Other (see text for further details)	4	5
Endocrine, metabolic and immunity disorders	6	7
Diabetes mellitus	4	3
Other (see text for further details)	2	4
Diseases of the gastrointestinal system	7	7
Intestinal obstruction	3	2
Pancreatitis	2	1
Other (see text for further details)	2	4
Diseases of the blood	4	2
Diseases of the circulatory system	2	3
Diseases of the renal system	0	3
Cause unknown	0	4
Total	75	90

It would not be surprising if pregnancy increased the risk of berry aneurysms bleeding, granted the general tendency noted below of blood vessels to aneurismal dissection and bleeding at this time. However, the data to confirm this risk are not available and the effect cannot be marked, given the tendency for bleeding to occur sometime after delivery rather than during pregnancy itself.

Intracerebral haemorrhage

There were four deaths from intracerebral haemorrhage. There were no cases of substandard care.

Cerebral thromboembolism

There were four deaths from cerebral thromboembolism. Two occurred after delivery: one in a woman with borderline hypertension and the other in a known diabetic who had severe vascular disease. The following vignette provides an example the lessons that should be learned from such cases:

> A woman developed headaches in early pregnancy, became unconscious and died the next day. She had had several previous deep vein thromboses and an operation for gangrenous bowel. Following an autopsy, death was certified due to cerebral infarction because of internal carotid artery thrombosis.

The consultant obstetrician reported she was seen just after booking and "all was well". In view of her history, the assessors considered that she must have had some form of thrombophilia and consideration should have been given to thromboprophylaxis; indeed, this should have been discussed with her before she ever became pregnant.

Epilepsy

There were 13 deaths from epilepsy. Four cases met the criteria for sudden unexplained death in epilepsy (SUDEP) and a further five were possibly due to SUDEP. It is not known whether pregnancy increases the risk of SUDEP.

Deaths from SUDEP are always very distressing to all concerned. This distress is encapsulated by the comments of one woman's midwife.

Aspiration of stomach contents during a seizure is another cause of death in women with epilepsy and was a factor in at least three of these deaths. A compounding factor is obesity, which made intubation difficult when one of these women with a BMI of 35 was admitted to hospital following a seizure during which she aspirated.

There is a conflict in the care of epilepsy in pregnancy. A reduction or cessation of therapy is probably better for the fetus. However, this does increase the risk of seizures and poorly controlled epilepsy increases the risk of SUDEP. Two women died having reduced or ceased anticonvulsant medication because of concern about its effect on the fetus. An example is given below:

> A woman who died from epilepsy had attended the antenatal clinic a few weeks before, complaining of seizures five times per day. No action was taken by the obstetric staff. This represents substandard care. Ideally, all women with epilepsy should be looked after by specialist combined obstetric and medical or neurological teams in pregnancy.

It may be very difficult, however, to treat women effectively, even in a specialist clinic. For example, a young woman with difficult social circumstances and a history of alcohol abuse attended the antenatal clinic infrequently and missed many appointments. She was a known epileptic taking carbamazepine. In the third trimester she was found dead at home. It is likely that this was following a fit because there were teeth marks in her tongue. Care has to be classified as substandard because she attended so little and was not followed up in the community. However, it was clearly very difficult to persuade her to come more frequently and attendance even at a specialist obstetric medicine/epilepsy clinic might have made no difference to the outcome.

Miscellaneous central nervous system disease

One death may have been due to epilepsy but it is counted in the miscellaneous section as it was caused by skull fracture following a fall, despite excellent treatment at a national centre of excellence. She had been diagnosed with epilepsy during childhood and had only one seizure as an adult. She received prepregnancy counselling from a consultant neurologist before her first pregnancy and he advised discontinuing sodium valproate because of the fetal risks. An earlier pregnancy was uneventful apart from a single generalised seizure in the puerperium. She restarted sodium valproate and had no further seizures. Her consultant again advised stopping valproate and she had had no seizures since discontinuing therapy for some years before her last pregnancy.

This case precisely illustrates the difficulty of counselling women with mild epilepsy regarding medication in pregnancy. It is unclear whether her fall was caused by a fit. Most fits are not fatal. There is no doubt that sodium valproate carries risks for the fetus. However, the puerperium does seem to be a time when women are at risk, as this woman had already demonstrated. In retrospect it is easy to suggest that she should have taken a course of valproate after delivery but a carefully considered opinion to the contrary does not represent substandard care.

Infectious diseases

There were 14 deaths due to infection not arising from the genital tract. Genital tract infection is considered as a *Direct* death in Chapter 7. Three cases involved substandard care.

Bacterial infection
There were six deaths from bacterial infection, including three deaths from meningitis. One of the deaths from meningitis was due to the meningococcus and another to the pneumococcus. The pneumococcus also caused one fatality from pneumonia and there was one case of staphylococcal pneumonia possibly secondary to viral pneumonia. A sudden death at the end of pregnancy was initially unascertained but it is counted in this section because postmortem blood cultures grew *Clostridia sordelli*, making it likely that septicaemia was the cause. One death was in early pregnancy from bilateral mastitis. This is very rare. Since the woman died from staphylococcal septicaemia it is likely that a staphylococcus was the causative organism.

The key features of these deaths were as follows:

- As with deaths from genital tract sepsis, these cases were characterised by the speed with which the women died, despite appropriate treatment. All four women who were admitted to hospital died within 2 days of admission, the majority within a few hours.

- Pregnancy may make women more susceptible to bacterial infection.

- In the case of meningococcal meningitis, the woman developed a rash; 2 days later she collapsed and was admitted and died soon after. Women with a rash that might be meningococcal should be treated with penicillin even before admission.

- Care was judged to be substandard in a woman who died of pneumonia. She attended her local accident and emergency department more than once with breathlessness and fever. She was eventually treated as if she had pulmonary embolism, for no good reason. The seriousness of her condition was not recognised until she was admitted to the maternity department, delivered of a dead baby and found to be in severe cardio-respiratory failure.

- In a case of mastitis, the junior doctors caring for the woman again did not appreciate the gravity of her condition. She was transferred to a hospital with gynaecology but no maternity unit without the knowledge of or consultation with senior staff. Advice from a consultant obstetrician was not sought until she was moribund in intensive care.

Fungal Infection

There was one death from aspergillosis. Aspergillosis usually occurs in immunocompromised patients. There was no evidence of this but the woman was emaciated at the time of her final admission. In retrospect, it was realised that she had been vomiting throughout pregnancy and this death may have been linked to her hyperemesis.

Viral infection

There were four deaths in this Report from HIV or AIDS and one in the last triennium; this is in marked contrast to the situation in some countries where AIDS is the leading *Indirect* cause of death in pregnancy. The following case illustrates the problems that women living with HIV/AIDS and their carers may face:

> An immigrant HIV-positive woman whose parents had already died of AIDS became pregnant following rape in her own country. She was admitted to hospital because of abdominal pain and found to have tuberculosis and cryptococcal meningitis. A few days after admission she refused all treatment or food and wanted to die. Such was her physical condition that she was referred to the psychiatric team and she received parental nutrition. She then developed thrombocytopenia and coagulopathy. The pregnancy was terminated in the interests of maternal health but she still died a few days later.

This woman was in a state of hopeless despair. She was totally alienated and her organic brain syndrome would have made matters worse. She was treated with skill and compassion. It is difficult to see what more could have been done for her.

Another recent immigrant who died of tuberculosis refused HIV screening, although the clinical diagnosis seemed clear. Two further women died of rare but recognised complications due to antiretroviral therapy, lactic acidosis and acute liver failure. It is, however, possible that the latter woman had acute fatty liver of pregnancy but this could not be verified at autopsy.

Other probable deaths from infection

To add to the number of cases in this triennium where prompt and appropriate treatment was not available in accident and emergency departments, a woman who had a splenectomy in the past and who also had had previous meningococcal meningitis and pneumococcal septicaemia attended casualty with "gastrointestinal symptoms". She waited for over 7 hours before she was eventually seen by a registrar who realised she was seriously ill. She subsequently miscarried and died later that day in the intensive care unit, probably from overwhelming sepsis.

As has already been commented on in other cases described elsewhere in this Report, the management of acutely ill pregnant women presenting to accident and emergency departments requires urgent review. She should not have been waiting so long only to be seen by junior staff when she was so seriously ill.

Diseases of the respiratory system

Asthma

There were five deaths from asthma. Asthma is still a life-threatening condition whether women are pregnant or not. One woman was not known to be pregnant by any healthcare attendants, including her general practitioner, before she was admitted to hospital in extremis in mid pregnancy. This case points to the need for ensuring that all women understand the need to book early in pregnancy and that booking is made as easy as possible.

Pneumonia, acute respiratory distress syndrome and fibrosing alveolitis

There were three deaths from pneumonia and one from adult respiratory distress syndrome. Care was substandard in one case of pneumonia because of a lack of intensive care beds. There was one death from fibrosing alveolitis.

Endocrine, metabolic and immunity disorders

This diverse group of conditions has been counted together for the sake of continuity with previous Reports. Some are discussed further here.

Diabetes

There were three deaths from diabetes and an additional death of a woman with diabetes from cerebral thrombosis has always been counted in this chapter, in the section on diseases of the central nervous system. The key learning points are summarised in the following table.

Deaths from diabetes; learning points

- All the maternal diabetic deaths were from hypoglycaemia or presumed hypoglycaemia. Hypoglycaemia has been the principal cause of death in diabetics in previous triennial Reports.

- There is no doubt about the benefit of good control in diabetic pregnancy. However, attempts to achieve this at the expense of recurrent maternal hypoglycaemia are misguided.

- In one case, care was judged substandard because the woman was not given glucagon by the paramedical team that was called to her home. This was because they were not informed about her diabetes.

Phaeochromocytoma

There were two deaths from phaeochromocytoma. This is a very rare tumour but it regularly results in a maternal death for one or two women in most triennia of this Report. The following vignette provides a typical example of such cases:

> A multigravid woman developed hypertension and was admitted near term with headache, blood pressure 210/100 mm/Hg, 4+ proteinuria and 3+glycosuria. She was thought to have pre-eclampsia and labour was induced. Fetal bradycardia led to a 'crash' caesarean section. She was noted to have pulmonary oedema before anaesthesia and collapsed during surgery. She had several cardiac arrests in the intensive care unit and died a few hours later.

The feature that suggested that this was not a simple case of pre-eclampsia was the occurrence of such severe hypertension for the first time in a multigravida. Glycosuria was also a clue.

> In another case, phaeochromocytoma had been discovered almost by chance when a computed tomography scan performed for a different reason showed a huge adrenal tumour. The major problem was hypotension. The autopsy showed marked contraction band necrosis in the heart.

Myocardial damage is a well-recognised complication of phaeochromocytoma. This is likely to have been a major cause of her hypotension although hypovolaemia (another complication of phaeochromocytoma) and which would have been exacerbated by her postpartum state was probably contributory.

Learning points: phaeochromocytoma

Although rare, phaeochromocytoma may present in pregnancy and is a regular cause of death in these Reports.

- Phaeochromocytoma should be excluded in multigravid women with severe hypertension with no previous history of pre-eclampsia.

- Glycosuria is a possible pointer towards phaeochromocytoma.

- Phaeochromocytoma can mimic all the features of pre-eclampsia.

- Myocardial damage is a well-recognised complication of phaeochromocytoma.

Disease of the gastrointestinal system

Intestinal obstruction, peritonitis, pancreatitis and ruptured oesophagus

There were three deaths from intestinal obstruction and/or perforation of the bowel. There was one death each from peritonitis, pancreatitis, a pancreatic cyst and ruptured oesophagus. The following problems were identified in one or more of these cases:

- One woman was discharged early following caesarean section, despite a rising pulse and falling blood pressure and without medical review.

- One woman had been admitted in pregnancy with abdominal pain, given intravenous fluids and discharged with no diagnosis.

- In one woman, symptoms were incorrectly ascribed to her known mental illness and abnormal biochemical test results were ignored.

- A woman with known bowel disease never saw a consultant obstetrician until she was admitted and then only after a few days. She had a potentially serious surgical complication, intestinal obstruction, yet was managed on an antenatal ward where the staff lacked experience in managing this surgical problem. She was given multiple doses of pethidine over several days without any diagnosis having been made as to the cause of the obstruction. She was also given betamethasone in case early delivery should be necessary. These drugs probably masked the signs of peritonitis, which are often obscure in pregnancy in any case.

- There was a delay for another woman before she had surgery. While some of the delay could be ascribed to communication difficulties, it was mainly due to the fact she was on an isolated site and required an ambulance to take her for X-ray (and come back) and another ambulance then had to be booked for her to go for surgery. This is an example of the problems faced by isolated maternity hospitals or hospitals that are not designed to allow the easy transport of patients from one department to another.

- Extreme obesity (over 200 kg) in another woman was a factor causing delay in diagnosis and caused problems with venous access in another whose BMI was around 85.

- In one case the consultant anaesthetist did not attend, despite being informed of the anaesthetic difficulties that were expected.

- One woman had major pulmonary problems as a result of her illness. No tertiary thoracic centre was able to take her, even though her doctors spent many hours on the telephone trying to find a bed.

Diseases of the blood

There were two deaths from thrombotic thrombocytopenic purpura (TTP). A further death from haemolytic uraemic syndrome is described later in the section on renal disease. The following vignette provides several learning points:

Poor communication:
The GP gave no details of the woman's part obstetric history of several previous pregnancies complicated by fetal losses. This may be because he/she did not know them, as there were difficulties with translation. Communication was only possible by translating from one dialect to another via several family members. Nevertheless, it is difficult to believe that in previous pregnancies no warnings were given to her of the risk of subsequent confinements.

Failure to appreciate severity:
She booked late in the second trimester, which was a problem in itself. However, she should have been seen by senior consultant staff when she

booked rather than a GP specialist, in view of her appalling obstetric history. Indeed, given the rarity and severity of her condition she should have been referred to a specialist centre once its nature had been diagnosed.

Failure to identify and follow up abnormal test results:
A low platelet count in the third trimester was not noticed.

Her TTP was diagnosed late because the blood film was not examined and she was treated with immunoglobulin and platelet transfusion for presumed immune thrombocytopenia (ITP). In patients with TTP, treatment for ITP with immunoglobulin and platelet transfusion is known to make the condition worse, as happened in this case.

Disease of the circulatory system

There were three sudden and unpreventable deaths from a ruptured iliac artery, a ruptured pelvic vein and a possible ruptured spleen. The last case may have been due to a ruptured splenic artery aneurysm, which is relatively more common in pregnancy than in the nonpregnant state. Other deaths from heart disease and those relating to dissection of the aorta and its branches in the thorax are counted in Chapter 10 Cardiac disease. All these cases demonstrate the frailty of blood vessels in pregnancy. The following case illustrates the potential danger of pregnancy for all disorders of collagen, whether or not they have specific diagnoses:

> A woman who died from ruptured iliac artery aneurysm had seen a rheumatologist who had diagnosed "benign joint hypermobility" due to a "benign" collagen disorder, a few years previously. This raises the possibility of Ehlers Danlos or Marfan's syndromes, although she was thought to have none of the phenotypic features of these conditions at autopsy or presumably during life. Both Ehlers Danlos and Marfan's syndromes are known to have a significant mortality in pregnancy.

Diseases of the renal system

There was one death from pyelonephritis, one from chronic renal failure and one from haemolytic uraemic syndrome. Lessons can be learned from all of these cases:

- Socially excluded or vulnerable women, including those known to social services, who regularly fail to attend antenatal appointments require outreach services and follow-up in the community. These women are at more risk of developing *Direct* or *Indirect* complications related to pregnancy.

- One woman died from complications of her renal disease on an obstetric ward and never saw a senior obstetrician, despite having been admitted for several days. Senior obstetric staff should personally review all sick patients.

- As already mentioned, women are dying of acute medical conditions without some midwifery or obstetric staff realising the serious nature of their problems. One of these women suffered a fatal cardiac arrest during anaesthesia because of multiple electrolyte disturbances secondary to undiagnosed chronic renal failure. She was known to be at risk of renal disease but no investigation had been made regarding her renal function at any time in pregnancy.

- The assessors are concerned that some current midwifery and obstetric staff do not have sufficient experience to recognise such sick patients as evidenced by the following example:

  > A woman miscarried at the end of the first trimester and about 2 weeks later was admitted with chest and epigastric pain. She was discharged with a significantly low platelet count. She was readmitted with fatal haemolytic uraemic syndrome, one of the features of which is thrombocytopenia. The low platelet count on her penultimate admission was either ignored or not seen. Had it been acted upon, she might have received treatment earlier and might have survived. This is a further example of a woman with problems outside the immediate framework of standard antenatal care.

- As in another cases in this Report, there were problems with resuscitation. One of these women suffered a cardiac arrest from which she could not be promptly resuscitated. This was due in part because the arrest team could not find either the patient or the defibrillator. Cardiac arrest drills must be practised in obstetric departments, particularly because cardiac arrest is an uncommon event.

Cases counted in other chapters

Some further cases from which lessons can be learned but which are counted in other chapters are discussed further to demonstrate key learning points.

Infection
The death of a woman from cerebral vein thrombosis (CVT) is counted in Chapter 2 Thromboembolism but mentioned here because she also probably had miliary tuberculosis, which would have increased her risk of CVT.

Endocrine, metabolic and immunity disorders
One woman who died from systemic lupus erythematosus has been counted in this chapter, but there are others in which immune disorders were predisposing factors. A woman whose undiagnosed autoimmune disease probably disposed her to sepsis died subsequent to chorioamnionitis. Her death is counted in Chapter 7 Sepsis. Two women with scleroderma and pulmonary hypertension are counted or discussed in Chapter 10, although one of these is a *Late* death, counted in Chapter 15, as is the death of a woman who developed cerebral lupus as part of a postpartum flare.

Disease of the blood
Lessons from the deaths of women with sickle cell disease (Hb SS) from myocardial fibrosis and Hb SC disease from pulmonary embolus are described in Chapter 10 and Chapter 2, respectively. The death of a woman from postpartum haemorrhage with factor XI deficiency is counted in Chapter 4 Haemorrhage.

Diseases of the central nervous system
Two *Late* deaths from epilepsy are counted in Chapter 15. Another death in a woman who suffered from epilepsy is counted as a death from substance abuse in Chapter 11.

A further death from cerebral haemorrhage is counted as a *Late* death and in one woman who was found to have Moya Moya disease, pre-eclampsia was thought to be the cause of death. This death is therefore counted as a *Direct* death in Chapter 3.

Renal disease

A woman who developed nephrotic syndrome in pregnancy is counted in Chapter 2 because she died from pulmonary embolism, having had inadequate thromboprophylaxis. Thromboembolism is a recognised complication of nephrotic syndrome.

Diseases of the respiratory system

A young woman developed pruritus in mid-pregnancy but her liver function tests were normal. A month later she was found to have a hydropic baby. Thalassaemia was excluded. She was transferred to a tertiary referral hospital and delivered by caesarean section of an anaemic baby in poor condition who died soon after. She quickly developed respiratory failure, which was unremitting. She died several weeks later so this is counted as a *Late* death, even though her fatal illness clearly started no later than the time of delivery; death was certified due to ARDS. At the relatives' request no autopsy of mother or fetus was performed. However, cytomegalovirus was found in the placenta and this may been responsible for the death of the baby; perhaps the episode of pruritus represented a primary maternal infection. The reason why the mother developed ARDS is unclear. Although women with fetal hydrops and a large placenta may develop pre-eclampsia and women with pre-eclampsia may develop ARDS, there was no other evidence for pre-eclampsia in this case.

Chromosomal abnormalities

One of the *Direct* maternal deaths in this Report occurred in a woman with Turner's syndrome who underwent IVF treatment. Although this was probably not a major contributory factor in her case, the estimated risk of maternal mortality in women with this condition is 2% and four maternal deaths, one in a twin pregnancy and all due to aortic dissection, have been reported.[1] Women with Turner's syndrome need to be fully informed of the risks of pregnancy. They are usually of very short stature and careful consideration should be given to the additional risks of multiple pregnancy before replacing more than one embryo. Before contemplating pregnancy, screening for cardiovascular malformations should be performed. Pregnancy should be managed in a major centre with a multidisciplinary approach and facilities, and it is recommended that the aortic dimensions should be monitored carefully during pregnancy.

Conclusions

Recurring themes in this Report that are also highlighted by the some of the cases in this chapter are summarised below.

Indirect deaths: key learning points

- Isolated maternity units without intensive care, advanced imaging and cardiology on site cannot look after sick women properly. There may even be a problem if hospitals are all on one site but an ambulance needs to be called for patients to be transported from one department to another. These facts must be taken into consideration both in terms of general healthcare planning and where to refer individual women with potential problems in pregnancy.

- Pregnant women with complications must be seen early in pregnancy by consultant obstetricians. If the complications are outside the experience of the local obstetrician, they should be referred to tertiary centres for a further opinion. This would not necessarily entail delivery at the tertiary centre.

- Women admitted with medical or surgical complications outside the experience of their obstetrician should be managed jointly with consultant physicians or surgeons. This may necessitate moving them to a medical or surgical ward, however great the pressure on these beds.

- Sick pregnant women should be anaesthetised by consultant anaesthetists.

- Tertiary units both in obstetrics and in medicine and surgery should be prepared to admit very sick women who have rare complications beyond the experience of their local hospital.

- Poor care has been given to pregnant women in accident and emergency departments. Women should not be discharged from accident and emergency departments without senior obstetric or midwifery review.

- Interpreters must be available for those who do not speak English. Family members should not be relied on. Their representation of both what the healthcare team and the woman are saying is likely to be biased.

- Tuberculosis is becoming increasingly common again particularly in immigrants whether or not they have HIV infection. Women with persistent chest symptoms must be referred for specialist review. Chest X-rays should not be withheld because a woman is pregnant.

- Pregnant women who are obese are at high risk in pregnancy and this risk should be made known to women in general.

- Pregnant women who do not attend antenatal clinic appointments are an at-risk group. Strenuous efforts must be made to contact them.

- It is very easy for abnormal pathology results to be ignored. Given the pressures under which most healthcare systems work, there is no easy solution to this problem except vigilance.

- From the cases assessed in this, and other chapters, it is clear there is too much pressure on intensive care unit beds.

- All women with epilepsy should be looked after by specialist combined obstetric and medical or neurological teams in pregnancy.

- Hyperemesis is a dangerous condition. It can cause severe malnutrition which can kill pregnant women.

- Blood vessels including pelvic blood vessels can rupture spontaneously in pregnancy.

- The assessors are concerned that some healthcare staff are not recognising medical conditions outside their immediate experience.

References

1. Karnis MF, Zimon AE, Lalwani SI, Timmreck LS, Klipstein S, Reindollar RH. Risk of death in pregnancy achieved through oocyte donation in patients with Turner syndrome: a national survey. *Fertil Steril* 2003; 80:498–501.

CHAPTER 13
Deaths from malignancy

GWYNETH LEWIS, JAMES O DRIFE and MICHAEL de SWIET,
on behalf of the Editorial Board

Deaths from cancer: key recommendations

These recommendations are also generally applicable for the management of pregnant women with other severe medical conditions.

Service provision

All maternity trusts should develop a protocol for the provision of multidisciplinary care should the need arise.

Pregnant women who are seriously ill from conditions not immediately related to pregnancy require exceptional care and routine referral patterns are not good enough for them.

The importance of planned multidisciplinary care for women with cancer and other serious problems cannot be over-stressed. Obstetricians, midwives, general practitioners, oncologists, surgeons, Macmillan nurses and palliative care services need to be involved, in conjunction with the woman and her partner, in planning a course of antenatal care that respects the wishes of the woman yet should optimise the outcome for the fetus.

Individual practitioners

Previous Reports have repeatedly stressed, and this Report does so again, that pregnancy is not a contraindication for radiological investigations for women with severe and unremitting pain or vomiting, including back, chest or epigastric pain, particularly if the pain is so severe that it requires management by major or epidural analgesia or prevents the woman from walking.

A clear medical and family history should be taken at booking to lower the threshold for the index of suspicion in women who complain of other symptoms during their pregnancy.

Clear, relevant and complete information must be passed from the general practitioner to the antenatal care team, at booking, accurately detailing any past medical history including previous malignancies, abnormal cervical smears, operations and any relevant family history.

When a woman says that she is or has been treated by an oncologist or any other consultant, such as a respiratory or cardiac physician, for an ongoing condition, these consultants should be contacted and up-to-date records made available. It should not be left to the woman to give her complete medical history or act as a go-between.

Pregnant women undergoing intercurrent treatment or investigation for medical or surgical conditions should be reviewed by a consultant obstetrician even though they may appear to be obstetrically well.

Women planning pregnancies after treatment for cancer, particularly breast or cervical cancer, should be counselled by an obstetrician or a clinician with specialist knowledge of obstetrics.

Pregnant (and all other) women should be encouraged to report breast lumps if they find them by chance.

Delivery needs to be planned with care and, if possible, performed at an optimum time with consultants in attendance. An anaesthetist should be involved at an early stage in the pregnancy. A written and agreed care plan should be in the woman's notes to pass this information on to colleagues who may have to attend for an emergency delivery.

If preterm delivery is planned to allow more radical therapy for the mother, a paediatrician should be involved antenatally, not only optimise the care of the baby but also to discuss with the parents what may happen afterwards in regard to neonatal care.

Cancer in pregnancy

The incidence of cancer in pregnancy is around one in 6000 live births. This is about 50% lower than the incidence in the nonpregnant population of a similar age. There are several possible reasons for this. A woman who already has cancer diagnosed may avoid pregnancy. A pregnant woman with occult cancer may have the diagnosis delayed because routine screening is not carried out or because symptoms are not investigated promptly (being attributed to the pregnancy) or because investigation is less thorough.

It is often thought that pregnancy accelerates the growth of cancer, particularly if the cancer is hormone-dependent, such as arising from the breast or cervix. For many types of cancer, the numbers of cases occurring in pregnancy are too small for reliable epidemiological studies to be carried out, but it appears that for most types, pregnancy does not alter the incidence or prognosis compared with cancer diagnosed at a similar stage in the nonpregnant patient. However, the Royal College of Obstetricians and Gynaecologists' 2000 Study Group on cancer in pregnancy[1] identified certain types of cancer that may be aggravated by pregnancy, as shown in Table 13.1, and deaths from these are classified as *Indirect* or *Late Indirect*. Further discussion of this can be found in the last Report[2] or the report of the RCOG Study Group.[1]

Although 14 of the 28 cases in this chapter are defined as *Indirect* or *Late Indirect*, in that the course of the disease was modified by the pregnancy or pregnancy masked its effects, the classification used by the UK CEMD does not accord with the International Disease Classification of Maternal Deaths (ICD10). The inclusion of these extra cases in

Table 13.1 Classification of causes of deaths from tumours or malignancy and type of death; United Kingdom 2000–02

Cause	Indirect	Late Indirect	Coincidental	Late Coincidental	Total
Central nervous system:					
Astrocytoma			1*		1
Glioma	2	2	1*		5
Cancer of the breast	2	3			5
Cancer of the lung			2	2	4
Cancer of the cervix	1	1			2
Hepatic cancer				2	2
Lymphoma or leukaemia		2			2
Cancer of unknown origin			1	1	2
Neurofibrosarcoma			1		1
Cancer of the oesophagus			1		1
Osteosarcoma				1	1
Pathathyriod adenoma			1		1
Cancer of the vulva		1			1
Total	5	9	8	6	28

* Known prior to pregnancy and therefore unaffected by pregnancy.

the overall maternal mortality figures helps to artificially inflate the UK *Indirect* maternal death rate when compared with *Indirect* and overall maternal mortality rates from other countries. An adjusted calculation for the UK maternal mortality rate, for comparative purposes, is given in Chapter 1.

Introduction

This chapter was introduced in the last Report because, in the past, the lessons from deaths from malignancy were difficult to draw together, as they were scattered throughout the Report and discussed in several different chapters. The chapter to which they were assigned depended upon the timing of the death and whether or not the assessors considered the course, diagnosis or treatment of the disease was modified by the pregnancy itself. As such, key recommendations may have been missed. However a death is categorised, it is the diagnosis and management, or lack of it that forms the most important part of case assessment. This chapter therefore aims to draw together all these deaths, irrespective of classification, to strengthen the impact and recommendations that can be drawn from them. It also provides an overview of both the key remediable factors as well as examples of outstanding care.

The overall number of cases reported to the Enquiry was 28, as shown in Table 13.1, with an age range of 15–41 years. As discussed in Chapter 15 *Late* deaths, a significant number of women who died of cancer some months after delivery were not reported to the Enquiry as they were no longer in touch with midwifery services.

Discussion

In general, a high and in some cases outstanding level of care was provided for women, babies and families once the diagnosis had been made. However, as has been discussed in several previous Reports, in many cases there were significant opportunities to have made the diagnosis earlier. While this may not have affected the eventual outcome, it would have enabled an appropriate degree of symptom relief to be provided to alleviate suffering as well as enabling earlier access to further medical care and the support services required. The messages and lessons to be learnt are summarised here.

Prepregnancy counselling

A few women who had previous episodes of cancer sought prepregnancy counselling. Women planning pregnancies after such a diagnosis, particularly of breast or cervical cancer, should be counselled by an obstetrician with a special interest in oncology or an oncologist with specialist knowledge of obstetrics. The latest guidance from the Royal College of Obstetricians and Gynaecologists recommends that pregnancy should be deferred for at least 2 years after treatment for breast cancer, as this timescale helps to differentiate those women with a better chance of long-term survival from those with more aggressive disease.[3] It further recommends that and that women with stage-IV disease (with a 5-year survival of less than 15%) should be advised not to have further pregnancies and women with stage-III disease should consider deferring pregnancy for 5 years.

Women not known to be pregnant

Two women who died of disseminated carcinomatosis late in pregnancy were unknown to the obstetric services. Both had concealed their pregnancies, perhaps from a misguided fear of being advised to consider a termination of pregnancy. One was an inpatient in the care of an oncology team.

Cases where poor communications between professionals led to a delay in diagnosis and treatment

As has been noted in past Reports, and in other chapters throughout this one, in some cases general practitioners failed to mention key aspects of the woman's past medical history to the obstetric team. In others, the obstetric or midwifery team did not communicate with other specialists providing her care and missed vital opportunities to alter her management plan. The following vignette provides an example:

> A woman with a history of cervical intraepithelial neoplasia grade 3 (CIN3) and lymphadenectomy was given an inadequate referral letter to the booking clinic by her GP which mis-stated the severity of her past disease (said to be CIN1) and omitted the fact she had had a cone biopsy and pelvic lymphadenectomy for presumed squamous cell cervical cancer. She herself was a poor historian but did mention to her antenatal care provider that she was still under the care of the oncology team; however, this was not followed up. The fact she had had cervical cancer was not highlighted anywhere in her notes and the operation for pelvic lymphadenectomy was only discovered when she was being prepared for an emergency caesarean section. She subsequently died.

Breast examination in pregnancy

As in previous Reports, cases of breast cancer continue to be detected late in pregnancy, usually in an advanced state. The practice of professional examination of the breasts as part of the routine antenatal care has been discontinued but women should be encouraged to examine their own breasts regularly.

Cases where a lack of investigation in pregnancy may have delayed the diagnosis

As has also been seen and repeatedly highlighted in previous Reports, there were a worrying number of cases where women were not investigated for severe sustained pain, vomiting, weight loss or other abnormal symptoms during pregnancy. Although earlier diagnosis would not have altered the course of the disease, appropriate pain relief and referral to the oncologists and support services could have been provided earlier.

A number of women made multiple presentations to hospital with chronic chest, abdominal and/or back pain. In several cases this necessitated several admissions for bed rest and analgesia, although no investigations were undertaken despite severe pain being recorded in the notes. Although the course of the disease could not have been altered by earlier diagnosis, more appropriate management would have enabled a better quality of these women's remaining life.

Women, whether they smoke or not, and who present with severe shortness of breath, chest pain and coughs, especially of the severity to necessitate one or more hospital admissions, require chest X-rays as part of the diagnostic investigation to help exclude embolism or lung cancer as a differential diagnosis. This was not undertaken in several cases, one in particular in the presence of a strong familial history of a genetically linked cancer. Even when the respiratory physicians are involved, as in a case of suspected embolism which failed to respond to treatment and which eventually was found to be due to non-Hodgkin's lymphoma, investigations were limited for several months and no contact was made with the obstetric team already caring for the woman.

Some women who required repeated antenatal admissions for chronic abdominal pain and vomiting were investigated for pre-eclampsia and fatty liver without imaging. When these conditions had been excluded there was little attempt to elucidate the underlying pathology, which only became apparent after delivery. Although the outcome may not have been different, an earlier diagnosis would have enabled an appropriate management and support plan to be implemented and would also have afforded the women symptomatic relief.

Severe back pain, sciatica and urinary incontinence continue to be under-investigated. A number of women in this triennium again had pain and symptoms so severe that they repeatedly attended accident and emergency departments or were admitted to hospital on a number of occasions. They often required complete bed rest and analgesia in hospital or at home, were unable to walk unaided and a few suffered urinary incontinence.

Previous Reports have repeatedly stressed, and this Report does so again, that pregnancy is not a contraindication for radiological investigations for women with severe and unremitting pain or vomiting, including back, chest or epigastric pain, particularly

if the pain is so severe it requires management by major or epidural analgesia or prevents the woman from walking.

Cases where 'social labelling' may have affected the diagnosis and management

Women with severe social problems, including drug dependency, can be challenging to care for, and sometimes their clinical symptoms may be dismissed as attention seeking, as demonstrated by the following case:

> A severely excluded drug-dependent woman, with a past history of abnormal cervical cytology, was admitted several times in pregnancy with severe abdominal and lower back pain. This was not investigated until after delivery, despite her past history and being noted to be in acute pain when visited at home during the antenatal period and also while in hospital. It was considered that she may have been attention seeking or wanting unnecessary pharmacological relief. A magnetic resonance imaging scan after delivery revealed a disseminated carcinoma, most likely to be cervical in origin, and thereafter she received excellent palliative care.

The importance of planned multidisciplinary care

When a woman with a malignancy is known prior to pregnancy, or as soon as it is diagnosed, planned multidisciplinary care is essential. It is heartening to note that this was the case for the majority of women in this Report, who, in the main, received excellent care. The multidisciplinary teams involved in their care comprised obstetricians, midwives, oncologists, radiologists, anaesthetists, paediatricians, Macmillan nurses, social services and others, as required. It is gratifying that it appears that the lessons from earlier Reports have been learned. Nevertheless, it is recommended that all maternity Trusts devise a formal protocol for the provision of such care should the need arise. The role of the midwife in such cases was summarised in the last Report and is reproduced here in Box 13.1.

Box 13.1 The midwife's role in supporting women suffering from malignancy or other serious medical conditions

- Acting as her advocate.
- Arranging familiarisation visits to the special care baby unit.
- Acting as the focal point for liaison with other health care teams.
- Providing information for her and her family.
- Ensuring time for rest and privacy.
- Ensuring the complex set of hand held-notes were transferred to all the professionals involved in her care.
- Teaching her partner parenting skills.
- Being involved with the first course of post-delivery treatment, if appropriate.

Cases of well-provided, thoughtful care, which supported the woman's dignity, wishes and beliefs

The majority of women received good multidisciplinary care once the diagnosis was made, but there were further instances of exceptional individualised care, which required an unconventional approach. These cases provide an excellent example of how sensitive but unconventional midwifery, obstetric and paediatric care can be the best option in the face of overwhelming illness and patient choice. Two short vignettes are given to demonstrate some of the variety of approaches that were adopted for such women and their families:

> A woman with an advanced malignancy actively sought alternative therapy during her pregnancy. She wanted no involvement from NHS professional services and wished to have a home birth under the care of an independent midwife. This request was supported and the midwife, in turn, liaised with and was supported by the supervisor of midwives. A number of family and professional meetings were held to discuss the prognosis and options with the staff respecting her choice to reject their care. She was helped to prepare a 'living will'. Eventually her condition required an early delivery, to which she agreed. The anaesthetist, while recommending a general anaesthetic for the necessary caesarean section, in view of her deteriorating condition opted for a slow-onset spinal block to provide a supportive environment with no aggressive interventions. Plans were made for her early discharge home but her condition rapidly deteriorated and she died peacefully with her family and friends in a specially prepared room at the hospital.

All the staff who were involved in this case commented that she taught them the true meaning of maternal choice. She was cared for in an exemplary manner throughout and died with dignity. Her wishes were respected at all times.

> A woman with known cancer developed secondary deposits in pregnancy. She was given appropriate highly specialised care but still required an early caesarean section. After a few weeks, and with the help of skilled multidisciplinary working, including the neonatal outreach team, she was able to help care for her premature baby at home until she died.

The neonatal team offered constant support and trained the family in neonatal resuscitation. All involved in her and her baby's care learned how to overcome routine obstacles such as transport and liability insurance, which, while put in place to support and protect patients and the organisation, can hinder optimum care in unforeseen circumstances. In the event, sensible decision making and the element of considered risk taking, such as enabling the baby to go home in an incubator, enabled the family to stay together as long as possible and to generate memories which should strengthen the father's ability to care for the child in the years to come.

References

1. Drife JO. The contribution of cancer to maternal mortality. In: O'Brien PMS, McLean AB, editors. *Hormones and Cancer*. London: RCOG Press; 2000. p. 299–310.

2. Lewis G, Drife J, editors. *Why Mother Die 1997–99. Report of the Fifth Confidential Enquiries into Maternal Deaths in the United Kingdom.* London: RCOG Press; 2001.

3. Royal College of Obstetricians and Gynaecologists. *Pregnancy and Breast Cancer.* Guideline No.12. London: RCOG; 2004.

Section

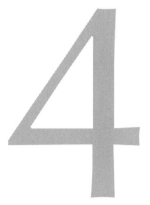

4

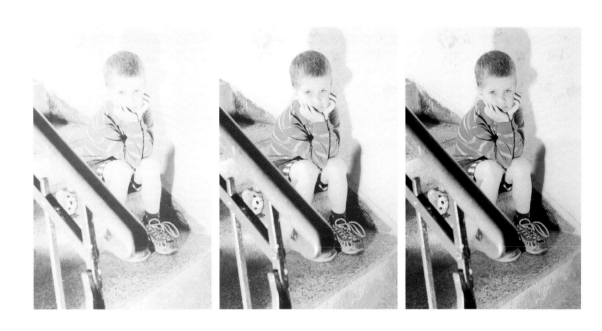

Coincidental and *Late* deaths

CHAPTER 14
Coincidental deaths and domestic violence

GWYNETH LEWIS on behalf of the Editorial Board

Domestic violence: key recommendations

Service provision

Enquiries about violence should be routinely included when taking a social history at booking or at another opportune point in the antenatal period.

Where possible, all women should be seen alone at least once during the antenatal period to enable disclosure more easily if they wish.

When routine questioning is introduced, this must be accompanied by the development of local strategies for referral to a local multidisciplinary support network to which the woman can be referred if necessary.

Local Trusts and community teams should develop guidelines for the identification of and provision of further support for these women, including developing multi-agency working to enable appropriate referrals or provision of information on sources of further help.

Information about local sources of help and emergency help lines such as provided by Women's Aid should be displayed in suitable places in the antenatal clinic, for example in the women's toilets or printed as a routine at the bottom of handheld maternity notes or cooperation cards.

It must be remembered that health professionals, too, may be victims of violence.

Individual practitioners

Women with known significant features of domestic violence should not be regarded as 'low risk' and should be offered multidisciplinary care in a supportive environment. If they choose midwifery-led care, the midwife should receive support and advice from an experienced superior.

All health professionals should make themselves aware of the importance of domestic violence in their practice. They should adopt a non-judgemental and supportive response to women who have experienced physical, psychological or sexual abuse and must be able to give basic information to women about where to get help. They should provide continuing support, whatever decision the woman makes made concerning her future.

> ### Training
>
> Programmes for the routine enquiry about violence must not be started until all local staff have received the appropriate training.
>
> Midwifery and obstetric staff should be aware of the role of social services and child protection issues and work in liaison with all appropriate support services.

Introduction

By international definition, deaths unconnected with pregnancy or the puerperium that occur before delivery or up to 42 days postpartum are called *Fortuitous*. They are not considered maternal deaths and do not contribute to maternal mortality statistics. However, as described in the last Report, in the opinion of the authors, the term *Fortuitous* is seen as out-dated, inappropriate and insensitive. Therefore definition was replaced with the term *Coincidental*. Even this word is an imperfect description for some such maternal deaths, which are related to pregnancy in the wider sense of public health, and which may have important implications for appropriate healthcare delivery.

Although many *Coincidental* deaths are considered unrelated to pregnancy it has long been standard practice to include them in this Report. These deaths may have important lessons for the management of certain nonpregnancy-related conditions, such as coincidental carcinomatosis (discussed in Chapter 13), and they also identify some wider public health issues of which health professionals need to be aware. Deaths from suicide following perinatal mental illness or deaths from domestic violence aggravated or directly caused by pregnancy cannot be regarded as coincidental. Neither can deaths where women were ill advised or unaware of the correct use of car seat belts during pregnancy. However, for the purposes of comparative data these deaths will continue, for the time being, to be counted as *Coincidental* and counted in this chapter.

Summary of findings for 2000–02

In this triennium 36 *Coincidental* deaths occurring during pregnancy or within 42 days of delivery or termination were notified to the Enquiry. These are shown in Table 14.1. Eight of these were from malignancies and these are discussed in Chapter 13. In addition, there 45 *Late Coincidental* deaths are counted in Chapter 15. The figures for the previous triennium were 29 *Coincidental* and 61 *Late Coincidental* deaths, respectively.

The majority of the deaths counted in this chapter again occurred among vulnerable and socially excluded women, and the general lessons to be drawn from these deaths are discussed in Chapter 1. The leading cause of death was murder, followed by road traffic accidents. These two causes of death are discussed further here.

Road traffic accidents: seat belts in pregnancy

Altogether, eight women died from road traffic accidents. Of these seven women died as a result of road traffic accidents while still pregnant and one died after delivery. Another

Table 14.1 *Coincidental* deaths; United Kingdom 2000–02

Cause of death	Deaths (*n*)
Neoplastic disease (see Chapter 13)	8
Infections:	
Meningitis	3
Pneumonia	1
Subdural abcess	1
Unnatural deaths:	
Murder	11
Road traffic accident	8
Overdose of street drugs	2
Carbon monoxide poisoning from faulty heater	1
Burns case unknown	1
Total	36

four cases are counted in Chapter 15 **Late deaths**. There was one death which, although due to a road traffic accident, is classified as psychiatric and counted in Chapter 11.

Four of the women who died were not wearing seat belts. Three of these were still pregnant and one died after delivery. Uterine rupture occurred in two cases where the woman was still pregnant. In contrast to the other women who died, and in whom death was unavoidable, the women who were not wearing seat belts, and whose lives might have been saved, were young girls or others with marked features of social exclusion.

A survey on pregnant women's knowledge and use of seat belts showed that, while 98% of pregnant front-seat passengers wore a seat belt, only 68% wore them in the back of the car.[1] The survey also found that only 48% of women correctly identified the correct way to use a seat belt, with only 37% reporting they had received information on the correct use of seat belts while pregnant. Although the survey was conducted several years ago, and the last two CEMD Reports have highlighted the need for pregnant women to be informed of the correct way to wear a seat belt in pregnancy, these findings in relation to young and socially excluded women cause concern and the recommendations made in the last Report are again repeated.

Recommendations for the use of seat belts in pregnancy

All pregnant women should be given advice about the correct use of seat belts as soon as their pregnancy is confirmed.

"Above and below the bump, not over it"

Three-point seat belts should be worn throughout pregnancy, with the lap strap placed as low as possible beneath the 'bump', lying across the thighs, with the diagonal shoulder strap above the bump lying between the breasts. The seat belt should be adjusted to fit as snugly as comfortably possible and, if necessary, the seat should be adjusted to enable the seat belt to be worn properly.

Domestic violence and murder

Domestic violence: summary of key points

- 11 women whose deaths were reported to the Enquiry were murdered by their partner during or shortly after pregnancy. One woman died later after delivery. Another 43 women had either voluntarily reported violence to a healthcare professional during their pregnancy or were already known to be in an abusive relationship.

- These 55 women represent 14% of the 391 women whose deaths were reported to this Enquiry. As none of the women in this Report had been routinely asked about violence as part of their social history, the 14% is probably an underestimate.

- All of the women who were murdered had one or more major characteristics of abused women, as shown in Table 14.1.

- 62% of the schoolgirls or young women under the age of 18 years whose deaths were considered by this Enquiry had suffered violence in the home.

- 71% of the women reporting violence booked late or were poor or non-attenders at the antenatal clinic. It was unusual for these women to be actively followed up.

- Nearly 50% the women who were murdered had very complex social circumstances yet had midwifery-led care with no referral or liaison between services.

- Women known to be in abusive relationships continue to been seen with their partners present at every visit.

- In many cases it appears that little or no help concerning the violence was offered to the woman.

- Family interpreters were used inappropriately.

- There was evidence of family 'secret keeping' in some cases.

Fourteen percent, 55 of the 391 women whose deaths were assessed this triennium, had either self-reported a history of domestic violence to a healthcare professional caring for them or the abuse was already known to health and social services.

Domestic violence was fatal for 12 of these women, all of whom were murdered by their partner. Of the 43 cases where the woman died of other causes, 29 were due to either *Direct* or *Indirect* causes, giving a known prevalence rate of 11%. Among *Coincidental* and *Late* deaths the rates were 6% and 10%, respectively. This percentage is undoubtedly an underestimate of the true prevalence of violence among this group of women as, in none of the 391 cases, was a history of violence actively sought through routine questioning as part of the social or family history at booking. Also the notes were incomplete for some of the cases assessed.

Of the 12 women who were murdered, all but one died either during pregnancy or within 6 weeks of delivery. Six of the eight girls or young women aged less than 18 years who died were in violent, dependent relationships and four had been sexually abused in the past. Three of the girls who had suffered sexual abuse were aged 16 years or under. Five women were living in, or had just left, women's refuges.

Currently, routine reporting of such cases to the Enquiry does not always take place, although the association between pregnancy and increasing domestic violence is well known. The cases described in this chapter should be regarded as being representative of other cases of murder and domestic violence that have not been reported to the Enquiry. From the cases that were reported, the warning signs were all too obvious in most cases. Several features of the women's cases illustrate the already described features of domestic violence as described in the Annex to this chapter. Some of these features will be illustrated by the cases in this Report.

Murder

Murder by a partner or ex-partner is the extreme end of the spectrum of domestic violence, an extremely important, but often overlooked, cause of maternal and child morbidity and mortality. Some of the cases in this Report are still *sub judice* so it is not possible to give details of the exact circumstances, but they underline the need for vigilance, especially when there may be a high index of suspicion.

In all the deaths there were readily identifiable risk factors of domestic violence. A summary of the characteristics of these women in shown in Tables 14.2 and 14.3.

The notable points are:

- All the women who were murdered had a known history of domestic violence.

- Nearly 50% the women who were murdered had low-risk midwifery-led care with no liaison between health professionals or services.

- All the women who were murdered after 20 weeks of gestation were either late bookers or poor attenders for care.

- Many had 'overbearing' partners who were present at all visits and sometimes disruptive.

Table 14.2 Deaths in women known to be suffering domestic violence (DV) and who were delivered or were 20 weeks pregnant or more; United Kingdom 2000–02

	Total deaths in women with DV (n)	Late booker >22 weeks (n)	Poor attender at ANC (n)	No antenatal care at all (n)	Total of late or non-attenders (n)	Total of all deaths in women with known DV (%)
Direct	14	6	4	2	12	86
Indirect	15	4	4	1	9	60
Murdered	12	4	3	3	10	83
Other						
Coincidental	4	1			1	25
Late	10	3	4		7	70
Total	55	18	15	6	39	71

Table 14.3 Characteristics of women who were murdered or suffered domestic violence (DV) during their pregnancy; United Kingdom 2000–02*

	Murdered (n = 12)		Other deaths associated with DV (n = 43)			Women with known DV (n = 55) (%)
	(n)	(%)	(n)	(%)	Total (n)	
Murdered while pregnant	9	75			12	22
Booking late (after 22 weeks)	4	33	16	37	20	36
Poor attendance	3	25	10	23	13	24
Concealed pregnancy/no attendance	3	25	3	7	6	11
Murdered before 20 weeks of gestation	3	25			3	5
History of severe depression/mental illness	5	42	13	30	18	33
Domineering partner present at all visits	8	66	4	9	12	22
Repeated miscarriage	4	33	6	14	10	18
Self discharge from hospital	2	17	3	7	5	9
Vaginal bleeding in pregnancy or PROM*	4	33	3	7	7	13
Admissions for minor complaints	3	25	4	9	7	13
Known to social services	7	58	6	14	13	24
Known to have been abused as child	3	25	7	16	10	18
Children known to child protection team or in care	5	42	4	9	9	16
Midwifery-led care	6	50	5	12	11	20

* Many had more than one characteristic

- Many women were known to social services and the local child protection team; some had all their previous children in care. One had a partner who, after her death, was found to have been a known juvenile sex offender and on the local sex offenders register.

- Several partners had visited the family GP alone, expressing their concerns about the woman's low self-esteem and jealousy.

- Some women appeared reluctant to give addresses but gave mobile phone numbers instead.

- Several had had episodes of gonorrhoea from their partner either just before or during pregnancy.

- Some had histories of multiple miscarriages or unexplained vaginal bleeding in pregnancy. The reasons for this were not followed up, despite the known history of violence.

The characteristics of domestic violence in relation to pregnancy were discussed in detail in an Annex to this chapter in the last Report and are not repeated here. Readers are referred to the last Report and the ever growing more updated literature on this important subject.[2]

What is of critical concern is that 71% of the women in abusive relationships who died found it difficult to access or maintain contact with antenatal care services. Over

---

Box 14.1 Indicators of domestic violence, relevant to maternity care

- Late booking.

- Poor/non attendance at antenatal clinics.

- Repeat attendance at antenatal clinics, the GP's surgery or accident and emergency departments for minor injuries or trivial or nonexistent complaints.

- Repeat presentation with depression, anxiety, self-harm and psychosomatic symptoms.

- Minimalisation of signs of violence on the body.

- Poor obstetric history.

- Recurrent sexually transmitted infections.

- Unexplained admissions.

- Non-compliance with treatment regimens/early self discharge from hospital.

- The constant presence of partner at examinations, who may answer all the questions for her and be unwilling to leave the room.

- The woman appears evasive or reluctant to speak or disagree in front of her partner.

85% of the women who were murdered or who were in violent relationships and died of *Direct* causes found it difficult to access care. Table 14.2 shows more the detailed characteristics of this. It also shows that the rates for late booking, poor or no attendance at all were even higher among women who were murdered or who died of *Direct* causes of maternal death.

Box 14.1, taken from the last Report, details some known indicators of domestic violence relevant to maternity care. Table 14.2 shows the characterises and percentages of the women who suffered violence in this Report against these and other indicators identified during the course of this triennial Enquiry. The findings are stark and point to the urgent need for health services to address these issues. The National Service Framework for Maternity and Children's Services in England has also recognised the importance of this, and many of its recommendations are similar to those in this Report.[3]

The circumstances of three women murdered by their partner while still pregnant illustrates many of the key features of abused women, and they are described further here:

> One woman who was murdered was already known to be in an abusive relationship by her GP, the child protection coordinator and her community midwives. She was booked for midwifery-led care but never provided with an opportunity to be seen without her partner being present. He was also present while she was admitted with vaginal bleeding some months into her pregnancy. The cause of this bleeding was not investigated, neither was she identified as being at any degree of risk. Her partner was described as "over possessive" in several of the healthcare worker reports. She was murdered by him shortly afterwards.

Another with a known history of partner violence booked for midwifery-led care. Again her partner seemed overbearing and was present throughout all visits. She had had several previous miscarriages and repeated episodes of sexually transmitted infections (STIs). Her midwife did not appear to appreciate the significance of her history and she was not offered further help or referrals.

Another woman who was murdered by her partner during pregnancy was booked for midwifery-led care. Again, her history of abuse was also well known and her existing children had all been taken into care by the child protection team. The notes say that these issues were not raised or discussed during her booking or subsequent visits.

Yet another women who had midwifery-led care and was known to suffer from both violence and a severe pre-existing mental illness was murdered by her partner shortly after delivery. The delivery was premature and possibly precipitated by a violet episode. She had booked late and again there was no communication between her midwife, the mental health services, the social services or the child protection team. Indeed, there is some doubt as to whether they knew she was pregnant. Further, on discharge her health visitor was not informed of her past medical or social history.

In all of these cases the clear warning signs were present but the midwife did not liaise with any other health or social care professionals.

References

1. Johnson H, Pring D. Car seatbelts in pregnancy: the practice and knowledge of pregnant women remain causes for concern. *BJOG* 2000; 107: 644–7.
2. Lewis G. Chapter 14: Coincidental (Fortuitous) deaths. Chapter 16: Domestic violence. In: Lewis G, Drife J, editors. *Why Mothers Die 1997–1999. Fifth Report of the Confidential Enquiries into Maternal Deaths*. London: RCOG Press; 2001. p. 225–30; 241–51.
3. Department of Health, Department for Education and Skills. *National Service Framework for Children, Young People and Meternity Services*. London: DoH; 2004 [www.doh.gov.uk].

CHAPTER 15
Late deaths

GWYNETH LEWIS on behalf of the Editorial Board

Introduction

Late maternal deaths are defined as deaths occurring in women more than 42 days but less than 1 year after miscarriage, abortion or delivery. The International Classification of Maternal Deaths (ICD10) only classifies *Late* deaths due to *Direct* or *Indirect* maternal causes, whereas this report also includes *Late Coincidental* (*Late Fortuitous*) deaths from which educational, public health or other messages and recommendations may also be drawn. For this reason all *Late* deaths reported to the Enquiry for 1997–99 are counted, and some are discussed, in this chapter, but none is included in the overall maternal mortality rate as defined in Chapter 1.

Some *Late Direct* deaths may occur in women who have received prolonged care in an intensive care unit, following the initial event. It is possible that this Enquiry may have missed some of these deaths because the immediate cause of death, as given on the death certificate, is not usually directly related to the pregnancy related event but relates to the final cause of death. These are therefore not currently picked up on death certificate data or currently notified by intensive care staff who may be unaware of this Report. The Enquiry is currently working with the Office for National Statistics (ONS) on a new record linkage system to enable these deaths to picked up more readily. Details of this are given in Chapter 1.

Late deaths often contain important messages for maternal health. For example, the majority of maternal deaths from suicide occur in this period and there are a number of other *Direct* and *Indirect* causes, for example from pulmonary embolism, cardiac disease and malignancies. These cases, although the deaths are counted in this chapter, are discussed in more depth in the relevant chapters of this Report to consolidate the key messages and recommendations in a more appropriate manner. Thus, for example, *Late* deaths from pulmonary embolism are discussed in Chapter 2, heart disease in Chapter 10, suicide and drug misuse in Chapter 11 and malignancies in Chapter 13.

The record linkage system described later in this chapter, and also in Chapter 1, identified a further 211 women who died within a year of giving birth. Apart from those women who died from suicide and have been counted as *Late Indirect* deaths, almost all of the others died of causes unrelated to their previous pregnancy and would be classified as *Late Coincidental* deaths.

Summary of findings for 2000–02

A total of 94 *Late* deaths were reported in this triennium compared with 107 in the last Report. Thirteen of these are discussed in Chapter 13 Deaths from cancer. Completed reports were available for all but ten cases. *Late* deaths are further classified as *Direct*,

Table 15.1   Interval between delivery and maternal death, *Late* cases reported to the Enquiry; United Kingdom 2000–02

Days after delivery	Direct	Indirect	Coincidental	Total
43–91	3	27	9	39
92–182	1	13	15	29
183–273	–	3	9	12
274–365		2	12	14
Total	4	45	45	94

Indirect or *Coincidental* (*Fortuitous*) although, as has already been stated, these are not included in the numerators for determining maternal mortality rates.

The interval between delivery and death for all *Late* deaths is shown in Table 15.1.

Direct causes

Four *Late* deaths were considered to be directly related to maternal causes and are discussed in the relevant chapters but counted here. There was one case each of thromboembolism, eclampsia, sepsis and volvulus of the bowel. A very late death, the antecedent events of which occurred before this triennium, is discussed in Chapter 9 Anaesthesia but not counted here.

Indirect causes

Table 15.2 shows the largest category of *Late Indirect* deaths are those due to mental illness (Table 15.2). In this triennium, 18 cases of suicide were reported and are discussed in full in Chapter 11 Deaths from psychiatric causes, where recommendations for the management of women suffering from postnatal mental illness are made. The ONS birth/maternal death record linkage study described in Chapter 1 identified that the majority of *Late* deaths from psychiatric illness and also deaths from subsistence misuse or due to accidental or violent means that might have been possibly due to suicide were not reported to this Enquiry. These data are also shown in Figure 15.1. This under-reporting is understandable in that these deaths, which occurred in the community, were not been recognised by this Enquiry until the last Report and the relevant health professionals or coroners are not used to reporting to this Enquiry. With the new ONS record linkage system in place in future, this degree of under-ascertainment should be

Table 15.2   *Late* deaths, *Indirect* causes; United Kingdom 2000–02

Cause of death	Deaths (*n*)
Neoplastic disease (see Chapter 13)	9
Suicide (see Chapter 11)	18
Cardiac causes (see Chapter 10)	13
Other causes:	
Epilepsy	2
Cytomegalovirus	1
Sudden adult death syndrome	1
Subarachnoid	1
Total	45

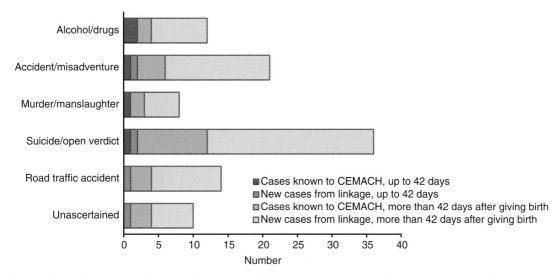

Figure 15.1 Maternal deaths idenitified by the ONS record linkage study from psychiatric, accidental, violent or unascertained causes; England and Wales 2000–02

reduced. It is hoped that a joint study might be undertaken with the National Inquiry into Death from Suicide and Homicide (NCISH) on these cases in the near future.

Lessons from deaths from cardiac disease or malignancies are discussed in Chapter 10 and Chapter 13, respectively. There appeared to be no cases of substandard care in the other causes of *Late Indirect* deaths.

Late *Coincidental* deaths

The causes of the 46 *Late Coincidental* deaths reported to this Enquiry are listed in Table 15.3. Six are also included in Chapter 13 Deaths from cancer. As with *Late Indirect*

Table 15.3 *Late* deaths, *Coincidental* causes; United Kingdom 2000–02

Cause of death	Deaths (*n*)
Neoplastic disease	6
Diseases of circulatory system:	
Subarchnoid	7
Myocardial infarction	3
Diseases of respiratory system:	
Asthma	3
Infectious diseases:	
TB	2
Pneumonia	2
Intracanial cyst	1
Haemophagocytosis	1
Other	2
Unascertained	2
Other	
Epilepsy	1
Scleroderma	2
Sudden unnatural deaths	
Road traffic accidents	6
Murder	1
Drug overdose in known drug users	4
Not stated	2
Total	45

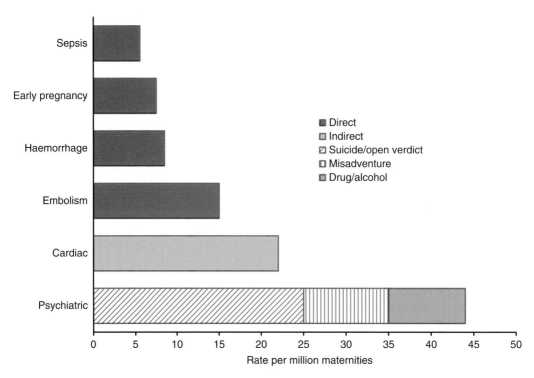

Figure 15.2 Maternal deaths from other *Indirect* or *Coincidental*, including *Late*, causes idenitified by the ONS record linkage study; England and Wales 2000–02

deaths, the vast majority of these cases were also unreported, as shown in Figure 15.2. The leading cause of death was, by far, malignancy.

It is worth noting, however, that the study described in Chapter 20, on the protective effects of pregnancy, showed that pregnant women or women who had delivered less than a year previously were five times less likely to die of all causes of mortality than women who were not pregnant.

Section

5

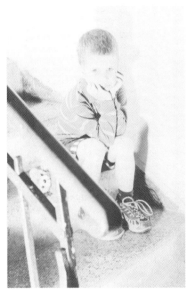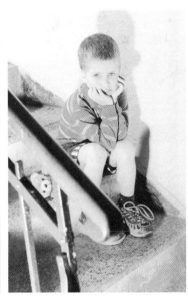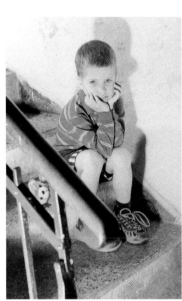

Other key issues

CHAPTER 16
Pathology

HARRY MILLWARD-SADLER on behalf of the Editorial Board

Pathology: recommendations

In all maternal deaths, if the autopsy cannot be performed by a pathologist with a special interest in these deaths then their help and advice should be sought.

As stated in the Royal College of Pathology guidelines, the autopsy report should include a summary correlating the clinical events and the pathological findings.

In all maternal deaths, histology should be undertaken unless there are positive reasons against such an action.

Amniotic fluid embolus should be carefully excluded as part of the differential diagnosis of all cases of disseminated intravascular coagulation, shock and haemorrhage.

In cardiac maternal deaths:

- All cases of cardiomyopathy diagnosed at autopsy should be supported by appropriate histological examination and, wherever possible, expert cardiac pathological opinion sought.

- The nature of the arterial pathology should be histologically confirmed.

- The severity of the cardiac and pulmonary pathology must be determined in all cases of congenital heart disease and in particular evidence for pregnancy induced accelerated pulmonary hypertension should be sought.

Toxicology should be performed not only in all unnatural deaths but also in deaths where epilepsy is the suspected cause.

50 years ago...

Although autopsies have been performed on the majority of maternal deaths evaluated in the Confidential Enquiries since their inception 50 years ago, it was not until the 1976–78 Report that there was a separate chapter on pathology. This was a direct result of criticism of the quality of the autopsy reports made in the preceding 1973–75 Report when the Chief Medical Officer wrote in the preface:

> "The importance of accurate diagnosis of the cause of death becomes greater as the number of deaths diminish. Postmortem examinations were carried out in 344 out of the 390 deaths investigated, but the authors and the Regional Assessors have all expressed concern that the reports available were not as helpful as they might have been. The assessors need full details of the

Table 16.1 Quality of autopsy reports in triennial reviews of the Confidential Enquiries into Maternal Deaths; England and Wales 1979–84, United Kingdom 1985–93

Triennium	Satisfactory		Unsatisfactory		Total (*n*)
	(*n*)	(%)	(*n*)	(%)	
1979–81	133	77	39	23	172
1982–84	150	80	38	20	188
1988–90	176	78	49	22	225
1991–93	141	77	42	23	183

postmortem and all histological examinations. More discussion between the clinicians and the pathologists as to the cause of death at the time of the examination might help to elucidate some of the problems."

The pathology assessor then recommended in the 1976–8 Report that:

"Autopsies on these patients should be regarded as specialised investigations. Coroners should be encouraged to consider maternal deaths as falling within a special category and as far as possible to ask pathologists with special interest or expertise in the field to perform them."

Since then there have been several triennial Reports in which the standard of the autopsy report has been analysed. The findings, shown in Table 16.1, have shown very little change despite being compiled by different assessors and sometimes including *Indirect* as well as *Direct* deaths.

The analysis for the last Report for 1997–99 was depressingly similar, with only 63 of the autopsies for 81 *Direct* maternal deaths (78%) being satisfactory. The reason for an apparent lack of progress in correcting a problem is usually multifactorial and was probably the case in this situation.

1. The standards required from the autopsy have changed as the clinical management of patients has become more complex. This may be true for some maternal deaths but overall, autopsies conducted according to Royal College of Pathology guidelines will be adequate.[1]

2. Most of the autopsies were, and even more so today, conducted for HM Coroners.

As stated in the 1976–78 Pathology Assessor's Report:

"The circumstances surrounding the arrangements for coroner's autopsies are often less than ideal. They are often undertaken in a mortuary at a distance from the maternity unit so that clinicopathological communication is poor; they are performed to discover causes of death rather than to make clinicopathological assessments and histological examinations are often not attempted. Inadequate histories may mean that careful search is not made for particular features or causes features to be missed or misinterpreted ..."

Sadly, this is still true today even though, apart from London, many public mortuaries have been integrated with hospital pathology departments. Many pathologists have claimed that they are limited by the local Coroner's instructions and it is true that some

Coroners have interpreted the regulations strictly. However, the personal experience of the author with Coroners from at least seven different districts (although none from London) is that they have accepted that the maternal death should be appropriately investigated.

3. The correct audiences have not been adequately addressed. The triennial Reports have been largely directed at those most directly involved in the care of pregnant women and as a generalisation, pathologists and Coroners have not been involved. As a consequence, pathologists with no experience or interest in maternal deaths are still conducting these autopsies.

As will be seen in the rest of this chapter, there are still problems with the quality of the autopsy in some cases of maternal death that must be addressed.

Summary of the findings for 2000–02

In the last triennial Report, the quality of autopsy reports for *Direct* maternal deaths was analysed. Eighteen of the 79 autopsy reports were considered to be deficient or appalling, not meeting the autopsy report standards identified by the Royal College of Pathologists. In this triennial Report, all *Direct* and *Indirect* maternal deaths for which an autopsy report was available have been reviewed using the same criteria.

The criteria used to categorise these autopsy reports were given in the last Report but for convenience are included here as Box 16.1.

The analysis for this Report shows a slight but gratifying improvement in the overall quality of autopsy reports: 136 reports on deaths classified as *Direct* or *Indirect* were analysed. Only 24 were considered to have significant deficiencies, as shown in Table 16.2.

Overall, in this triennium, 82% of these autopsies were considered adequate or better, which is a slight improvement over the last triennial report, when 77% of reports were in this category. This small improvement is matched by a reduction in the number of autopsy reports categorised as appalling, as shown in Figure 16.1. Nonetheless, of the three appalling reports for this triennium, two again came from the London area.

Some reports were downgraded because the documentation was incomplete and the missing components were critical to the conclusions or clinicopathological correlation. The following vignette gives an example:

> A parous women who was known to have an anterior placenta (but not a placenta praevia) was admitted with an antepartum haemorrhage and hypotension. She was taken to theatre and a placenta percreta was identified. Despite hysterectomy, her bleeding continued and despite massive transfusions of blood and colloids she died in intensive care. The autopsy was thorough and detailed but there was no review of the hysterectomy specimen to confirm the placenta percreta nor was the histology report included for review purposes. Also, the bladder was adherent to the uterus at the site of the percreta during the operation. Haemorrhage was noted in the dome of the bladder at autopsy but was not examined histologically.

Box 16.1 Criteria for assessing a maternal death autopsy

Excellent

A thorough, detailed autopsy report with comprehensive histology and appropriate microbiological, toxicological or other specific directed investigations, with careful exclusion of alternative diagnoses and clarification of a complicated clinical history.

Good

Many of the above features are included but a more straightforward clinical problem with no significant differential diagnoses. Met all the recommendations of the Royal College of Pathologists (RCPath).

Adequate

Established the cause of death but did not necessarily address all the clinical issues. Sometimes there was a lack of supporting evidence because of inadequate documentation. Recommendations of RCPath not necessarily completely fulfilled but deficiencies not apparently affecting the conclusions.

Deficient

Report consistent with clinically suspected cause of death but lacks detail. Lack of supporting investigations, no evidence of clinical correlation or attempt to exclude differential diagnoses. Does not comply with RCPath guidelines in more than one area.

Appalling

All of the 'deficient' criteria but worse. Often, the total report including patient details and stated causes of death occupies one side of A4 paper or less. There are discrepancies between the minimally described pathology and the pathological conclusions, there are no supporting investigations and there is no evidence of any knowledge of the clinical problems or of any attempt to exclude differential diagnoses.

Table 16.2 Quality of autopsy reports for *Direct* and *Indirect* maternal deaths; United Kingdom 2000–02

Quality	Reports (*n*)
Excellent	28
Good	44
Adequate	40
Deficient	21
Appalling	3
Total	136

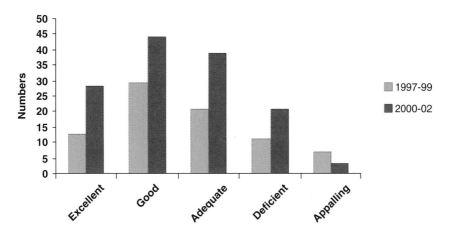

Figure 16.1   Quality of maternal death autopsies by number of autopsies; United Kingdom 1997–2002

Substandard autopsies

The major reasons why the quality of the autopsy report was considered poor or worse fell into three broad categories: technically substandard autopsies, inappropriate conclusions and lack of supportive investigation.

In 24 autopsy reports there is evidence that the performance of the autopsy was substandard and/or the conclusions drawn from the observations were inaccurate or demanded necessary supportive evidence. Combinations of these categories were inevitably present, as shown by the following representative example:

> A woman presented ill after a termination of early pregnancy. The clinical diagnoses were presumed sepsis and acute renal failure. She also had unexplained hypercalcaemia. She developed ARDS and died. The autopsy report gave the cause of death as multiple organ failure on the basis of very heavy lungs weighing more than 1 kg each and mottled liver and kidneys but no histology. The report commented that the vaginal bleeding that had continued since her termination of pregnancy could be associated with ARDS and subsequent multiple organ failure. This seems a rather strange conclusion, given that her haemoglobin a few days before death and approximately 1 week after her termination was 13.2 g/l and that bleeding was not a significant clinical feature. A second autopsy was subsequently performed, whereupon a large 5-cm diameter parathyroid adenoma was found. This was confirmed by histology and the cause of death appropriately adjusted.

The following vignettes concerning cases inappropriately attributed to cardiomyopathy point out the need for careful histology:

> A woman with a longstanding history of essential hypertension was being treated with methyldopa and labetalol. She also had a history of pre-eclampsia in previous pregnancies. Near term, she was admitted with rising blood pressure and proteinuria and labour was induced because of severe pre-eclampsia. After delivery she collapsed and died. At autopsy, the heart was enlarged, weighing 530 g and the pathologist concluded from the gross findings that death was due peripartum cardiomyopathy. There was no histology though the heart was sampled.

A woman was admitted with vaginal bleeding and lower abdominal pain near term. The bleeding subsided but owing to fetal distress an emergency caesarean section was performed. She was well for a few days but readmitted later too weak to walk. After investigations, a diagnosis of infection was made and antibiotic therapy started. She had a sudden cardiac arrest with some chest discomfort and shortness of breath from which she could not be resuscitated. Clinically, she was thought to have either pulmonary embolus or overwhelming sepsis.

The pathologist's report is confined to one side of a sheet of A4 paper and there was no histology. The heart was described as enlarged (404 g) with marked right ventricular hypertrophy and a dilated left ventricle. The conclusion was congestive cardiomyopathy. The weight of the individual ventricles was not established, there was no histology and no cultures were taken to exclude sepsis. The obstetrician attended the autopsy and subsequently commented that he was greatly dismayed by the service from the pathologist because the diagnosis of the cardiomyopathy had not been followed up with any histological studies and the main suspected diagnoses of infection and thromboembolic disease had not been pursued in any detail.

It is inappropriate to make a diagnosis of peripartum cardiomyopathy without the appropriate supportive histology and particularly when there are clear alternative causes of cardiovascular disease.

Clinical correlation

The failure to correlate postmortem findings adequately with the clinical history was a common problem. For instance, a woman who had postpartum haemorrhage associated with a large cervical laceration died. The report totally failed to mention any search for trauma in the genital tract, although, ironically, a careful search for amniotic fluid embolus was made. However, this failing was most common with deaths from pulmonary embolus.

Pulmonary embolus

Of the 25 deaths from pulmonary embolus only nine autopsy reports are available for review. Five of these were poor reports, three were adequate and only one was good. The major reason why reports were regarded as poor was the failure to correlate the postmortem examination with the clinical history. The following vignettes act as examples:

A mother had a major primary postpartum haemorrhage with disseminated intravascular coagulation (DIC) shortly after a caesarean section. The clinical diagnosis was of amniotic fluid embolism but the differential diagnosis included a heparin-induced thrombocytopenia. Some hours after delivery she suddenly collapsed and died. The autopsy demonstrated impacted coiled thromboemboli in both main pulmonary arteries with residual thrombi in the deep calf veins. The uterine veins were clear. No histology was performed so the cause of the primary postmortem haemorrhage and her DIC was not adequately investigated and the clinical diagnosis of amniotic fluid embolism was not adequately excluded.

Another mother had been investigated for a tachycardia and shortness of breath in her second trimester without any firm diagnosis being reached.

Postpartum she had a mild pyrexia and a few days later she collapsed and died. The autopsy established the cause of death as massive pulmonary embolism occluding both main pulmonary arteries. Thrombi were present within the pelvic veins but not the calf veins. There was no description of the peripheral pulmonary vascular tree and no histology was undertaken of any organs. Although the appearances in one kidney were "suggestive of a degree of pyelonephritis", no histology was undertaken.

This mother had been treated as low risk for thromboembolism but the assessors consider that her risk was much higher. An opportunity was missed at autopsy to determine whether there had been previous thromboemboli causing the clinical episodes of tachycardia and shortness of breath. There was also failure to confirm a pyelonephritis as the probable cause of the post delivery pyrexia.

As stated in the Royal College of Pathology guidelines,[1] the autopsy report should include a summary correlating the clinical events and the pathological findings.

Alternative diagnoses

Sometimes there was inadequate investigation to determine or exclude another cause of maternal death. Most frequently, this was the failure histologically to confirm the cause of death and exclude alternatives.

The best example of this is in the investigation of antepartum and postpartum haemorrhage. In five cases of amniotic fluid embolus, two women had suffered a major postpartum haemorrhage and two others antepartum haemorrhage. The fifth presented with DIC and collapse and died very quickly. One of the cases presented with massive postpartum haemorrhage after caesarean section and the strong clinical presumption was of amniotic fluid embolus but no autopsy was performed. In at least two of the remaining four cases there were possible alternative causes of death and the amniotic fluid embolus would have been missed without adequate investigation. One of these was postpartum haemorrhage (PPH) associated with genital tract trauma and the other was an antepartum haemorrhage in a road traffic accident with multiple injuries.

Not all cases were sufficiently investigated. For example:

A woman was found dead at home having delivered her baby on her own. There was evidence of massive postpartum haemorrhage. This was the diagnosis given at autopsy but there was no attempt to identify or exclude the presence of amniotic fluid embolus. While the findings may have been adequate in excluding a forensic cause of death, the pathologically process(es) resulting in the blood loss were not investigated in detail.

It is recommended that in all maternal deaths histology should be undertaken unless there are positive reasons against such an action.

The added value of the autopsy

Attention has been given to deficiencies in the autopsy report but, as is evident from Table 16.2, the overwhelming majority of the reports were good or excellent. Some autopsies have revealed unexpected pathology or cause of death and even when findings have been essentially negative some autopsies, by excluding many of the differential diagnoses, have had a major positive contribution.

Amniotic fluid embolism

The value of negative findings from a well-conducted autopsy must be emphasised. The Assessors accept that a diagnosis of amniotic fluid embolus can be made on clinical criteria. This is valid when there is no autopsy and permissible when there is a badly conducted autopsy but the diagnosis should otherwise be supported by histological evidence. It is therefore imperative that pathologists carefully exclude amniotic fluid embolus in difficult cases. In the current triennium, amniotic fluid embolus was clinically diagnosed in two women which the assessors consider to have been anaesthetic deaths and in two cases of DIC where the differential diagnoses were respectively eclampsia and postpartum haemorrhage. In all of these cases, there was careful examination of multiple blocks of lung for fetal squames supplemented by the use of immunohistochemistry: all were negative as shown by the following example:

> A mother had been normotensive throughout a normal pregnancy and had a spontaneous labour with a retained placenta. She then complained of central chest pain and was given oxygen. However, a short while later, prior to induction of anaesthesia for removal of the placenta, her blood pressure was elevated and she had a grand mal seizure. The diagnosis was considered to be amniotic fluid embolus or pulmonary embolus and she was transferred to the intensive care unit. It was noted that her platelets and fibrinogen levels had fallen and at this stage she had massive vaginal bleeding. Despite a subtotal hysterectomy and massive transfusion of blood and blood products she had a cardiac arrest from which she could not be resuscitated. The autopsy was detailed and thorough. In particular multiple blocks of lung were stained immunocytochemically for fetal squames with the antibody LP34 and also stained for fetal mucins. These results were also reviewed and repeated by the local pathology assessor and were again negative. In addition histology of the uterine bed showed the features of an acute atherosis which, although not diagnostic, are typical of pre-eclamptic change.

This difficult case illustrates not only the need for careful detailed analysis of maternal deaths but it also highlights what is not known about amniotic fluid embolus. Although fetal squames in the lungs are the hallmark of diagnosis, we do not know whether other components of amniotic fluid can precipitate the syndrome in the absence of squames. Fetal squames have been identified in the pulmonary arterial blood of pregnant mothers but the threshold above which the syndrome is precipitated is unknown. The length of survival of fetal squames in the maternal lung is also unknown and could be a critical factor in determining the diagnosis where prolonged survival in an intensive care unit has occurred. For all these reasons, it is imperative that a thorough detailed search is conducted in all autopsies where there is any clinical suspicion of amniotic fluid embolus.

It is therefore recommended that amniotic fluid embolus should be carefully excluded as part of the differential diagnosis of all cases of DIC, shock and haemorrhage.

Other specific conditions

Cardiac disease

After suicide, cardiac disease is the leading cause of maternal death in the UK. The causes of cardiac disease are many and varied but again in this triennium include cardiomyopathy, dissecting aneurysms and congenital heart disease, as well as a miscellany of causes ranging from ischaemic heart disease to scleroderma.

Cardiomyopathy

Of the eight cases of cardiomyopathy reviewed in this triennial Report, only four are known to have had an autopsy and the autopsy report was not available for one of these deaths. Two have already been identified and discussed as examples of poor autopsy examination and interpretation. In each of these, there was evidence of pre-existing heart disease, which, in the opinion of some authors, should exclude the diagnosis.[2] In one *Late* death from cardiogenic shock due to dilated cardiomyopathy, the autopsy report was very good. At autopsy, the heart was enlarged and dilated and there was endocardial fibroelastosis in the left atrium and ventricle. There was also evidence of severe DIC with changes in the liver, pancreas and kidneys and evidence of extensive soft tissue bleeding. There was detailed histology, which not only confirmed the macroscopic findings but together with microbiological sampling of the heart excluded an active or preceding myocarditis.

Another case falls broadly into the category of cardiomyopathy, highlighting the importance of a good autopsy for the health of the remaining family:

> A woman collapsed and died while exercising in mid-pregnancy. She had no relevant medical history and her pregnancy had been problem-free. At autopsy the macroscopic findings were minimal. The heart weighed 350 g but showed mild dilatation of both ventricles and there was a straw-coloured right pleural effusion. There was no coronary artery atheroma. However, histology showed myocyte disarray, myocyte damage and fibrosis within the heart. There was no active myocarditis. A specialist cardiac opinion was obtained, which identified idiopathic myocardial fibrosis. Screening of direct family members was advised and was subsequently undertaken.

Aneurysms

There were ten autopsy reports in this category of maternal death. Five deaths were due to dissecting aortic aneurysm and five due to dissecting coronary artery aneurysm.

Aortic aneurysms

The cases of dissecting aortic aneurysm all started in the ascending aorta usually just above the aortic valve cusps and in all five there was rupture into the pericardium producing cardiac tamponade. One case was unusual in that the tear originated in a 5-cm diameter saccular aneurysm at the origin of the ascending aorta and thought to be congenital in origin.

Another woman had a dissecting aortic aneurysm which extended along the aorta to the bifurcation into the common iliac arteries. She had had hypertension and proteinuria attributed to pre-eclampsia in the later part of her pregnancy and had then had several admissions complaining of chest pain. She had collapsed and died shortly after her last admission. The extensive dissection in this case suggests that the dissection had started several days before the final events though the vigorous attempts at resuscitation could also have contributed. As the pathologist had been requested to limit the examination to determining the cause of death, these possibilities were not further investigated nor was the clinical diagnosis of pre-eclampsia confirmed by histology.

In another case there was also evidence from histology that the dissection had started at least 48 hours before death. In this particular instance, the woman had been admitted with breathlessness clinically diagnosed as pulmonary embolus and had a cardiac arrest from her cardiac tamponade while being investigated for pulmonary embolism. This is the only case in which Marfan's syndrome was suspected.

Cystic medial necrosis of the arterial wall is the common pathology in dissection. Nonetheless, this should be confirmed by histology and, where positive, family members offered screening. An attempt should also be made to determine when the dissection started. The problems of pregnancy in Marfan's syndrome have been reviewed.[3]

Dissecting coronary artery aneurysms

Each triennial Report records an occasional death from a dissecting arterial aneurysm not related to the aorta. Of these dissecting coronary artery aneurysms are the most common and in this triennium there were five deaths from this cause. Four of these involved the left anterior descending coronary artery, starting at its origin or immediately distal to it. The fifth case was a dissection of the right coronary artery, starting from close to its origin. In four of these cases death occurred in the puerperium and one death during pregnancy. All the autopsies were performed to a very good standard. In one autopsy the dissection was only diagnosed on histology. This emphasises the value of postmortem histology even when the macroscopic findings may seen clear cut.

In this triennium, three other maternal deaths were attributed to myocardial infarction and ischaemic heart disease but no postmortem histology was undertaken. One other case died from rupture of the right iliac artery while in labour. The mother was described as having a collagen disorder not otherwise specified. No histology was undertaken. While many of the collagen disorders have no specific arterial pathology, failure to exclude vasculitis and dissection must be considered a deficiency.

Congenital heart disease

Nine women died from varieties of congenital heart disease or primary pulmonary hypertension. Four had pulmonary hypertension and one of these was associated with dissection of the pulmonary artery. In one woman with Eisenmenger's syndrome, a very well-performed autopsy produced evidence suggesting that the pulmonary hypertensive changes had accelerated during pregnancy:

> A young woman had a ventricular-septal defect (VSD) repaired in childhood because she was thought to have developed slight right ventricular hypertrophy and pulmonary hypertension. After surgery, these findings improved but she still had some pulmonary hypertension. An echocardiogram was reported as normal only months before her pregnancy. During her pregnancy she was seen by a cardiologist who found nothing unusual and she then had a normal vaginal delivery. Shortly after this she collapsed with cyanosis and died. The autopsy confirmed that the VSD had been successfully repaired but found marked right ventricular hypertrophy. Both lungs showed moderate acute congestion and focal pulmonary artery atheroma. The histology of the lungs was dramatic. There was very well established and advanced pulmonary hypertension with medial hypertrophy and focal atheroma of the larger pulmonary arteries, marked fibrointimal thickening of the smaller pulmonary arteries many of which contain microthrombi and many angiomatoid and plexiform lesions. Many of the latter were hypercellular and also contained thrombi. The histology of the lungs and the heart

were referred for specialist opinion and the findings were confirmed. The features were felt to be compatible with an accelerated process during pregnancy as has been described by Brach Prever.[4]

This contrasts with another autopsy on a woman with congenital pulmonary artery stenosis who died. The macroscopic description was reasonably detailed but despite describing the right ventricle as hypertrophied the ventricles were not weighed separately. Furthermore, there was no histology performed so the state of any pulmonary arterial disease is unknown.

It is recommended that in cardiac maternal deaths:

a. all cases of cardiomyopathy diagnosed at autopsy should be supported by appropriate histological examination and wherever possible expert cardiac pathological opinion sought

b. the nature of the arterial pathology is histologically confirmed, and

c. the severity of the cardiac and pulmonary pathology must be determined in all cases of congenital heart disease and in particular evidence for pregnancy induced accelerated pulmonary hypertension should be sought.

Suicide

Suicide is the largest cause of maternal death. The unusual feature of such deaths is the high proportion due to hanging, jumping from high buildings or other violent modes. While the Office of National Statistics is able to provide the linkage to the Enquiry to identify such deaths, frequently the major source of clinical information lies in the pathology report. It is clearly understood that there are situations where this information may be confidential or *sub judice*. Nonetheless, the pathologist can have a crucial role to play in ascertaining the relevant clinical details and providing valuable information relevant to the chain of events. The evidence adduced from these triennial Reports is that these women are no longer in contact with the maternity services. The pathologist's report is therefore a key source of information with regard to the clinical circumstances prior to death and their relationship to death. Also the toxicological analysis can represent further key evidence, for example:

> A woman with a long history of depression became severely depressed but refused inpatient care. On the day of her death she seemed better but while her husband was out of the house, she hanged herself. Although she was supposed to have been taking her drug therapy regularly, there was no trace of these drugs on toxicological examination.

While there were instances where toxicology was inappropriate – particular after major transfusions from the suicides due to multiple injuries, toxicological analysis of the drugs used in therapy is very helpful even when the cause of death is not obviously related to an overdose.

Epilepsy

Autopsy reports were available for ten deaths attributed to epilepsy. Of these, one was substandard and two others were deficient because drug levels were not analysed.

The substandard autopsy attributed death to epilepsy, even though the drug levels of methadone in the blood were well within a range associated with death. Although there is considerable individual variation in susceptibility to the effects of methadone it seems perverse to make a diagnosis that is essentially one of exclusion, in the absence of any witnesses to the death, in the absence of circumstantial autopsy evidence of epilepsy, and in the presence of another cause frequently associated with death.

The drug levels were analysed in the other seven cases. Two women who died in their second trimester had no trace of drugs in their blood at postmortem. In one, a consultant neurologist had advised continuation of sodium valproate but had also warned of the risks of fetal malformation. While the reasons why these two women did not take their anti-epileptic treatment are not known for certain, the possibility that they were concerned about fetal malformation cannot be discounted.

It is difficult to draw conclusions from these small numbers, especially as epilepsy is controlled by clinical response to therapy and not by the drug levels, but it is possible that some mothers are unilaterally stopping their drugs against medical advice because of their fears for their baby.

Toxicology is an important tool in the investigation of the chain of events leading to maternal death and particularly in epilepsy.

It is therefore recommended that toxicology should be performed not only in all unnatural deaths but also in deaths where epilepsy is the suspected cause.

Diabetes mellitus

There were three deaths in diabetic pregnant mothers: two of these were declared unascertained after the autopsy and the third was attributed to acute heart failure from a diabetic nephropathy. In all three, the circumstantial evidence implicated hypoglycaemia as the precipitating cause. Vitreous humour glucose was measured in all cases and was always less than 1 mmol/l. While compatible with hypoglycaemia, this level falls rapidly after death and therefore is not diagnostic:

> A known insulin-dependent brittle diabetic woman was found dead at home. She had a history of severe hypoglycaemic attacks in previous pregnancies and had been provided with home glucagon. An outstandingly good autopsy included specialist opinions on the heart, brain and liver, extensive histology, virology and toxicology. There was no ascertainable cause of death from these investigations. The vitreous glucose was zero but the autopsy was three days after death. Serum insulin and C-peptide levels were measured, however. They were within normal limits but the sample was haemolysed, which usually results in readings below the true level. While insulin overdose seems unlikely the results would be compatible with death from hypoglycaemia.

In difficult cases serum insulin assay can be helpful though the result still has to be interpreted in relation to the clinical history.

Ogilvie's syndrome

In this triennium, there were four cases of death from Ogilvie's syndrome. This is pseudo-obstruction leading to perforation of the large bowel. Two cases of perforation occurred in the caecum and in one case perforation occurred in the sigmoid colon. Perforation usually occurs 7–12 days after caesarean section. In one case there was marked pseudo-obstruction but no perforation:

> A woman who had had a caesarean section collapsed and could not be re-suscitated around eight days after delivery. At autopsy, conducted less than 24 hours later, the abdomen was markedly swollen and tympanic and this was due to gross distension of small and large bowel. There was no evidence of volvulus or mechanical obstruction and there was no perforation or necrosis of either the small or the large intestine. There was no evidence of inhaled vomit or of pulmonary emboli. This was confirmed on examining multiple blocks of lung and no significant pathological features were found in the heart, liver, kidneys, uterus or pancreas. Death was attributed to an arrhythmia secondary to the electrolyte disturbance associated with the pseudo-obstruction.

Pregnancy and, in particular, caesarean section, are among the most common causes of pseudo-obstruction, although it is also well described in other postoperative states. In one study of 212 cases of pseudo-obstruction, 74 were associated with pregnancy and, in particular, caesarean section. It has been postulated that the normal parasympathetic outflow from sacral segments 2, 3 and 4 are disrupted, causing a functional obstruction where the proximal and distal nerve supplies to the colon overlap.[5]

Conclusion

The Royal College of Pathologists produced guidelines for postmortem reports in 1993[1] and have updated them in 2004.[6] The pathology of maternal deaths has also been reviewed in 2003 and will also be of benefit.[7] Although there are some specific requirements in maternal death autopsies, adherence to these College recommendations will produce reports that are of value to the Enquiry and its assessors in evaluating these sad and tragic cases.

References

1. Royal College of Pathologists. *Guidelines for Post Mortem Reports*. London: RCPath; 1993.
2. Mehta NJ, Mehta RN, Khan IA. Peripartum cardiomyopathy: clinical and therapeutic aspects. Angiology 2001;52:759–62.
3. Lind J, Wallenburg H. The Marfan syndrome and pregnancy: a retrospective study in a Dutch population. *Eur J Obstet Gynecol Reprod Biol* 2001;98:28–35.
4. Brach Prever S, et al. Fatal outcome in pregnancy in Eisenmenger syndrome. *Cardiology in the Young*, 1997;7:238–40.
5. Spira IA, Rodrigues R, Woolf WI. Pseudo-obstruction of the colon. *Am J Gastroenterol* 1976;65:397–408.
6. Royal College of Pathologists. 2004 [www.rcpath.org/index].
7. Millward-Sadler GH. Pathology of maternal deaths. In: Kirkham N., Shepherd N, editors. *Progress in Pathology Volume 6*. London: Greenwich Medical Media; 2003. p. 163–84.

CHAPTER 17

Trends in intensive care

TOM CLUTTON-BROCK on behalf of the Editorial Board

Intensive care: key recommendations

Service provision

High bed occupancy rates in intensive care reduce the availability of emergency beds. It is sometimes possible to create a bed for an emergency and this should be facilitated by early consultant-to-consultant referral.

Early warning scores should be used more often on obstetric wards; they may need modifying for pregnant women.

Elective admissions should be prearranged and this may require the cancellation of other booked intensive care admissions on the day.

Intensive care consultants should be part of the multidisciplinary team planning care for patients with serious co-morbidity.

Intensive care should start as soon as it is needed and does need to wait for admission to an intensive care unit. It is possible to provide the majority of immediate intensive care in an obstetric theatre. Where available outreach staff should be used.

Individual practice

Arterial lines should be inserted early and samples taken for blood gases, haemoglobin, electrolytes and clotting on a regular basis. Where indicated, fluids and inotropes should be started without delay.

Consideration should be given to improved stabilisation and elective intubation prior to transfer.

Blood gases should be done earlier and a metabolic acidosis should always be taken seriously and investigated.

Fifty years ago...

Fifty years is a long period in any medical specialty; in intensive care medicine it is a lifetime. The first chapter dedicated to intensive care issues in maternal deaths appeared in the 1991–93 triennial Report. Mothers have, of course, made use of intensive care for much longer than this and intensive care as we would recognise it today traces its origins back almost exactly 50 years. Developed in response to a poliomyelitis epidemic in Copenhagen in 1952, intensive care medicine in Europe has grown from the poorly understood province of a small number of dedicated enthusiasts to a major medical speciality in its own right.[1]

Early intensive care units were primarily created around concentrations of particularly sick patients; such a process was adopted by Florence Nightingale and became common practice in military hospitals. We have advanced well beyond this today and modern intensive care thrives on the ability to deliver expert and evidence-based care to critically sick patients from any number of sources and increasingly to commence the process in a variety of different locations. Nevertheless, dedicated intensive care areas are an important feature of modern hospitals if the most efficient use of resources for staffing, equipment and support services is to be made. There are many principles of care common to all critically ill patients and patients are increasingly being classified according to nursing dependency rather than by diagnosis.

Patterns of disease have changed as well; 50 years ago intensive care units were mainly concerned with the ventilation of patients with respiratory failure from poliomyelitis and tetanus. The Copenhagen epidemic saw the introduction of positive pressure ventilation via tracheostomy as a highly effective alternative to tank ventilators (iron lungs). The introduction of effective vaccines changed the population of patients presenting to intensive care units to those we would recognise today, patients with multiple organ dysfunction often secondary to major surgery or sepsis.

50 years ago the critically sick mother could have been ventilated but without access to blood gases or pulse oximetry. Invasive cardiovascular monitoring was entirely experimental with rat-tailed manometers and complex dye dilution methods of estimating cardiac output. Effective renal support was 25 years away and enforced starvation would continue for even longer. Blood transfusions were a complex affair and our understanding of clotting and clotting products was in its infancy. Had she suffered a cardiac arrest then the outlook was bleak, external cardiac massage had yet to be introduced and defibrillation with a pair of insulated spoons connected to the mains electricity supply was a far cry from today's sophisticated biphasic devices.

The 1960s and 1970s were the dawn of the digital era, albeit in forms we would not recognise today. Microprocessor-controlled medical devices began to appear as did the widespread use of cardiopulmonary bypass for open heart surgery. Pulmonary artery catheterisation and thermodilution cardiac output monitoring, although described in London in the 1960s,[2] would wait until the 1970s to be popularised as a monitoring tool.[3] The intra-aortic balloon pump, described in 1958,[4] only really became an effective tool in the late 1970s with the introduction of a percutaneous version.[5] This remains an important tool today in the management of peripartum dilated cardiomyopathy. In 1969, intensive care in the United Kingdom was still very much in its infancy but at least the recovering patient, unable to sleep, could have sat up and watched a man land on the moon!

The next 20 years would see intensive care develop into the complex and sophisticated specialty we recognise today. The now widely accepted principles behind the pathogenesis and treatment of critical illness really began to take shape in the 1980s. They began with a marked increase in the understanding about systemic inflammatory processes, cell signalling and the pivotal role of nitric oxide. This led in turn to a proliferation of clinical trials searching for 'silver bullets' with the power to reverse the devastating effects of severe systemic sepsis. This remains an elusive goal with particular relevance to severe sepsis associated with pregnancy. Despite these disappointments significant progress has been made in the field of organ system support and it is now common for patients to survive periods requiring respiratory, cardiovascular, renal and nutritional support.

The acute respiratory distress syndrome in adults (ARDS) has featured in all the intensive care chapters to date. This complex inflammatory process has a clear association with pre-eclampsia, sepsis and massive haemorrhage. Our understanding of the pathogenesis has increased significantly but treatment remains essentially supportive. Care with this support is important and the last decade has seen an emphasis on the damage that poorly controlled mechanical ventilation can cause. Trials into inflammatory moderators, surfactant and extracorporeal support continue to the present day.[6]

As intensive care moved from the province of the dedicated enthusiast into an important acute service so the complex problems of bed numbers, training and severity scoring came to the fore. Knaus and others introduced APACHE scoring in 1981[7] and the second version is now widely used as part of a national audit scheme in the UK. Competing interests between anaesthesia, medicine and surgery delayed the introduction of formal intensive care training in the UK. Joint training posts were introduced in 1986 and, since 2000, intensive care training has been supervised by the Intercollegiate Board for Training in Intensive Care Medicine.[8] The recognition in 2002 of intensive care as a specialty in its own right is an important milestone in a long struggle.

The provision of sufficient intensive care beds is an essential component in minimising the delays in the admission of critically sick emergencies. In 1998, there were just over 1,400 adult beds available for general intensive care for the whole of England and Wales.[9] By January 2002, this had risen to 1,711 intensive care beds and 1,319 high-dependency beds. Increasingly, these high-dependency beds are to be found on obstetric units. The provision of specially trained staff and a suitably equipped area improves the care of patients while allowing for continued contact between mother and baby.

To the occasional visitor, intensive care in the 21st century is all about sophisticated technology. Bed spaces are filled with computer-controlled ventilators, multichannel monitoring systems and several different methods of measuring cardiac output with varying degrees of invasiveness. Most drugs are given by infusion and ten or more syringe drivers are common. Other, equally important developments in intensive care are less obvious; highly evolved nursing training and in-service development programmes have given us a nursing workforce unrivalled anywhere in the world. Our eventual understanding that intensive care is exactly that, intensive care provided by an experienced member of the nursing staff has encouraged us to take intensive care out of the dedicated unit and to deliver it to a much wider patient base. This is an extremely important development for obstetric services in particular and has yet to reach full potential. Remote obstetric units make this approach more difficult but by no means impossible.

Intensive Care 2000–02

In contrast to many of the other chapters in this Report, intensive care is usually a consequence, rather than a cause, of serious illness and death. As in previous Reports approximately one in three of all maternal deaths have some involvement with intensive care; a detailed analysis of the causes of death in mothers admitted to intensive care has not been included in this chapter, as it is difficult to draw meaningful conclusions from such data. Either an increase or a decrease in admissions from a particular cause could represent an improvement in the quality of care, and in common with many other chapters denominator data are required.

Recognising sick women

A recurring issue in a significant number of women referred to intensive care is an apparent delay in the recognition of the severity of their illness. Accepting that it always easier with hindsight to recognise serious illness earlier, there are nonetheless a number of cases in which readily recognisable signs of significant physiological abnormality were either missed or ignored.

Young, previously fit pregnant women have significant physiological reserve in most major organ systems. They make use of some of this reserve to survive the stresses of normal pregnancy but it is evident that a considerable amount remains unused. The effect of this is to mask the physiological signs of a number of important pathological conditions, most notably hypovolaemia and systemic sepsis. A modest tachycardia, mild hypotension and warm well-perfused peripheries are all normal signs in late pregnancy but are also the signs of sepsis. There is no absolute method of distinguishing these in the early phase but a high index of suspicion must be maintained if serious illness is to be diagnosed and treated in time.

Many of the woman went on to become critically ill were tachypnoeic before they deteriorated. This has been described previously and is an important sign worthy of extensive investigation in every case. Pulse oximetry is universally available and any sustained reduction in saturation should be investigated with arterial blood gas analysis. A metabolic acidosis is a serious, always significant, sign and should never be ignored.

Communication issues continue to figure in women becoming unexpectedly critically ill and diagnosis and treatment may be delayed in women from ethnic minorities. Stoicism combined with significant physiological reserve further exacerbates the recognition of impending critical illness. In a small number of cases, significant physiological disturbance appears to have been attributed to anxiety and cultural differences, with tragic sequelae.

Medical student and junior doctor training programmes have started to appreciate the need for improved training in the recognition and management of the acutely sick and deteriorating patient as a separate entity to the management of cardiac arrests.[10,11] The relative rarity of such women presenting to obstetric services makes the need for effective education and training at all levels, from the most junior healthcare assistant through to senior consultant staff, an important area for improvement.

Early referral and outreach

In some cases, women presented with catastrophic life-threatening disease and were appropriately referred and transferred to an intensive care unit after resuscitation and stabilisation. There were, however, some cases in which the involvement of intensive care and eventual transfer was much delayed.

Early referral and involvement of the intensive care consultant from the start is essential. Most intensive care units in the UK operate at very high bed occupancy rates, often in excess of 90%. The effect of this is to reduce the chance of an intensive care unit having an empty bed for any unexpected emergency. Some units still reserve a bed for 'in-house' emergencies and the case may need to be made at a senior level if this bed is to be released. Early consultant-to-consultant referral also facilitates decisions about discharging or transferring other patients to make space. There can be few patients more deserving of efforts to make a bed than the critically sick mother.

In a small number of cases, women with significant coexisting cardiac disease, for example, the need for an intensive care bed could have been predicted prior to their delivery. Here, a bed must be booked in advance and a management plan agreed between intensive care, obstetric, anaesthetic and cardiology consultants. Bed booking and subsequent cancellation of major surgery is an all too common activity on busy intensive care units. The situation is clearly different here and intensive care units must appreciate that the bed will be required irrespective of other pressures from in-house emergencies and other reasons.

The level of support provided between delivery and eventual admission to an intensive care unit varied enormously between cases. A feature, by no means confined to obstetric emergencies, is that referral to intensive care is almost seen as a treatment in itself and the support provided while waiting for admission is often left to very inexperienced staff.

There is, however, little that is done on an intensive care unit that cannot be performed in an obstetric theatre. Invasive monitoring should be available in all obstetric theatres and the anaesthetists and assistants who work there should be conversant with its use. Intensive care staff are, however, much more comfortable with the use of inotropic infusions, measurements of cardiac output and so on, and so need to be involved as early as possible. Arterial blood gases, haemoglobin levels, electrolytes and clotting profiles all change rapidly in these women and should be taken at regular intervals.

Early involvement of the intensive care consultant should allow for earlier, more effective use of advanced support measures. Increasingly intensive care units are staffing outreach teams and, where available, these can supply invaluable support to the stabilisation of patients prior to transfer. There were several cases in which women deteriorated very rapidly immediately after admission to the intensive care unit requiring emergency intubation and ventilation. While unavoidable in some cases, this does support the view that patients can deteriorate significantly while waiting for transfer. Consideration should be given to elective intubation and ventilation for transfer, done early this will allow for a period of stabilisation in the operating theatre prior to transfer. Obstetric theatres are well equipped to manage difficult intubations, most intensive care units are not; these patients may seriously challenge the intubating abilities of junior intensive care staff, not all of whom have anaesthetic training.

Massive haemorrhage

The management of major blood loss is discussed in a number of other chapters in this Report. Nevertheless, it remains an important event leading up to some of the intensive care unit admissions reported. Significant blood loss is not a rare event in an obstetric theatre and yet there still appears to be areas for improvement in management. Significant blood loss leads to a disastrous fall in oxygen delivery to mitochondria both from the reduction in capillary blood flow and from the reduced oxygen content as the haemoglobin falls. The effects of this in some patients is to trigger the immuno-inflammatory cascade; if intense this cascade may lead to the acute respiratory distress syndrome, acute renal failure and a cardiovascular collapse identical to that seen in severe systemic sepsis.

The conventional management of severe haemorrhage has been questioned recently in the setting of out-of-hospital trauma and has led to a set of recommendations from the National Institute for Clinical Excellence (NICE).[12] Although clearly not intended for use in the bleeding obstetric patient, the physiological basis for the recommendations may prove to be highly relevant.

Evidence from a number of sources suggests that excessive resuscitation with either crystalloid or non-blood colloids may increase the mortality from severe haemorrhage. Faced with significant blood loss the body responds with a number of well-intentioned physiological manoeuvres. Increased sympathetic tone and the release of endogenous catecholamines lead to an appropriate tachycardia in an attempt to maintain cardiac output and intense vasoconstriction diverting blood towards vital organs. From simple physics, the fall in blood pressure both in the arterial and venous circulations reduces the loss of blood from damaged vessels. Clearly, if haemorrhage continues then death from hypovolaemic cardiac arrest will occur.

Transfusing readily available sodium containing crystalloids or non-blood colloids seems an attractive solution and has been widely practised in a variety of arenas, including during obstetric emergencies. The physiological effects of this approach are, however, more complex; restoring circulating volume in this way produces a reassuring rise in blood pressure and a reduction in heart rate. Unfortunately, however, the oxygen carrying capacity of the circulating blood is seriously reduced and oxygen delivery to the tissues will not be restored leaving mitochondria profoundly hypoxic. In addition, the clotting factors in the blood become rapidly diluted leading to further haemorrhage from small vessels and the restoration of arterial and venous pressures will encourage further blood loss from larger vessels. This, in turn, leads to a vicious cycle of events and the effects are compounded.

The NICE recommendations for out-of-hospital trauma are intended to reduce this effect by restricting the amount of non-blood fluid that is given prior to admission. Is this relevant to obstetric emergencies? In the usual situation in which only a small amount of crossmatched blood is available and clotting products may be an hour away then the similarities are apparent. There is no ideal solution but the emphasis should be placed on stopping the bleeding at the earliest opportunity and restoring haemoglobin levels and clotting as early as possible. Trauma anaesthetists are having to learn to anaesthetise patients who are still significantly hypovolaemic so that the sites of blood loss can be controlled before circulating blood volume is restored with transfusions of blood and clotting factors. Anaesthesia for the bleeding obstetric patient is a highly skilled task and senior anaesthetic help must be obtained as early as possible. Several pairs of hands are needed to manage the case properly.

In many of the women admitted to the intensive care unit after severe haemorrhage a marked coagulopathy was still present. It is still common to see clotting factors being withheld until the results from a clotting screen are available; in the presence of significant blood loss, the delay caused by waiting for these results combined with the delay in obtaining and defrosting fresh frozen plasma will lead to a serious dilutional coagulopathy.

In at least one reported case, simple organisational problems led to a protracted delay in obtaining blood and blood products and there is much to recommend the development of in-house, scenario-based training for the management of severe haemorrhage within the obstetric theatre. In particular, the delays involved in getting blood and blood products actually to the patient need to be built in to the scenario, so that these are ordered much earlier. It is not possible to tell from the records provided how often fluids are being warmed prior to infusion but again it is still common to see large volumes of cold fluids being administered. The relatively high frequency of cardiac arrest following induction of anaesthesia may, in part, be due to this.

The emphasis must be placed on stopping the bleeding and senior surgical input, if necessary from a consultant vascular surgeon, must be obtained as early as possible. It may be necessary to temporarily control the bleeding by pressure alone until more experienced help arrives and until blood and blood products and a blood warmer are available.

Accident and emergency departments

A significant number of women admitted to intensive care came through accident and emergency departments rather than from obstetric units. Almost without exception, the management of cardiac arrest within accident and emergency units was excellent and pays tribute to the highly successful implementation of Advanced Life Support training. In the non-arrested patient, however, the situation is far less satisfactory. Other chapters have alluded to the poor management of these women by some accident and emergency departments and it is apparent in those admitted to intensive care that some accident and emergency departments continue to miss serious illness in the pregnant patient or to put abnormal physical signs down to pregnancy alone.

Pulmonary embolus

The difficulties in diagnosing pulmonary embolus are not exclusive to obstetric patients but there are still cases in which the diagnosis should have been excluded or confirmed much earlier. Pulmonary embolus remains a life-threatening condition, which tends not to be taken seriously enough. Urgent steps should be taken to confirm or exclude the diagnosis including high resolution spiral computed tomography scanning, pulmonary angiography and echocardiography, as available. The management of a significant pulmonary embolus remains a complex and controversial process and death, primarily from right ventricular failure, remains an all too common sequel. Early anticoagulation is essential if further emboli are to be prevented and consideration should be given to thrombolysis if possible. If significant clots can be demonstrated in the lower limbs or inferior vena cava then expert advice about the use of umbrellas etc should be sought.

Intensive care: key learning points

- Abnormal physical signs are masked in young people due to physiological reserve; this reserve is increased further during the second and third trimester.

- Tachypnoea is an important sign of serious illness and should always be investigated.

- Just because someone cannot speak English does not mean that they are not seriously ill.

- Referral to the intensive care unit is not of itself a treatment. Early intensive care admission will not cure everybody but delays cannot help.

- The variable management of massive haemorrhage in obstetric theatres continues and delays still exist in getting senior help: surgical, anaesthesia and pairs of hands. There is also failure to take account of the delay in getting blood and blood products, especially in remote sites and women still arrive on intensive care with severe dilutional coagulopathies. There is a need to practice major haemorrhage drill in obstetric units and it is likely that the theory behind the National Institute for Clinical Excellence (NICE) guidelines for management of 'out-of hospital haemorrhage' will be relevant in obstetric haemorrhage as well.[12]

Conclusions

This Report only deals with mothers who have died and so inevitably gives a distorted view of what can be achieved by modern intensive care. In many cases, detailed records of outstanding intensive care were provided and yet death was still the final outcome. There were also cases in which little or no information was available about the intensive care provided. This is inexcusable and inevitably raises questions about the quality of intensive care actually provided.

Fortunately less than 1:1,000 mothers will end up in intensive care but they still represent an important and challenging group of patients. Often young, previously well and unexpected admissions, these women are very stressful to care for and are not unlike young trauma victims in their effect on intensive care staff, especially when they die.

Mothers who become brainstem dead, usually from intracerebral disasters, can donate organs and it is very encouraging to see this either occurring or at least being discussed.

Intensive care and obstetric units are often remote from each other and present a significant challenge to shared care processes. Obstetric patients on intensive care often need continuing obstetric and midwifery input throughout their stay and arrangements for this should be discussed proactively.

The tragedy of an avoidable death is all too apparent in this Report, none more so than from airway management disasters under general anaesthesia. Intensive care has come a long way in 50 years but it has a long way still to go. We continue to introduce new therapies; the recent introduction of activated protein-C into the treatment of severe sepsis is an exciting step with obvious relevance to maternal deaths.

Even with excellent management and early referral and admission, we still cannot cure all patients, especially those with multi-organ failure from severe sepsis. Despite this, delays in referral, inadequate resuscitation and the late recognition of severe illness cannot be expected to improve survival.

References

1. [www.ics.ac.uk/downloads/icshistory.pdf].
2. Bradley RD. Diagnostic right heart catheterisation with miniature catheters in severely ill patients. *Lancet* 1964; 2: 941–2.
3. Swan HJ, Ganz W, Forrester J, Marcus H, Diamond G, Chonette D. Catheterization of the heart in man with use of a flow-directed balloon-tipped catheter, *N Engl J Med* 1970; 283: 447–51.
4. Harken DE. Presentation at the International College of Cardiology, Brussels, Belgium, 1958.
5. Bregman D, Casarella WJ. Percutaneous intraaortic balloon pumping: Initial clinical experiences. *Ann Thorac Surg* 1981; 29: 153–5.
6. [www.cesar-trial.org/].
7. Knaus WA, Zimmerman JE, Wagner DP, Draper EA, Lawrence DE. APACHE: acute physiology and chronic health evaluation: a physiologically based classification system. *Crit Care Med* 1981; 9: 591–7.
8. [www.rcoa.ac.uk/ibticm/].
9. Department of Health. *Comprehensive Critical Care: A Review of Adult Critical Care Services.* London: DoH; 2000 [www.doh.uk/nhsexec/compcritcare.htm].
10. [www.rcseng.ac.uk/ewtd/earlywarning_html].
11. Stenhouse C, Coates S, Tivey M, Allsop P, Parker T, Prospective evaluation of a modified early warning score to aid earlier detection of patients developing critical illness on a surgical ward. *Br J Anaesth* 2000; 84: 663P.
12. [www.nice.org.uk/pdf/ta074guidance.pdf].

CHAPTER 18

Issues for midwives

KATE SALLAH on behalf of the Editorial Board

Introduction

This chapter highlights the issues that have arisen in this Report which relate to the care and services for pregnant or recently delivered women that are provided by midwives. Although, in the majority of deaths, midwifery practice did not directly contribute to the woman's loss of life, there are still many examples of what indirect effects midwives can have on influencing care and outcomes. There were also a number of examples of truly outstanding midwifery care.

The aim of this chapter is to stimulate debate on what lessons can be learned from the management of the women who died during this triennium, 2000–02, and how midwives can further help in the development of maternity services to improve the health of all pregnant women and their babies. In England, the findings of this Report are particularly timely, as they coincide with the publication of the National Service Framework for Maternal and Child Health, which gives impetus both to design and implement maternity services that equally meet the needs of all pregnant women and places an increasing emphasis on midwifery-led care.[1]

This chapter cannot provide an exhaustive overview of all the key findings and recommendations contained within this Report and, although many midwives will want to read the whole Report, all should read and act on the findings and recommendations contained both in this chapter and:

- highlighted in Chapter 1, which details the overall risk factors for maternal deaths and the underlying rationale for many of the recommendations made here

- given in the summary of key overall recommendations and those for the management of particular conditions provided at the start of this Report, and

- provided in Chapter 11 and Chapter 14 relating to psychiatric illness, drug and/or alcohol misuse and domestic violence.

Summary of overall key findings for 2000–02

- The maternal mortality rate for both *Indirect* and *Direct* causes of death shows a slight increase for this triennium as compared with the last Report, although this is not statistically significant.

- As with the previous Report, the overall maternal death rate for *Indirect* causes of death is higher than for deaths from *Direct* causes.

- The most common cause of *Direct* deaths was again thromboembolism, the rates for which remain largely unchanged since 1997–99. There have been increases in the mortality rates from haemorrhage and those associated with anaesthesia and no significant decreases in deaths from other causes. There was no under-reporting of these deaths.

- The most common cause of *Indirect* deaths, and the largest cause of maternal deaths overall, was psychiatric illness, although not all of these were reported to the Enquiry and many were identified from linkage with the Office for National Statistics (ONS) as discussed later in this chapter. Cardiac disease remains the second most common cause and most of these cases were reported to the Enquiry.

Summary of risk factors for maternal deaths

Social disadvantage

Women living in families where both partners were unemployed, many of whom had features of social exclusion, were up to 20 times more likely to die than women from the more advantaged groups. In addition, single mothers were three times more likely to die than those in stable relationships.

Poor communities

Women living in the most deprived areas of England had a 45% higher death rate compared with women living in the most affluent areas.

Minority ethnic groups

Women from ethnic groups other than White were, on average, three times more likely to die than White women. Black African women, including asylum seekers and newly arrived refugees, had a mortality rate seven times higher than White women and had major problems in accessing maternal health care.

Late booking or poor attendance

Twenty percent (50) of the women who died from *Direct* or *Indirect* causes booked for maternity care after 22 weeks of gestation or had missed over four routine antenatal visits.

Obesity

Thirty-five percent (78) of the all women who died were obese: 50% more than in the general population.

Domestic violence

Fourteen percent (51) of all the women who died self-declared that they were subject to violence in the home.

Substance abuse

Eight percent (31) of all the women who died were substance misusers.

Suboptimal clinical care

Sixty-seven percent of the 261 women who died from *Direct* and *Indirect* causes were considered to have some form of suboptimal clinical care.

Lack of interprofessional and/or inter-agency communications

In many cases, the care provided to the women who died was hampered by a lack of crossdisciplinary working. There were a number of cases in which crucial clinical information, which may have affected the outcome, was not passed from the general practitioner to the midwifery or obstetric services at booking or shared between consultants in other specialties, including staff in accident and emergency departments and the obstetric team. There were also cases where significant information, particularly regarding a risk of self-harm and child safety, were not shared between the health and social services.

Summary of findings and recommendations in relation to midwifery practice

Antenatal care

Key finding
In some instances the clinical antenatal care provided did not follow best practice guidance or meet the needs of individual women. There were also many examples of poor follow-up arrangements for women known to be at higher risk of medical or complex social problems who found it difficult or hard to attend arranged antenatal appointments.

Recommendations
- The National Institute for Clinical Excellence (NICE) for England and Wales, has recently produced evidence-based clinical guidelines for the management of antenatal care for healthy pregnant women, which also supports the development of individual care plans to meet each women's own needs.[2] NICE has also recently published guidelines for caesarean section[3] and are in the process of producing guidelines for the management of intrapartum and postnatal care. All NHS health professionals, including midwives, should include the recommendations from these guidelines, or their other country equivalents, as a routine part of clinical practice.

- Many of the women in this Report found it difficult to access or to maintain access with the services and follow-up for those who failed to attend was poor. Midwives have an important role in ensuring that local maternity services reach and maintain contact will all pregnant women. It is important that women who find it difficult to attend appointments should be actively followed up. This may require imaginative solutions in terms of the timing and setting for antenatal clinics and the provision of outreach services. As a large number of women appear to change their address during pregnancy, the midwife should re confirm contact details at every consultation.

- Women with complex pregnancies and who receive care from a number of specialists or agencies should receive the support and advocacy of a known midwife throughout their pregnancy. Her midwife will help with promoting the normal aspects of pregnancy and birth as well as supporting and advocating for the woman through the variety of services she is being offered. Midwives should be able to directly refer women they are concerned about to a consultant obstetrician or other specialist.

- Flexible programmes of care should be based on available evidence with clear protocols agreed and communicated across acute and primary care settings. These should include the early detection and management of pre-eclampsia, other medical or psychiatric needs and social problems. These may result in referrals for specialist medical and psychiatric care as well as liaison with social services, other local government services and the voluntary sector.

- Midwives should advocate for professional interpreters to be provided for women who do not speak English. The use of family members, including children and partners as interpreters, should be avoided if at all possible.

At booking

Key finding
Women who booked late appeared to have increased risks of complications and maternal mortality. Other women had an inadequate initial risk assessment and therefore inadequate care planning, of whom some were booked for midwifery-led care although risk factors clearly indicated the need for their care to be shared with an obstetrician and other specialist medical or social services.

Recommendations
- At booking, a risk and needs assessment should take place to ensure every woman will be offered the type of care that most suits her own particular requirements. This chapter contains the key recommendations made in the Report concerning women with a past history of mental illness, those who have a problem with substance misuse or who are experiencing violence at home.

- Women should be encouraged to book at the earliest opportunity. Midwives should explore ways of educating hard to reach, vulnerable women to book as soon as they suspect or are aware of their pregnancy.

- Booking provides a unique opportunity for midwives to advise and support women on developing healthy lifestyles as mothers and their partners are often most receptive to health messages at this time. Midwives will need to ensure they are up to date with current health promotional information and can utilise the skills of other specialist staff to obtain the best outcomes for woman and baby; for example, smoking cessation services.

- Midwives must apply clear risk assessment criteria when booking women for midwifery-led care. These criteria should not only relate to the identification of women who by virtue of their medical or previous obstetric history may be at higher risk of complications but also those women with complex social needs. Particular attention should be taken in those cases where women have poor knowledge of, or difficulty in communicating, their previous obstetric or medical history. Where English is not the woman's first language independent interpreting services should be planned and used.

- Pregnant women with significant problem drug and/or alcohol use may have other social problems and their care should reflect this. They should not be managed in isolation but by maternity services that are part of a wider multi-agency network, which should include both addiction and social services.

- Women with problems with substance misuse, mental illness or known domestic violence and their babies also require close multidisciplinary follow-up in the postnatal period.

- The strengthening or development of robust and effective communication systems to increase interdisciplinary working will help to address some of the problems identified in this Report. Part of this should include ensuing all relevant information is passed between the midwife, the obstetric or other professional staff, the woman's GP and local social services, if appropriate. This will help to provide a full health and social profile on which to base the most appropriate care plan for the individual woman. Midwives should access and have direct access to the woman's GP's records for details of any previous medical, psychiatric or social history that may have a bearing on the type of care she should receive during and after her pregnancy. It is not fair on the woman to expect her to relay all such information and there are a number of cases in this Report where, should such background information have been provided, the care plan and outcome may have been different.

- All mothers should have their body mass index (BMI) calculated and recorded at booking. This should then lead to a full risk assessment and advice for women with BMI scores over 30 (the definition of obesity as described in Chapter 1). Obese women will require additional advice and information on managing their increased risks of deep vein thrombosis and pulmonary embolism, diabetes and any intercurrent cardiac or other conditions. A full family medical history taken at booking is also important for the risk management of these women. Due to the heightened maternal risk associated with obesity it is advised that very obese women with a BMI of, or greater than, 35 may be unsuitable for entirely midwifery-led antenatal care and should be recommended to give birth in a consultant unit with appropriate emergency facilities on hand should they be required.

  The risk assessment should also include an accurate weight recording so that hospital equipment (such as operating tables and overhead hoists) can be checked for their weight-bearing capacity. Where the weight capacity of the equipment does not match the woman's requirements, alternative plans must be made to hire specialist equipment for any pending admissions and/or birth.

- Midwives need adequate education and training on perinatal mental health, domestic violence, substance abuse and child protection issues both during their preregistration and continuing professional development to ensure that they have the knowledge and skills to perform the appropriate assessment in the antenatal period.

- As a contribution to improving assessment and providing support or information, all women should be routinely asked if they have previously or currently experienced domestic violence. Such systematic enquires should only be undertaken once midwives have received the appropriate training and local multidisciplinary support services are in place.

As this is a sensitive area, midwives should stress the routine nature of the question and the reasons for approaching the subject. It may be that abused women may not wish to discuss their circumstances at this stage but the midwife should demonstrate an open approach to encourage contact as the pregnancy develops, giving the woman opportunity for individual and confidential support when required. This should include opportunities for the woman to meet with the midwife without the presence of her partner and providing links with other statutory and non statutory organisations.

- Midwives should also ask all women about their consumption of alcohol, cigarettes and use of prescribed or recreational drugs. Although these have a strong correlation with social exclusion factors, it is important to note that many more affluent groups are increasingly viewing this as normal recreational behaviour.

As an individual practitioner

Key finding
The midwives who contributed to this Report often acknowledged gaps in services that prevented or delayed appropriate care. This was a particular issue in the development of care plans for women with complex needs or chaotic lifestyles.

Recommendations
- Midwives need to be at the forefront of service design to ensure that appropriate skills, knowledge and expertise are available to meet women's changing needs. This will require midwives to examine their own role and develop new ways of working in collaboration with other staff groups and local communities to the benefit of women in their care.

- Where gaps in the skills or knowledge base of local midwives are identified, heads of midwifery will need to develop local training programmes in conjunction with other professional and educational colleagues and provide time for midwives to attend.

- Midwives, as professionals, are responsible for their continuing professional development and so should adopt a lifelong learning approach to their care provision. This will require commitment to seek new knowledge and evidence through research and audit in order to challenge existing paradigms of care.

- Midwives may need to be aware of their professional obligations and limitations as they develop services to meet the needs of the most disadvantaged groups. Where medical intervention is required but either is not available through current care systems or is against the women's wishes, the midwife should seek alternative routes to ensure provision of appropriate care. In some cases, this may require the development of more flexible antenatal care systems and access to medical services; for instance, arranging home visits by obstetricians or using family, friends or religious leaders to influence compliance with care plans. In these complex cases it is essential that the midwife has close contact with her statutory supervisor of midwives.

- Midwives should be fully conversant with statutory supervision of their care provision and use this mechanism in their everyday practice. Supervisors of midwives should be supportive of practitioners delivering care within current service pressures and receptive to their needs following tragic outcomes such as maternal deaths.

General lessons to be learned from the findings for 2000–02 as they apply to midwifery practice

Although midwifery practice did not directly contribute to many women's deaths, there are still lessons that can be dawn from the findings. There were also a number of examples of truly outstanding midwifery care.

As midwives are often the most senior professionals having initial contact with pregnant women, it is vital that they have the skills to assess and communicate risk and support women in all aspects of the progress of their pregnancy, whether this be normal or complicated. With the additional challenges of deprivation, poverty and difficulty in accessing services, the midwife may often be the only professional who is able to build an element of trust with the woman, even when risk factors clearly indicate the need for medical intervention. In this triennial Report, this is of even greater importance owing to the increase in refugees and asylum seekers requiring the use of maternity services.

Deciding which women may be appropriate for midwifery-led care was a key factor in this Report and some women received inappropriate midwifery-led care. It is important to recognise that some women presenting with social and medical complexities are often those who do not feel able to seek or actively resist medical advice, and may rely in the midwife to act as their advocate through the services.

Pressures such as national shortages of practising midwives, the reduction in junior doctors' hours and changes in medical training will continue to challenge NHS professionals and managers alike as NHS modernisation progresses. However, with these challenges also come opportunities to review current service provision and explore what workforce and skills will be required to deliver the desired changes. Women as service users will need to be closely involved in service development to ensure their perspective of good care provision is adequately reflected in future service design.

Midwifery involvement in this Enquiry is increasing, with comments and lessons learned being documented by midwives at all stages of the process. In many instances, midwives have played a major part in the organisational review of cases as part of the Trust's risk management and clinical governance strategies. There are some exemplary records from midwives who demonstrate through their accounts the need to reflect on their practice and learn from their experiences. However, in some cases this commitment was sadly lacking with midwives contributing very little or no insight into the events leading to the woman's death.

Overall themes

Several key themes emerged as a result of the detailed midwifery assessments of the maternal deaths which occurred during 2000–02. These themes for midwifery practice are similar to those in the last Report. However, evidence of the new challenges posed by workforce and training shortfalls is also apparent. The main themes are:

- **developing care to meet individual needs**: this means addressing inequalities, both in terms of enabling all women to access high quality maternity services as well as improving maternal and perinatal outcomes. Particularly in relation to:
  - the socially excluded, including women who live in poverty and/or areas of deprivation

- women from minority ethnic groups
- women who live with obesity
- mental health concerns
- drug and/or alcohol use
- domestic violence

- **communication**
- **professional accountability**
- **challenges for future care delivery and improvement**.

Developing care to meet individual needs

Deprivation and social exclusion
This Report has highlighted yet again the stark differences in maternal death rates between women living in comfortable circumstances compared with those who were economically and/or socially excluded.

Many of the most vulnerable women did not access or feel able to maintain access with maternity care services. This was in some instances due to violence in the home, previous mental illness or drug or alcohol abuse but was also linked to ethnicity, particularly for recent arrivals as immigrants or refugees. However, there were some cases where women with financial stability also did not regularly attend for care as they were victims of physical abuse in the home or had problems with substance misuse.

Women with complex social needs require a comprehensive history taken at booking with GPs, midwives and social services sharing relevant information of the woman's background. As part of multidisciplinary and multi-agency working midwives will need to be aware of the range and types of service provision in their localities, how these may benefit women in their care and to be able to refer women to them as required. Some women who died attended local addiction services or local social services but there appeared to be no record of this at booking or throughout the pregnancy. Indeed, in some cases, it appeared that the midwife had little or no knowledge of other crucial factors in the woman's pregnancy including substance abuse or issues relating to child protection.

Midwives can and often are key players in addressing these wider issues as they impact on the woman's health. However, more needs to be done. Ensuring better inter-agency links and communications may require the development of new roles to meet these women's needs and to help support midwives in their professional role. The development of different care providers can also assist in the regeneration of local communities, as local people can become involved in providing support and friendship. One way in which this can be achieved, as suggested also in the National Service Framework,[1] is through the development of integrated care pathways for vulnerable women and their families. Local women and health professionals, including midwives, should help in their design.

Minority ethnic groups
Women from minority ethnic groups are again over represented in this Report. There is a particular risk for those women who are new to this country and who have little or no

command of the English language. There were several cases where women who were unable to communicate their symptoms were not provided with prompt and appropriate treatment. This also applied to poor history-taking at booking where women could not communicate relevant medical or obstetric histories either through lack of interpreting services, knowledge, and understanding or perhaps fears. Regardless of the recommendations made in previous Reports, there were still some instances where family members were used as interpreters. This was a particular issue in localities where minority ethnic groups made up a small percentage of the local population or where services had not been able to respond quickly enough to a changing ethnic mix.

Cultural beliefs and practices also played a part in adverse outcomes, as demonstrated by the following vignette:

> A woman who died of a pulmonary embolism made clear her intention to rest in bed for 1 month post-delivery. Although the midwife provided her and her family with advice about the risks of deep vein thrombosis and pulmonary embolism, it would appear that the woman's traditional belief, which on investigation did not accord with those of her religious leader, proved stronger than Western medicine.

Many cultures mark the first month following childbirth as a significant time for women to recuperate after childbirth enhancing her wellbeing and that of her baby. However, in some cultures this is wrapped in mystique, religious belief and traditional practices. In reality, it is a time when the needs of mother and baby are central to family life to ensure they are free from external stresses and distractions. Several cultures believe the mother and baby should remain indoors and rest for the whole month, while some Chinese traditionalists also believe that the mother should stay in bed as much as possible to assist in straightening the back bone after carrying the baby for nine months.[9] These practices would not be seen as efficacious with current medical knowledge of the risks of deep vein thrombosis. However, although these traditional beliefs may be hard to define they should not be generalised as being linked to any one religious group or nationality as the reality may be much more to do with folklore linked to the individual family and birthplace. Therefore, midwives should make every effort to ascertain such traditions in the antenatal period and clarify the woman's intentions to rest following the birth of the baby. Where the mother and her family decline advice on the benefits of mobilisation this must be respected and prophylactic measures incorporated into the individual woman's care plan.

Interpreting services

Women who spoke little or no English seemed to be at increased risk due to poor history-taking and the reliance of family and friends to communicate their needs. The following two cases act as examples of the consequences of this:

> A woman who spoke no English relied fully on her husband to interpret throughout her labour. However, when a spinal anaesthetic was required prior to a caesarean section her husband did not feel able to attend. This resulted in an extremely frightening time for the patient, the need for general anaesthesia, a failed intubation and subsequent cardiac arrest. The case, however, was fully reviewed by the Trust and an excellent report with action plan produced.

The key action points included the following:

- Reviewing the use of women's relatives as interpreters, especially where clear instructions are required in an emotionally pressured situation.

- Developing systems and protocols for accessing appropriate independent interpreters.

- Raising staff awareness and understanding of cultural issues.

Similar issues were raised with a newly arrived immigrant who spoke no English and relied upon her family to interpret. She booked very late and no medical history was disclosed. She was booked for low-risk midwifery-led care in an isolated unit. No medical examination appears to have been undertaken by either the midwife or the GP who referred her. During labour, a high systolic blood pressure and tachycardia were noted and an ECG requested. However, this was not undertaken, nor was her pulse checked in the postnatal period. She subsequently died of severe pre-existing cardiac disease.

Even if she had known of any existing cardiac problems or previous family history, she may not have wanted to disclose this information for her personal desire to become a mother to conform to her role in her wider family. She may also have had a lack of understanding of the significance of her cardiac disease in pregnancy. There are several examples of such cases in preceding Report of this Enquiry.

With hindsight, this woman would have benefited from a full medical examination and having her care and delivery managed in a consultant-led unit for ease of specialist referral and further investigations. Indeed, this should probably be the standard for all women booking with an unclear medical history. With regard to interpreters, again, an independent service with clinical and cultural understanding may have identified any risks and helped with further advice.

There were a number of other complex cases where women with pre-existing medical and psychological conditions required additional clinical and social support. In many of these the midwives were, in hindsight, able to reorganise local service provision as the helpful reflection from one midwife involved such a case included the following statement: "I realise now just how important it is to provide specialist care to vulnerable groups. Perhaps more support in the community could have been arranged to help the client with her family. This area is now a Sure Start area".

These cases highlight the need for midwives to view women in context of their lives, not just their pregnancy, and to develop services to meet these needs.

Trusts that have small minority ethnic populations may experience more difficulties in providing responsive interpreting and link worker services. This may be due to a limited number of local interpreters to recruit from or the growing diversity of languages required. All healthcare providers will need to review changes in immigration patterns and review their local needs on a regular basis to ensure availability of appropriate language skills and cultural knowledge.

Following up women who failed to attend antenatal clinics
The active follow-up of women who failed to attend antenatal care was an issue in a number of cases. Although most maternity services have follow up procedures for women who do not or are unable to attend antenatal appointments, these are often not robust enough or are seen to take up too much scarce midwifery time. What the findings of this Report show is that among the women who died there was a high rate of non-attendance in the socially excluded and minority ethnic groups. This may reflect the fact that these women considered the current services were unapproachable or did not reflect their perceived wishes. The reasons for this may vary but it is clear that in some areas the existing, often long-held, patterns of service provision do not meet the needs of these women and are unable to attract them to seek care in the first place or to want them to maintain contact with services. Therefore, women from all groups who find it difficult to use the current services should be fully involved in the design of services to meet their needs. This is likely to challenge some current patterns of service delivery and lead to more flexibility and ease of access to ante natal care. In addition, health information about the importance and availability of different models of antenatal care should be reviewed for appropriateness, format and accessibility.

Advocacy
Where services are not meeting the medical or cultural needs of women midwives should act as advocates for their clients and ensure that appropriate services are delivered, interpreting services are available and cross organisational communications are of the highest standard. The need for this appeared a number of times in several of the cases reviewed, where midwives may have made a difference to the outcome if they had voiced their obvious concerns. The following is an example:

> A pregnant woman was in obvious pain and distress but unable to communicate due to her limited understanding of English. Although the midwives were concerned and raised these with junior medical staff, her care plan remained unchanged. The midwives could see that the woman's condition deteriorating but took no further action. She died shortly afterwards.

In instances like these, where language is a real barrier, midwives should either call for appropriate and urgent interpreting services to get a clear history of symptoms and or report up to a higher level of medical authority. Midwives must feel confident and enabled to contact a consultant obstetrician or anaesthetist directly when they are concerned their professional expertise is not being heeded.

Recommendations for midwives caring for women newly arrived in the UK and/or those who are unable to speak English

Midwives should:

- ensure that all pregnant women recently arrived in the UK have a full health screen as part of the booking process

- advise shared midwife/consultant-led care where the woman's medical history is vague or absent, or if there is any index of suspicion that she may be unwell

- err on the side of caution and investigate further or refer for a medical opinion when women cannot communicate their degree of illness or describe their pain levels

- act as advocates for women to ensure the appropriate investigations, treatment and care are delivered

- ensure that care plans reflect the cultural and traditional beliefs of the individual as far as known

- Help in assessing the needs of the local population for interpreting services and link workers

- help with the development of strategies to ensure 24-hours-a-day, 7-days-a-week access to interpreting services.

Obesity

In this Report, over 35% of the women who died were obese (estimated as having a BMI of greater than 30), representing a disproportionate number of deaths associated with obesity in childbearing women. Obese women of every age died from a variety of causes of maternal death because either their physical size precluded the availability of optimum care or their obesity had clinical implications for their health.

The current epidemic of obesity is of growing concern in this country as well as many other countries in the world. As described by the Office for National Statistics in Chapter 21 Trends in reproductive epidemiology, in 2002 over one-third of all women were overweight and almost one-quarter of all women were classified as obese. This is a dramatic rise from the 16% reported in a similar survey in 1993. These figures provide an indicator of future healthcare needs, the possible clinical impact of obesity on the individual and the cost to health economies. In terms of obstetric care, it is of importance not only because of the increased risks to the pregnant woman and her baby but also the expected increase in numbers of obese pregnant women as obese teenagers reach childbearing age. This requires a review of current services and risk management strategies including the provision of appropriate health education and support. The Government is currently developing strategies to tackle obesity and unhealthy lifestyles but recognises the need for cross-government working and collaboration with many other agencies. In addition, the need to increase public responsibility for health is also being highlighted.

As obesity rates rise, it will be of even greater importance to communicate health messages regarding prepregnancy weight and healthy eating during pregnancy. Health information will therefore require review, as will service provision to support women in developing healthy lifestyles and reducing weight.

A number of the women who died and were classed as obese also had elements of social exclusion, unemployment and low income. This raises the question of the affordability of a healthy diet and the effect of psychological pressures on eating patterns. Midwives need to provide advice and support to women in these situations and where necessary refer to dieticians.

The effect of obesity in pregnancy is well documented, with a range of risks for mother and baby.[5,6] However, in addition, there will be considerable impact on service delivery such as associated cost of complications and provision of specialist equipment, which includes beds, hoists and chairs.

Hospital and community risk assessment should be undertaken as part of the care plan for each obese woman. This will include accurate weight monitoring of the woman and ensuring beds, theatre tables, hoists, chairs, and so on, have the appropriate weight capacity. Where this is not the case, arrangement will need to be made to hire or purchase specialist equipment for subsequent admission or clinic examination. The following representative vignette illustrates many of the problems encountered in caring for 'super weight' women:

> Although a woman had several risk factors for a high-risk delivery in addition to her gross obesity, there seemed to be no preparation for her admission. Once in labour, it became apparent that she would require a caesarean section; however, the theatre table was not of the capacity to take her weight. This resulted in the operation being undertaken on two normal hospital beds placed side by side, which would have further increased the woman's risk and also the risk to staff. Although this, in itself, did not contribute to the woman's death, it is unacceptable not to have planned for and managed the situation more appropriately.

To ensure that the risks for severely overweight woman are reduced it is important midwives be involved in developing a care plan which includes a risk assessment for all stages of pregnancy, the birth and postnatal period. It is recommended that, owing to the increased health risks to mother and baby, obese women with a BMI of greater than 35 should be booked for shared care and delivered in a consultant obstetric unit.

Obesity: midwifery recommendations

Midwives should

- ensure that all women have their height and weight measured and their BMI calculated at booking

- encourage healthy eating in pregnancy and offer referral to a dietician

- organise the availability of appropriate equipment that can take the weight of very obese women before delivery

- advise very obese women with a (BMI of 35 or more) to book for shared care with a consultant and to deliver in a consultant unit.

Mental health

The mental health and wellbeing of women in pregnancy is pivotal to ensuring good clinical, social and other outcomes for both mother and baby and a healthy start to family life. Modern-day stresses effect many women either through their working lives, emotional situations or through elements of social exclusion. Therefore, maternity services should focus on reducing to a minimum the stress levels of pregnant women by providing support and communicating with other specialist services if necessary.

Mental illness continues to carry considerable stigma, as does the inability to cope with the everyday stresses of modern life. However, it is important that maternity service users and their families are aware of the importance of providing an accurate medical and social history to the midwife at booking. To ensure this understanding and encourage compliance, midwives must provide clear information on why the information is important and the relevance to the woman's care and future wellbeing. It may also be appropriate to include this health information in maternity services booklets and education programmes within schools and colleges.

Of the cases reviewed in Chapter 11 Deaths related to psychiatric causes, the vast majority of women had some type of social or emotional bearing on their daily lives. Emotional influences included ongoing marriage difficulties, the recent experience of stillbirth, family bereavement or termination of pregnancy. The social aspects included unemployment, being single and unsupported, drug abuse and homelessness. Additionally, 55 women were known to have had some form of mental health problem in the past or during the current pregnancy.

Several women withheld information about their mental health history and in some cases their families colluded in this. There were also examples of the families of women who did not want to take advice from professionals about the urgent need to section the woman to a place of safety under the Mental Health Act.

The lack of identification of risk, multidisciplinary service planning and intra-agency working is one of the main areas of concern identified in this Report. Another is the lack of professional knowledge and training in the area of perinatal mental health. Further, communication between organisations and sharing of patient information was often very poor and this suggests a need for reconfiguring services to meet the needs of these, often vulnerable, women.

As in previous Reports there were several women married to men serving in the Armed Forces who appeared to be very isolated. This was especially the case when living overseas, where they may experience language difficulties and have little family support. Further, and has been reported before, in some cases there was the added issue of domestic violence. Therefore, services available to these women should be reviewed and mechanisms developed to provide appropriate support and care mechanisms.

Although there is much to be learned from the deaths of women who committed suicide, as discussed in Chapter 11, there were some excellent examples of service delivery and intra agency working. These included well-planned and coordinated care across professional groups and organisations, exemplary record keeping and report writing by midwives, reflective practice with midwives and health visitors contributing to the learning outcomes for local service provision and professional practice. It is sad to note that some midwives who provided exemplary care still blamed themselves for the woman's death, although they had done everything and more to support them. Counselling or debriefing for midwives and other health professionals in these situations should be available if required.

Midwives with a specialist interest and training in the care of vulnerable women appear to be effective in streamlining services and enhancing cross-organisational communication. This was demonstrated in some cases where specialist midwives in drug abuse provided excellent continuity and support in the care for women who died but for whom the highest standard of care had been delivered and documented.

There is a need for maternity services to review their current care pathways for women with previous mental health problems. Support may also be required for women with stressful lifestyles or life events. Service reviews should include involvement of women, their families and other major stakeholders. They should also address the effectiveness and availability of specialist mother and baby units.

Links with higher education, further education and local regeneration schemes will be required to develop training, education and manpower strategies to ensure appropriate skills and staff to deliver new service design. Some women who died had little social support or service coordination to meet their needs. Midwives, health visitors and community psychiatric nurses cannot always provide support in this way owing to workload and manpower issues. However, service redesign may result in new ways of working and the development of new support roles that will fill any existing service gap. Midwives should lead these developments within the maternity services in collaboration with psychiatric professionals to identify how future generic support workers could provide effective services across current organisational boundaries while maximising professional time and skills.

It is apparent from the cases reviewed that some professionals involved in delivering maternal health services are unaware of the significance of recognised risk factors for mental illness. The pre- and post-registration curriculum for midwives, nurses and health visitors, practice nurses and community psychiatric nurses should include these aspects. It is also important that general practitioners, obstetricians and psychiatrists have similar input into their undergraduate and postgraduate training.

Mental health: recommendations for midwives

Midwives can help to provide general health education on mental health issues as they affect pregnant and the postpartum period for pregnant women and their families.

A systematic enquiry about previous psychiatric history, its severity, care received and clinical presentation should be routinely made at the antenatal booking visit.

The term 'postnatal depression' or 'PND' should not be used as a generic term for all types of psychiatric disorder. Details of previous illness should be sought and recorded including what, if any, treatment the woman had required, including medication, specialist help or inpatient treatment.

Women who have a past history of serious psychiatric disorder, postpartum or non-postpartum, should be assessed by a psychiatrist in the antenatal period. A management plan, regarding the high risk of recurrence following delivery, should be agreed with the woman and her maternity team and GP and placed in her handheld records.

Self-medication on wards should be underpinned with systems and controls, including the provision of secure bedside lockers for storage.

Obstetricians and midwives should be aware of the laws and issues that relate to child protection and when and to whom to refer if concerned.

Domestic violence

A more detailed description of the issues that emerge from this Report concerning domestic violence and the recommendations arising from them are discussed in Chapter 14. In summary, 14%, 55 of the 391 women whose deaths were assessed this triennium had either self-reported a history of domestic violence to a healthcare professional caring for them or the abuse was already known to health and social services. Domestic violence was fatal for 12 of these women. The 14% is undoubtedly an underestimate of the true prevalence of violence among this group of women as in none of the cases was a history of violence actively sought through routine questioning as part of the social or family history at booking.

The characteristics of domestic violence in relation to pregnancy were discussed in detail in an annex to this chapter in the last Report and are not repeated here. Midwives are referred to the last Report and the ever-growing more up-to-date literature on this important subject.

The findings for this triennium show that:

- all of the women who were murdered had a known history of domestic violence

- nearly 50% of the women who were murdered had low-risk midwifery-led care with no liaison between health professionals or services

- all of the women who were murdered after 20 weeks of gestation were either late bookers or poor attenders for care

- many had 'overbearing' partners who were present at all visits and were sometimes disruptive

- many women were known to social services and the local child protection team; some had all their previous children in care; one had a partner who, after her death, was found to be a Schedule One offender

- several partners had visited the family GP expressing their concerns about the woman's low self-esteem and jealousy

- some women appeared reluctant to give their address but gave mobile phone numbers instead

- several had had episodes of gonorrhoea from their partner either just before or during pregnancy

- some had histories of multiple miscarriages or unexplained vaginal bleeding in pregnancy; the reasons for this were not followed up, despite the known history of violence.

What is of critical concern is that 70% of the women whose deaths are considered in this Report and who were in abusive relationships found it difficult to access or maintain contact with antenatal care services. Over 85% of the women who were murdered or who were in violent relationships and died of *Direct* causes found it difficult to access care. The rates for late booking, poor or no attendance at all were also higher among women who were murdered or who died of *Direct* causes of maternal death.

Domestic violence: key recommendations for midwives

Enquiry about violence should be routinely included when taking a social history at booking or at another opportune point in the antenatal period. Programmes for the routine enquiry about violence must not be started until all local staff have received the appropriate training and be underpinned by a local multidisciplinary support service to whom the woman can be referred if necessary.

Where possible, all women should be seen alone at least once during the antenatal period to enable disclosure more easily if they wish.

Local trusts and community teams should develop guidelines for the identification of, and provision of further support for, these women, including developing multi-agency working, to enable appropriate referrals or provision of information on sources of further help.

Information about local sources of help and emergency help lines such as provided by Women's Aid should be displayed in suitable places in antenatal clinic, for example in the women's toilets or printed as a routine at the bottom of handheld maternity notes or cooperation cards.

Women with known significant features of domestic violence should not be re-garded as 'low risk' and should be offered multidisciplinary care in a supportive environment. If they choose midwifery-led care, the midwife should receive sup-port and advice from an experienced superior.

All health professionals should make themselves aware of the importance of domestic violence in their practice. They should adopt a non-judgemental and supportive response to women who have experienced physical, psychological or sexual abuse and must be able to give basic information to women about where to get help. They should provide continuing support, whatever decision the woman makes made concerning her future.

Drug and/or alcohol misuse

Thirty-one women who died this triennium were known to have problems with drug and/or alcohol use. The issues that arise from these cases are discussed in a new sec-tion, Chapter 11B, of this Report. Many have been counted as deaths from psychiatric disorders, or in Chapter 15 as *Late* deaths, but some died from other *Direct* or *Indirect* causes. Seventeen deaths were associated with drug use, seven with alcohol use and seven with drug and alcohol use. In nine cases, insufficient information was available to allow detailed examination.

The huge increase in problem drug use that has occurred nationally and internation-ally since the 1980s has been disproportionately large among women of childbearing age. Consequently, there has been a large increase in numbers of pregnant drug-using women. No such change has occurred in numbers of pregnant women with problem alcohol use. There is under-identification of both groups of women in maternity services. Additionally, drug-related deaths that occur within a year of pregnancy are often not identified as such and not reported as maternal deaths.

Problem drug use is usually illegal and is socially unacceptable and therefore women may be reluctant to admit to an activity that could lead to loss of custody of their child or children. Alcohol consumption is legal and socially acceptable but levels of consumption are often underestimated by pregnant women or not recognised as problematic. A further source of underestimation is the frequent failure by healthcare professionals to take an adequate history. Nevertheless, there is increasing awareness of the need to provide specialised services for such women and specialist care is increasingly provided to varying degrees in many maternity units throughout the UK. The almost trebling of numbers in the current compared with the last triennium no doubt indicates a true increase in numbers but may also reflect better identification.

Drug and/or alcohol related deaths: key recommendations for midwives

Staff providing antenatal care for pregnant women should ask sensitively, but routinely, about all substance use, prescribed and non prescribed, legal and illegal, including tobacco and alcohol.

Pregnant women with significant problem drug and/or alcohol use may have other social problems and their care should reflect this. They should not be managed in isolation but by maternity services that are part of a wider multi-agency network, which should include both addiction and social services.

Women with problems with substance misuse, and their babies, also require close multidisciplinary follow-up in the postnatal period.

Women with problem drug and/or alcohol use have potentially high-risk pregnancies and an obstetrician should supervise their management. However, most of their care can be usually be delivered by midwives.

Midwives require opportunities to update their knowledge and skills to identify substance misuse, assess its severity and refer women to specialist services.

Professional accountability

Communication

In a number of cases, poor communication of either patient need or between professionals resulted in poor care management and adverse clinical outcomes. On occasion, midwives were well placed to communicate this need and provide a coordinated approach to the necessary care plan but failed to do so. Midwives are well placed as clinical experts and equal members of the care team to challenge decision-making around effective care planning and apply their knowledge in the coordination of care, especially in emergency situations. An example of this is illustrated in the following case:

A woman with placenta praevia presented with vaginal bleeding before term. She was managed conservatively for a number of days but eventually an emergency caesarean section and an urgent blood transfusion was required. However, the crossmatched blood that had been available was found to be out of date and had been removed from storage. In this case, the urgent need for crossmatched blood was predictable at some stage during pregnancy or delivery and therefore should have been a basic requirement in this woman's care plan.

In another maternal death, the local Midwifery Assessor documents her disappointment in the standard of both written and verbal communication. She states that, although the events were unpredictable, she had serious concerns about the lack of attention to detail in the woman's care. For example, there was little evidence of contemporaneous notes, timings of events were difficult to explain, delays were apparent in recognising and communicating severity of symptoms and there was a failure to take and record appropriate observations.

If maternal deaths are to be further reduced, it is vital that communication of care needs are a high priority, if lessons are to be learned from these events it is essential that clear and accurate records are produced and maintained.

Continuing professional development

There were several instances where midwives did not appear to have the skills and knowledge required to deal with a given situation. Midwives have an individual responsibility for recognising shortfalls in their knowledge base and updating their skills as part of lifelong learning. In conjunction with this, employing authorities should facilitate the continuing professional development of midwives to enhance care delivery and clinical risk management. Statutory supervision of midwives provides a unique and independent tool to ensure safe practice and regular updating of midwives' skills. In addition, supervisors of midwives can support midwives in complex care dilemmas and in instances where poor care outcomes can be reviewed, reflected upon and lessons learned.

The future may hold many challenges for midwives, as services are redesigned and professional roles redefined. However, the most important aim must be to ensure the safest outcome of care and not the protection of professional boundaries. This point may be illustrated by the perceived shortfall of midwifery skills in postoperative care that is referred to in several cases in this Report. This was not only apparent in high-dependency or critical care situations but also more worryingly in the routine post-caesarean section care of some women. When considering preregistration and post-qualification requirements for midwives, this aspect of care must be considered of paramount importance to midwifery education and training.

Recognising deviations from the norm

Midwives are trained as practitioners in normal pregnancy, childbirth and postnatal care. However, they work in a team with other professional groups to ensure that women receive appropriate and safe care. It is therefore important that midwives use their skills and knowledge in recognising and reporting apparent deviations from the normal. In a number of cases, midwives appeared not to recognise obvious risk factors or early warning signs of ensuing complications, such as rise in blood pressure, tachycardia or a raised temperature. In some of these cases the appropriate medical care was delayed. Other women with known risk factors were sometimes inappropriately booking under midwifery-led care.

Advocacy

Midwives are perfectly placed as advocates for the safe delivery of maternity care. Not only are they skilled professionals but they are also accessible, viewed by many as approachable and have an understanding of women's needs. These attributes are particularly important to those women who are socially excluded or from minority ethnic background, as they often find accessing services more intimidating. As an advocate for women, midwives should be able to assess need and provide navigation through health and social care systems. This is of particular importance for vulnerable groups such as ethnic minority groups, lone parents and low-income groups.

In some instances in this Report, midwives appeared to have missed the opportunity to question the decisions made by other professionals and advocate for the women in their care. To achieve this, midwives must have a sound knowledge base and be able and have the confidence to voice their concerns. These concerns should also be clearly documented. Where the necessary changes fail to be made, midwives should voice their concerns higher up the line. This can be in the form of a supervisor of midwives, head of midwifery services, a senior obstetrician or the medical director of the Trust. Clear reporting mechanisms in such situations should be a major part of individual and organisational risk management strategies.

Challenges for future care delivery and improvement

Today's NHS is rapidly changing. The NHS plan sets out challenging targets for improving care and clinical outcomes but also highlights the necessity to maximise the skills and knowledge of the current workforce while recognising future manpower and skill shortages. The current shortage of healthcare professionals is well recognised. Nearly 25% of all practising midwives are aged 50 years or above.[8] Further, changes in training for junior doctors will impact on the level of skills available in clinical areas. Some of these challenges, however, can be viewed as opportunities to review custom and practice services to ensure appropriate use of skills and knowledge to meet future patient needs. There are many different initiatives now being undertaken that test new models of care and new ways of working. These initiatives require a two-pronged approach to ensure services meet individual needs of the users and to maximise the skills of an effective workforce. These include projects where the role of para-professionals are being developed, professional skills extended and local women being trained to work in their own communities as breastfeeding 'buddies'. Midwives should play an active role in the planning and design of future services for women, to ensure safe and effective practice but also to test their own paradigms of the appropriate use of their vital skills.

References

1. Department of Health, Department for Education and Skills. *National Service Framework for Children, Young People and Maternity Services.* London: DoH; 2004 [www.doh.gov.uk].

2. National Collaborating Centre for Women's and Children's Health. *Antenatal Care; Routine Care for Healthy Pregnant Women*. London: RCOG Press; 2003. [www.nice .org.uk; www.rcog.org.uk].

3. National Collaborating Centre for Women's and Children's Health. *Caesarean Section*. Clinical Guideline. London: RCOG Press; 2004[www.nice.org.uk; www.rcog .org.uk].

4. Pillsbury B. Doing the Month: Confinement and Convalescence of Chinese Women after Childbirth in Health and Disease. In: Kay MA. *Anthropology of Human Birth*. Philadelphia, PA: FA Davis; 1982.

5. Sebire NJ, Jolly M, Harris JP, Wadsworth J, Joffe M, Beard RW, *et al*. Maternal obesity and pregnancy outcome: a study of 287,213 pregnancies in London. *Int J Obes Relat Metab Disord* 2001; 25: 1175–82.

6. Galtier-Dereure F, Boegner C, Bringer J. Obesity and pregnancy: complications and cost. *Am J Clin Nutr* 2000; 71(5 Suppl): 1242S–8S.

7. Lewis G, Drife J, editors. *Why Mothers Die 1997–1999. Fifth Report of the Confidential Enquiries into Maternal Deaths in the United Kingdom*. London: RCOG Press; 2001.

8. Nursing and Midwifery Council. Data on practising midwives for 2002–2003. *Employing Nurses and Midwives* 2004; (82).

Section

6

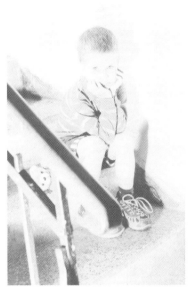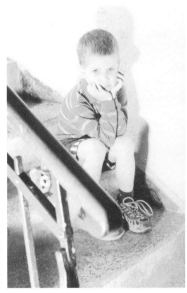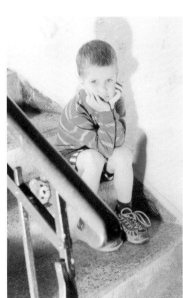

Epidemiology

CHAPTER 19

'Near misses' and severe maternal morbidity; the Scottish experience

GILLIAN PENNEY and VICTORIA BRACE on behalf of the Editorial Board

For the first time, a chapter on 'near misses' and severe maternal morbidity was included in the 1997–99 edition of this Report. That chapter outlined the rationale behind extending our traditional review of maternal deaths to include cases of severe morbidity; summarised the international literature on the topic; and described early pilot work in Scotland. In this present chapter, we describe our more recent experience with a national confidential audit of severe maternal morbidity in Scotland.

There is debate surrounding what constitutes the optimum definition of severe obstetric morbidity. The aim is to identify a group of women who were very ill and whose lives were threatened. In the international literature, the terms 'near miss' and severe morbidity are used interchangeably. We favour the latter term, as it carries no implication that the woman's life-threatening condition was due to negligence or poor care. There is also debate around the working definitions for inclusion criteria for a study of 'near miss' events. We chose to use a combination of pathophysiological (or clinically based) and management-based definitions.

Methods

The Scottish Confidential Audit of Severe Maternal Morbidity is funded by NHS Quality Improvement Scotland: the body which now has responsibility for the Scottish Maternal Deaths Enquiry. Although initiated with ring-fenced funding, the hope is to continue the Enquiry within the core funding allocated by NHS Quality Improvement Scotland to the Scottish Programme for Clinical Effectiveness in Reproductive Health.

Since October 2001, all consultant-led maternity units in Scotland have participated in data collection for this audit. We began with 22 units but, due to amalgamations or closures, the number of units has now decreased to 19. Definitions for categories of life-threatening maternal morbidity were developed from the published literature,[1–4] taking into account the views of participants. Each month, each unit reports the number of women meeting one or more of the agreed definitions to the central office of the Scottish Programme for Clinical Effectiveness in Reproductive Health. A minimal dataset on each case is collected, comprising: a unique identifier, age, date of event and limited clinical information to verify that the case definitions are being met. In the first year of national data collection these monthly returns were collated centrally and used to calculate national and unit-level rates of 'near miss' events.[5]

For the second year, and following consultation with participants, both the case definitions were refined and the number of categories was increased from 13 to 14. In addition, a case assessment pro forma relating to the most common category of 'near miss' event, severe obstetric haemorrhage, was developed. This pro forma comprised both condition-specific (that is, assessing adherence to national guidance on the management of haemorrhage) and general (that is, root-cause analysis) sections. This national pro forma was used by local clinical risk management teams during assessment of cases of severe obstetric haemorrhage. It served to guide local teams through a systematic and structured assessment of each case. The risk management teams were required to make an overall assessment of quality of care using the definitions of substandard care similar to those used by the Confidential Enquiries into Maternal Deaths and they were also required to formulate an action plan. The completed pro formas were collated centrally in order to identify recurrent themes and draw generalisable lessons for Scotland as a whole. Thus, during the second year, both case ascertainment (permitting the calculation of rates of events) and case assessment (permitting the learning of clinical lessons) took place.

Results

The case definitions in use at the time of publication of this Report for the 14 categories of 'near miss' event are summarised in Table 19.1.

Table 19.1 Definitions for the 14 categories of severe maternal morbidity currently in use by the Scottish Confidential Audit 2003–04

Code	Category	Definition
1	Major obstetric haemorrhage	Estimated blood loss ≥ 2500 ml, or transfused 5 or more units of blood **or** received treatment for coagulopathy (fresh frozen plasma, cryoprecipitate, platelets; includes ectopic pregnancy meeting these criteria)
2	Eclampsia	Seizure in presence of pre-eclampsia
3	Renal or liver dysfunction	Acute onset of biochemical disturbance, urea > 15 mmol/l, creatinine > 400 mmol/l, aspartate aminotransferase/alanine aminotransferase > 200 u/l
4	Cardiac arrest	No detectable major pulse
5	Pulmonary oedema	Clinically diagnosed pulmonary oedema associated with acute breathlessness and O_2 saturation < 95%, requiring O_2, diuretics or ventilation
6	Acute respiratory dysfunction	Requiring intubation or ventilation for > 60 minutes (not including duration of general anaesthesia
7	Coma	Including diabetic coma. Unconscious for > 12 hours
8	Cerebrovascular event	Stroke, cerebral/cerebellar haemorrhage or infarction, subarachnoid haemorrhage, dural venous sinus thrombosis
9	Status epilepticus	Unremitting seizures in patient with known epilepsy
10	Anaphylactic shock	An allergic reaction resulting in collapse with severe hypotension, difficulty breathing and swelling/rash
11	Septicaemic shock	Shock (systolic blood pressure < 80 mm/Hg) in association with infection. No other cause for decreased blood pressure. Pulse of 120 bpm or more
12	Anaesthetic problem	Aspiration, failed intubation, high spinal or epidural anaesthesia
13	Massive pulmonary embolism	Increased respiratory rate (> 20/minute), tachycardia, hypotension. Diagnosed as "high" probability on V/Q scan or positive spiral chest CT scan. Treated by heparin, thrombolysis or embolectomy
14	Intensive care admission Coronary care admission	Unit equipped to ventilate adults. Admission for one of the above problems or for any other reason. Includes coronary care unit admissions

Table 19.2 Overall assessments of quality of care assigned by local risk management teams after assessing cases of severe obstetric haemorrhage using a standard proforma

Quality of care category	No.
1. Appropriate care; well managed	91
2. Substandard care, incidental. Lessons can be learnt, but may not have changed outcome.	21
3. Substandard care, minor. Different care **may** have altered outcome.	17
4. Substandard care, major. Management contributed significantly to morbidity. Different management **might well** have resulted in a more favourable outcome.	4
Total	133

During the first year of national data collection, 'near miss' events (identified using definitions which differed in minor respects from those shown in Table 19.1)[5] occurred in 196 women (of 51,165 deliveries in Scotland) (rate 3.8/1000 deliveries, 95% CI 3.3/1,000–4.4/1,000). Of these, 30% fell into more than one of our defined categories. Sixty-four women (33%) were admitted to an intensive care unit during their care. Severe haemorrhage was the most common category of event, occurring in 98 women (50%). During the year, there were four maternal deaths in Scotland due to causes related to one of our severe morbidity categories. Thus, the ratio of severe morbidity (as defined in our study) to maternal mortality was 49:1. The findings of our first year of national data collection are presented in full elsewhere.[5] Because of the frequency of 'haemorrhage' events, this topic was chosen for development of our first case assessment pro forma.

During the second year, 167 cases of severe obstetric haemorrhage were reported (meeting the refined and expanded definition shown in Table 19.1). At the time of writing, 133 (80%) of these had been assessed by local clinical risk management teams using the national case assessment pro forma. Overall assessments of quality of care are summarised in Table 19.2.

National collation of the case assessment pro formas allowed the identification of learning points applicable to all maternity units in Scotland. National learning points comprised examples of both suboptimal care and good practice and comprised both recurrent themes and solitary, but important, instances. Examples of learning points distilled from the case pro formas are summarised in Table 19.3.

Discussion

The Scottish experience has confirmed that ascertainment and assessment of defined categories of severe maternal morbidity, on a national basis, is feasible. We have found that the 'system-based' definitions originally proposed by Mantel *et al.*[1] have proved eminently usable, with minimal adaptation. Our strategy for case ascertainment involves consultant-led maternity units only. A small proportion of women in Scotland deliver in midwife- or general practitioner-led units, or at home. We are aware that some cases of severe morbidity might be missed, as we have no case ascertainment mechanisms in place in these settings. However, any woman being managed in such a setting who develops severe morbidity would usually be transferred to a consultant-led unit; so we assume that missed cases, if any, would be few in number. Continuing collection of 'case ascertainment' data will allow examination of time trends in rates of 'near miss' events at local and national levels. Continuing collection of 'case assessment' data will

Table 19.3 Generally applicable learning points distilled from local risk management assessments of 133 cases of severe obstetric haemorrhage

Suboptimal care		Good practice	
Recurrent themes	**Important instances**	**Recurrent themes**	**Important instances**
Documentation	Check 'group and save' sample at laboratory before elective operation	Use a postpartum haemorrhage 'checklist'	Use of prophylactic Syntocinon infusion for high-risk case
Call senior staff early	Do not ignore post-operative tachycardia	Have interventional radiologist present at high risk elective operations	Elective insertion of pelvic drain at caesarean section in anticoagulated patient
Use protocols		Hold regular 'fire drills' on emergency procedures	Allocate a designated 'scribe' during emergency management
Check under theatre drapes for bleeding		Give positive feedback when job well done	Post a notice by the telephone reminding staff of availability of 'O negative' and 'group-specific' blood
Use 'O negative' blood if cross match delayed			
There is no such thing as a woman with 'no risk' Consider hysterectomy early			
Ensure staff can operate equipment			
Investigate medical conditions antenatally			

allow examination of time trends in rates of suboptimal care and collation of further learning points.

A formal, qualitative focus group exercise has shown that this approach to learning from adverse events is acceptable to, and indeed welcomed by, local risk management teams. However, a small-scale study of interobserver variability has indicated that, even using a structured pro forma, assessment of 'substandard' or 'suboptimal' care may be somewhat subjective and of limited reproducibility. We plan further development and evaluation of this approach to adverse event audit in order to improve the validity and rigour of our methods.

For further information on the Scottish Confidential Audit of Severe Maternal Morbidity, contact Gillian Penney (g.c.penney@abdn.ac.uk).

References

1. Mantel GD, Buchmann E, Rees H, Pattinson RC. Severe acute maternal morbidity: a pilot study of a definition for a near-miss. *Br J Obstet Gynaecol* 1998;105: 985–90.
2. Bouvier-Colle MH, Salanave B, Ancel PY, Varnoux N, Fernandez H, Papiernik E, *et al.* Obstetric patients treated in intensive care units and maternal mortality. *Eur J Obstet Gynecol Reprod Biol* 1996;65:121–5.

3. Baskett TF, Sternadel J. Maternal intensive care and near-miss mortality in obstetrics. *Br J Obstet Gynaecol* 1998;105:981–4.

4. Waterstone M, Bewley S, Wolfe C. Incidence and predictors of severe obstetric morbidity: case–control study. *BMJ* 2001;322:1089–93.

5. Brace V, Penney G, Hall M. Quantifying severe maternal morbidity: a Scottish population study. *BJOG* 2004;111:481–4.

CHAPTER 20

Mortality in pregnant and nonpregnant women in England and Wales 1997–2002: are pregnant women healthier?

CARINE RONSMANS, GWYNETH LEWIS, LISA HURT, NIGEL PHYSICK, ALISON MACFARLANE and CAROLE ABRAHAMS

Introduction

Pregnancy and the postpartum are thought to be vulnerable periods in a woman's life either because pregnancy directly leads to increased morbidity and mortality (*Direct* obstetric causes) or because pregnancy aggravates underlying disease conditions (*Indirect* obstetric causes). It is generally accepted that the adverse effects associated with pregnancy extend up to 6 weeks postpartum, although longer-term effects have also been suggested. The Tenth International Classification of Diseases, Injuries and Causes of Death (ICD10) revision added the category of *Late* maternal deaths, implying that the risks associated with pregnancy may extend up to 1 year after the termination of pregnancy.[1] Few studies have compared mortality during pregnancy with mortality at other times, however, and little is known about the actual length of the postpartum period during which women experience pregnancy-associated mortality risks.

While there is no doubt that deaths from *Direct* obstetric causes are attributable to pregnancy, less certainty exists about the so-called *Indirect* obstetric causes. The very nature of diseases aggravated by the pregnancy remains uncertain, and the extent to which deaths coinciding with the pregnancy are in effect caused by it has not been clearly appreciated.[2] According to ICD10, any death that occurs during pregnancy or within 42 days, and even within 1 year, potentially qualifies as an *Indirect* cause, except for accidents. In practice, those responsible for classifying maternal deaths often decide on a case-by-case basis whether or not they categorise certain diseases as indirectly attributable to or incidental to the pregnancy. It is not surprising, therefore, that definitions vary.[3]

Although deaths from injuries are not generally considered maternal deaths, some studies suggest that intentional injuries, and possibly unintentional injuries, may be more common among women when they are pregnant then when they are not. In New York City, for example, the risk of homicide was found to be higher among pregnant black women than among the general population of black women.[4] In the UK, suicide has been reported as a leading cause of maternal death,[5] although suicide rates appear to be much lower during pregnancy and in the first year after childbirth than in women without a recent pregnancy.[6] Some authors have even supported the idea that women may be more prone to accidents during their pregnancy.[7]

One way to gain a better understanding of the contribution of indirect and injury-related causes to pregnancy-related mortality is to compare death rates from these causes in pregnant and nonpregnant women. If certain causes are more common or more severe in pregnancy, then mortality from these causes should be higher among pregnant than nonpregnant women. The objective of this study is to compare all-cause and cause-specific death rates in women during pregnancy and up to 42 days postpartum with all-cause and cause-specific death rates between 43 days and 1 year postpartum and in women without a recent pregnancy.

Methods

We computed death rates in women aged between 15 years and 44 years in the years 1997–2002 in England and Wales (E&W) in three exposure periods: during pregnancy and within 42 days after the end of pregnancy; between 43 and 365 days after the end of pregnancy and outside these two periods.

Numerators

Numbers of deaths of women aged between 15 years and 44 years in England and Wales were obtained from the Office for National Statistics (ONS). Deaths during pregnancy and within 1 year after birth were available through the Confidential Enquiry into Maternal Deaths (CEMD) 1997–2002 and a maternal death linkage study between 1997 and 2002 conducted by the ONS. In each of the four countries of the United Kingdom, any death of a woman who is either pregnant or within 1 year following delivery, termination of pregnancy, ectopic pregnancy or miscarriage should be reported to the local director of public health and/or directly to the country's Confidential Enquiry. To update deaths that may not have been notified to the Enquiry, all death records of women of reproductive age who died between 1997 and 2002 in England and Wales were matched with birth registrations up to 1 year previously.

Since this linkage study was restricted to data from England and Wales, we used only deaths registered in England and Wales in this analysis. These could not be extracted directly from the Enquiry database, as information on the country in which the death occurred is removed from the database following the publication of each Enquiry report. The total number of deaths from 1997 to 2002 was therefore estimated by assuming that cause-specific death rates in England and Wales were the same as cause-specific death rates in the UK overall.

Deaths reported to the Enquiry are assigned an underlying cause of death by a team of central assessors who review each case. Their assessment may occasionally differ from the underlying cause of death as recorded on the death certificate. We used the Enquiry causes of death for deaths during pregnancy and within 42 days after birth and ONS causes for all other deaths. Deaths were classified using the ninth revision of the International Classification of Diseases, Injuries and Causes of Death (ICD9) for deaths in 1997 to 2000 and the tenth revision (ICD10) for deaths in 2001 and 2002.

Deaths were subdivided into *Direct* obstetric, accidents and violence, and other causes. Deaths from *Direct* obstetric causes were classified separately because they occur only as a direct consequence of pregnancy. We also separated deaths from accidents and violence and, within those, deaths attributed to suicide, to clarify the possible relationship between pregnancy and mortality from intentional or unintentional injuries. Deaths attributed to accidents and violence were defined using ICD codes E800.0 to E999.9 in ICD9; and V01 to Y98 in ICD10. Deaths attributed to suicide were defined using ICD codes E950.0 to E959.9 in ICD9 and X60 to X84 in ICD10. All deaths for which it had not been possible to determine whether they had been accidental or purposefully inflicted were grouped with the suicides (codes E980.0 to E989.0 in ICD9 and Y10 to Y34 in ICD10). The same was done for the Confidential Enquiry deaths.

Denominators

The mid-year population estimates of women aged 15–44 years in England and Wales in each of the years 1997 to 2002 were obtained from the ONS. The total women-years spent during pregnancy or within 1 year of birth were derived from the number of pregnancies, assuming a fixed gestational age by pregnancy outcome. The ONS provided data on maternities (live and still births), induced abortions, spontaneous miscarriages and ectopic pregnancies. Gestational age for live births, stillbirths, miscarriages and abortions, and ectopic pregnancies was assumed to be 280, 196, 84, and 84 days, respectively. To estimate the person time exposed for the 'during pregnancy and within 42 days after birth' category, each pregnancy was assigned the above period of gestation plus a puerperal period of 42 days. For the 'between 43 and 365 days' category, deaths during pregnancy or within 42 days of birth were deducted from the total number of pregnancies, and each remaining pregnancy assigned 323 days.

Death rates were expressed as deaths per 100,000 years of exposure. Death rates were compared using exact confidence intervals for the rate ratio. The heterogeneity of rate ratios across age groups was assessed using the Mantel–Haenszel test.

Results

All-cause mortality in women aged 15–44 years was 58.4 deaths per 100,000 women per year, increasing from 25.2 per 100,000 in women aged 15–19 years to 123.8 per 100,000 in women aged 40–44 years. Deaths during pregnancy and within 1 year after birth represent a small proportion of all deaths in women of reproductive age (1.3% of all deaths in women aged 15–44 years occur during pregnancy and within 42 days after birth and 1.7% occur between 43 and 365 days after birth).

All-cause death rates in the three exposure periods are shown in Table 20.1 and Figure 20.1. Death rates during pregnancy and within 42 days after birth were remarkably similar to those between 43 and 365 days after birth. Surprisingly, however, mortality during pregnancy or within 1 year after birth was between four and five times lower than mortality in women without a recent pregnancy. The rate ratios comparing the pregnancy–42 day and the 43–365 postpartum periods with nonpregnant women were 0.21 and 0.22, respectively.

Death rates by cause are shown in Figure 20.1, with the corresponding rate ratios shown in Table 20.2. *Direct* obstetric mortality was substantially higher during pregnancy and within 42 days postpartum (37.6% of all deaths) than between 43 days and 1 year postpartum (4.2% of all deaths).

Deaths attributed to accidents or violence represented 11.8%, 26.6% and 20.1% of all deaths in the three exposure periods, respectively. Death rates from accidental or violent

Mortality in pregnant and nonpregnant women

Table 20.1 All-cause death rates per 100,000 women-years, by age and exposure period; England and Wales 1997–2002

Age group (years) and exposure period	Death rates	Rate ratios (95% confidence interval)
15–19		
Pregnant and 42 days	10.56	0.40 (0.27, 0.56)
43 days to 1 year	8.37	0.31 (0.22, 0.43)
Not pregnant	26.66	1.00
20–24		
Pregnant and 42 days	9.85	0.29 (0.22, 0.37)
43 days to 1 year	11.69	0.34 (0.28, 0.42)
Not pregnant	34.15	1.00
25–29		
Pregnant and 42 days	12.08	0.29 (0.24, 0.35)
43 days to 1 year	11.55	0.28 (0.23, 0.33)
Not pregnant	41.27	1.00
30–34		
Pregnant and 42 days	14.41	0.25 (0.21, 0.29)
43 days to 1 year	15.17	0.26 (0.23, 0.31)
Not pregnant	57.74	1.00
35–39		
Pregnant and 42 days	19.96	0.24 (0.20, 0.30)
43 days to 1 year	23.06	0.28 (0.23, 0.33)
Not pregnant	82.39	1.00
40–44		
Pregnant and 42 days	26.21	0.21 (0.13, 0.31)
43 days to 1 year	29.60	0.24 (0.16, 0.33)
Not pregnant	125.73	1.00
All (15–44)		
Pregnant and 42 days	13.56	0.21 (0.19, 0.23)
43 days to 1 year	14.17	0.22 (0.20, 0.24)
Not pregnant	64.74	1.00

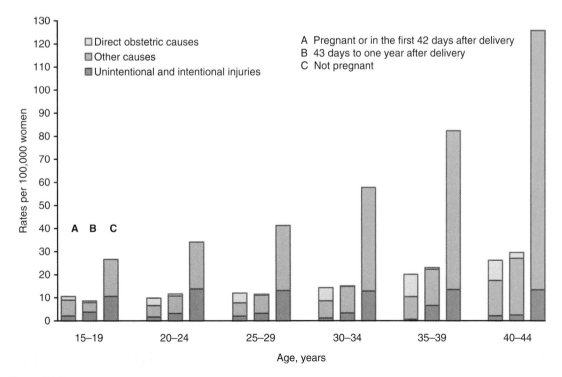

Figure 20.1

Table 20.2 Rate ratios (95% confidence intervals) comparing death rates during pregnancy and within 42 days and between 43 days and one year postpartum with those in nonpregnant women, by cause and age; England and Wale, 1997–2002

Age group (years) and exposure period	Direct obstetric causes	Accidents or violence*	Suicides	Other causes
15–19				
Pregnant and 42 days	3.43 (0.56–36.04)	0.20 (0.08–0.42)	No deaths	0.43 (0.27–0.65)
43 days to 1 year	1.00	0.36 (0.21–0.58)	0.21 (0.04–0.63)	0.25 (0.15–0.40)
Not pregnant	–	1.00	1.00	1.00
20–24				
Pregnant and 42 days	3.64 (1.57–9.40)	0.12 (0.06–0.21)	0.05 (0.01–0.17)	0.24 (0.17–0.34)
43 days to 1 year	1.00	0.23 (0.15–0.34)	0.16 (0.07–0.32)	0.37 (0.29–0.48)
Not pregnant	–	1.00	1.00	1.00
25–29				
Pregnant and 42 days	8.78 (3.74–25.20)	0.16 (0.10–0.24)	0.15 (0.08–0.27)	0.20 (0.15–0.26)
43 days to 1 year	1.00	0.25 (0.18–0.34)	0.30 (0.20–0.45)	0.28 (0.22–0.34)
Not pregnant	–	1.00	1.00	1.00
30–34				
Pregnant and 42 days	22.54 (7.35–112.36)	0.10 (0.05–0.17)	0.07 (0.02–0.17)	0.17 (0.13–0.21)
43 days to 1 year	1.00	0.26 (0.19–0.36)	0.32 (0.21–0.48)	0.26 (0.21–0.31)
Not pregnant	–	1.00	1.00	1.00
35–39				
Pregnant and 42 days	13.66 (5.00–52.22)	0.05 (0.01–0.13)	0.03 (0.00–0.16)	0.14 (0.10–0.19)
43 days to 1 year	1.00	0.49 (0.34–0.67)	0.51 (0.32–0.79)	0.23 (0.18–0.28)
Not pregnant	–	1.00	1.00	1.00
40–44				
Pregnant and 42 days	3.44 (0.83–20.15)	0.16 (0.02–0.58)	0.33 (0.04–1.20)	0.14 (0.07–0.23)
43 days to 1 year	1.00	0.19 (0.04–0.55)	0.13 (0.00–0.72)	0.22 (0.15–0.31)
Not pregnant	–	1.00	1.00	1.00
All (15–44)				
Pregnant and 42 days	8.65 (5.72–13.59)	0.12 (0.09–0.16)	0.09 (0.06–0.14)	0.13 (0.12–0.15)
43 days to 1 year	1.00	0.29 (0.25–0.34)	0.31 (0.25–0.38)	0.19 (0.17–0.21)
Not pregnant	–	1.00	1.00	1.00

* including suicide

causes were slightly higher between 43–365 days after birth than during pregnancy but were still substantially lower compared with women without a recent birth (rate ratios comparing the pregnancy–42 day postpartum and 43–365 day periods with nonpregnant women were 0.12 and 0.29, respectively).[1]

Deaths attributed to suicide accounted for 4.3%, 13.6% and 9.6% of all deaths in the three exposure periods, respectively. Death rates from suicide were very low during pregnancy or within 42 days postpartum (Figure 20.1) but trebled after 6 weeks postpartum (compared with during pregnancy). However, death rates from suicide within a year after birth remained substantially lower than in the period beyond that (rate ratios comparing the pregnancy–42 day postpartum and 43–365 day periods with nonpregnant women were 0.09 and 0.31, respectively).[1]

After excluding *Direct* obstetric and accidental or violent causes, death rates during pregnancy and 42 days postpartum and between 43 and 365 days postpartum were seven and five times lower than death rates beyond a year after birth (rate ratio 0.13 and 0.19, respectively). As expected, death rates from non-obstetric or non-injury-related causes increased with age, but the magnitude of the increase was much smaller among pregnant or recently delivered women than among women without a recent birth

(Figure 20.1). Rate ratios differed significantly with age when comparing women during pregnancy and within a year after birth with nonpregnant women, with the magnitude of the protective effect increasing as the women's ages increased.

Discussion

As observed elsewhere in industrialised countries, we found a lower risk of death during pregnancy and within a year after its termination. The magnitude of the protective effect was greater than that reported in three other studies. In Canada, mortality rates during pregnancy or within 42 days of its termination and between 43 and 225 days postpartum were about half those of nonpregnant women.[8] In Finland, the age-adjusted risk of a natural death within a year after birth or a miscarriage was half that of women without a pregnancy.[9] In the USA, women who had delivered a live or stillborn infant in the previous year were half as likely to die as women who had not recently delivered.[10]

After excluding *Direct* obstetric and injury-related causes, the protective effect of pregnancy was even greater, particularly among older women. The rise in mortality with age was much more marked among women without a recent birth, widening the gap between the pregnant and the nonpregnant as age increases. This is strongly suggestive of a 'healthy pregnant woman effect', i.e. that women suffering ill health are less likely to become pregnant then their healthier peers, resulting in an over-representation of healthier women among those who are pregnant.[2,11] Although better access to health care or enhanced preventive behaviour among pregnant women or those with a small child may have partly contributed to their lower mortality, this is unlikely to reduce mortality to the extent seen here. Similarly, there is as yet little evidence of a direct protective effect against certain diseases during pregnancy or immediately after birth and, if any, most of the evidence points to a harmful effect.

Data quality and, in particular, under-reporting of deaths, is a recurrent concern with maternal mortality data. However, record linkage of female deaths with registered births will have ensured that almost all deaths following childbirth were identified in this population. In addition, any death of a pregnant or recently pregnant woman is reported to the Enquiry in the UK, and the numbers of *Direct* and *Indirect* deaths identified by the Enquiry, always exceeds those identified from an examination of the causes of death on death certificates. Nevertheless, a small number of deaths may have been missed, although this is unlikely to explain the huge differential mortality between pregnant and nonpregnant women.

The lower risk of suicide during pregnancy or in the year after its termination confirms previous findings from the UK,[6] Canada[8] and New York City.[4,12] Under-reporting of maternal suicides is unlikely to explain the findings, though it may affect their magnitude. The lower risks of suicide during pregnancy and in the year after birth remain largely unexplained.[13] Although postpartum depression is common, it does not seem to result in an increased incidence of suicide compared with the general population.

Some authors have suggested a re-examination of the definition of maternal mortality, for example by categorising injury-related deaths as maternal[4] or by considering diseases of the arteries, arterioles and capillaries in the category of *Direct* obstetric deaths.[8] The interaction between pregnancy and disease or injury is complex however, and whether or not a cause is attributable to the pregnancy is likely to be influenced by the social, epidemiological and healthcare context of the population under study. Whatever the statistical definition of maternal mortality, careful scrutiny of all deaths among pregnant and recently pregnant women, as currently carried out in the Enquiry, should continue. The design of appropriate public health interventions requires knowledge of the magnitude of all causes of death during and after pregnancy, whether or not these causes are thought to be attributable to or incidental to the pregnancy.

References

1. World Health Organization. *Statistical Classification of Diseases and Related Health Problems*. Tenth Revision. Geneva: WHO; 1992.
2. Khlat M, Ronsmans C. Deaths attributable to childbearing in Matlab, Bangladesh: indirect causes of maternal mortality questioned. *Am J Epidemiol* 2000; 151: 1–7.
3. Salanave B, Bouvier-Colle MH, Varnoux N, Alexander S, Macfarlane A. Classification differences and maternal mortality: a European study. MOMS Group. Mothers' Mortality and Severe morbidity. *Int J Epidemiol* 1999; 28: 64–9.
4. Dannenberg AL, Carter DM, Lawson HW, Ashton DM, Dorfman SF, Graham EH. Homicide and other injuries as causes of maternal death in New York City, 1987 through 1991. *Am J Obstet Gynecol* 1995; 172: 1557–64.
5. Oates M. Perinatal psychiatric disorders: a leading cause of maternal morbidity and mortality. *Br Med Bull* 2003; 67: 219–29.
6. Appleby L. Suicide during pregnancy and in the first postnatal year. *BMJ* 1991; 302: 137–40.
7. Fortney J. Measurement and levels of maternal mortality. In: Demographie: analyse et synthèse-causes et conséquences des évolutions démographiques. Actes du séminaire de San Miniato (Pise), 17–19 Décembre 1997, Vol. 1, Rome, Paris: Louvain-la-Neuve; 1997.
8. Turner LA, Kramer MS, Liu S. Cause-specific mortality during and after pregnancy and the definition of maternal death. *Chronic Dis Can* 2002; 23: 1–8.
9. Gissler M, Berg C, Bouvier-Colle MH, Buekens P. Pregnancy-associated mortality after birth, spontaneous abortion, or induced abortion in Finland, 1987–2000. *Am J Obstet Gynecol* 2004; 190: 422–7.
10. Jocums SB, Berg CJ, Entman SS, Mitchell EF. Postdelivery mortality in Tennessee, 1989–1991. *Obstet Gynecol* 1998; 91: 766–70.
11. Ronsmans C, Khlat M, Belco K, Ba M, de Bernis L, Etard J-F. Evidence for a "healthy pregnant woman effect" in Niakhar, Senegal? *Int J Epidemiol* 2001; 30: 467–74.
12. Marzuk PM, Tardiff K, Leon AC, Hirsch CS, Portera L, Hartwell N, *et al*. Lower risk of suicide during pregnancy. *Am J Psychiatry* 1997; 154: 122–3.
13. Kleiner GJ, Greston WM, editors. *Suicide in Pregnancy*. London: John Wright; 1984.

CHAPTER 21

Trends in reproductive epidemiology and women's health

JESSICA CHAMBERLAIN and TANIA CORBIN,
Office for National Statistics

Introduction

The purpose of this chapter is to place in context the data on maternal deaths given earlier in this Report. Changes in the population at risk could change the number of deaths expected if rates remain at the same level. This chapter provides an overview of trends in reproductive epidemiology by discussing conceptions, terminations, embryonic deaths (miscarriages) and births. It discusses the fertility of women in different age groups and at different parities, and presents relevant information about problems around the time of delivery. The chapter also discusses other aspects of women's health highlighted in this Report, in particular obesity, smoking and use of alcohol in pregnancy.

Maternal deaths identified by the Registrars General

As described in the section of Aims and Methodology, the numbers of *Direct* and *Indirect* deaths identified by the Enquiry always exceeds those identified from an examination of the cause of death given on death certificates. The Office for National Statistics (ONS) death certificates are examined to select deaths where there is a mention anywhere on the certificate of a pregnancy-related condition, such as eclampsia. Women who die while pregnant but where no mention of the pregnancy is made on the certificate will not be identified in this way. In Scotland, however, there is a box on the certificate that can be ticked to identify that a woman was pregnant or had recently given birth at the time of her death.

In 2000–02, 148 deaths in the UK were identified from death registrations as having a pregnancy-related condition mentioned on their death certificates. This represented a rate of 4.0 per million women aged 15–44 years and contributed 0.7% of all deaths in the age group. The Enquiry identified 106 *Direct* maternal deaths and 155 *Indirect* maternal deaths, suggesting that only 57% of maternal deaths mention the pregnancy at death registration (Tables 21.1 and 21.2). Work is currently being undertaken to assess the feasibility of identifying further deaths by linking women's death certificates with recent birth registrations.

Overall trends in reproductive epidemiology

Maternities and estimated pregnancies

Maternities are pregnancies that result in a live birth at any gestation or a stillbirth occurring at 24 weeks of completed gestation or later. Statistics on these outcomes can

Table 21.1 *Direct* and *Indirect* maternal deaths and mortality rates per 100,000 maternities as reported to the Registrars General (ONS) and to the Enquiry; United Kingdom 1985–2002

Triennium	Maternal deaths known to Registrars General (ONS)		Direct deaths known to the Enquiry		Indirect deaths known to the Enquiry		Total Direct and Indirect deaths known to the Enquiry		Total maternities
	(n)	Rate	(n)	Rate	(n)	Rate	(n)	Rate	(n)
1985–1987	174	7.7	139	6.1	84	3.7	223	9.8	2,268,766
1988–1990	171	7.2	145	6.1	93	3.9	238	10.0	2,360,309
1991–1993	149	6.4*	128	5.5	100	4.3	228	9.8	2,315,204
1994–1996	175	8.0**	134	6.1	134	6.1	268	12.2	2,197,640
1997–1999	142	6.7**	106	5.0	136	6.4	242	11.4	2,123,614
2000–2002	148	7.4**	106	5.3	155	7.8	261	13.1	1,997,472

Source: Office for National Statistics; General Records Office, Scotland; General Records Office, Northern Ireland.
* Final ONS revised figures for 1991–93. The rate available at the time for the publication of the 1991–93 Report was 6.0.
** England and Wales figures for 1994 onwards now include underlying cause and mentions (ICD9 630–676); the rate for 1994-96 in the previous Report was 7.4.

be given with great confidence, since they are required by law to be registered. However, since not all pregnancies result in a registrable live or stillbirth it is impossible to know the exact number of pregnancies that occurred during this or any preceding triennium. Other outcomes of a pregnancy can be a legal termination (which is also registrable by law), an embryonic death (at less than 24 weeks) or an ectopic pregnancy.

Therefore, the number of pregnancies is estimated from a combination of the number of maternities, together with legal terminations, hospital admissions for embryonic death and ectopic pregnancies, and an adjustment to allow for the period of gestation and maternal ages at conception. The estimated number of pregnancies and the components of this estimate are shown in Table 21.3. Data in earlier Reports were given for England and Wales only and these are included for comparison. The resulting total is still an underestimate of the actual number of pregnancies, since these figures do not include other pregnancies that miscarry early, those where the woman is not admitted to hospital or, indeed, those where the woman herself does not know she is pregnant. Studies have estimated that up to 50% of all pregnancies may result in a spontaneous miscarriage (a miscarriage before 24 weeks of gestation) and the majority of these are lost prior to implantation or within the first 4 weeks of pregnancy. Therefore, estimates differ

Table 21.2 Mortality rates per million female population aged 15–44 years, all causes and maternal deaths; United Kingdom 1979–2002

Triennium	All causes	Maternal deaths	Deaths in age group due to maternal causes (%)
1979–81	697.2	6.6	1.0
1982–84	641.7	4.7	0.7
1985–87	622.5	4.2	0.7
1988–90	625.9	4.1	0.7
1991–93	608.1	4.0	0.7
1994–96	610.3	4.8	0.8
1997–99	599.2	3.9	0.6
2000–02	583.9	4.0	0.7

1994–2002 England and Wales includes underlying cause and mentions (ICD9 630–676, ICD10 O00–O99).
Sources: Office for National Statistics, General Records Office: Scotland, General Records Office: Northern Ireland.

Table 21.3   Estimated pregnancies (in thousands); England and Wales 1976–93 and United Kingdom 1991–2002

Triennia	Maternities	Legal abortions	Spontaneous abortions	Ectopic pregnancies	Total estimated pregnancies
England and Wales					
1976–78	1781.3	324.6	158.3*	11.6	2275.8
1979–81	1910.9	380.5	134.3**	12.1	2437.8
1982–84	1905.8	393.1	113.6**	14.4	2426.9
1985–87	1987.9	451.1	N/A	N/A	2439.0
1988–90	2073.0	512.7	277.2**	24.0	2886.9
1991–93	2045.3	485.7	233.8**	27.0	2791.8
United Kingdom					
1991–93	2315.2	525.7	266.4**	30.2	3137.4
1994–96	2197.6	518.8	164.7**	33.5	2914.6
1997–99	2123.6	564.1	153.6**	31.9	2873.3
2000–02	1997.5	568.8	143.1***	30.1	2739.4
Percentage	72.9	20.8	5.2	1.1	100.0

N/A = not available.
*   ICD (8th revision) 640–645.
** ICD (9th revision) 634-638.
*** ICD (9th revision) 634 and ICD (10th revision) O03.
Sources: Birth statistics Series FM1, Abortion statistics Series AB, Department of Health: Hospital Episodes Statistics, Welsh Office: Hospital Activity Analysis, Scottish Morbidity Records (SMR) 1 Inpatients and Daycases Acute, Scottish Morbidity Records (SMR) 2 Inpatients and Daycases Maternity, DHSS Northern Ireland.

between studies because fetal loss before 4 weeks in particular is very hard to estimate. It has been estimated that up to 35% of fertilised ova may be lost before the first missed period.[1]

Using the available sources of data, ONS estimated that 73% of pregnancies in the UK between 2000 and 2002 led to a maternity resulting in one or more registrable live or stillbirths. A further 21% of pregnancies were legally terminated under the 1976 Abortion Act. The remaining 6% of known pregnancies were admitted to hospital following an embryonic death or an ectopic pregnancy. Embryonic deaths that resulted in a day stay or in women who were not admitted to hospital are not included in this data. The absolute numbers and the percentage distribution of the outcomes of the estimated pregnancies during 2000–02 are very similar to those in the previous triennia. The striking changes in the estimated number of embryonic deaths and ectopic pregnancies between 1982–84 and 1988–90 are most likely due to the different ways the data were collected during these triennia and the different sampling and grossing up procedures used. There appears to be no obvious change in clinical patterns over this period that could have contributed to this increase in number.

Trends in legal abortion

Some women die following legal (and in the past, illegal) abortion. Since the introduction of legal abortion in 1968, following the 1967 Abortion Act in England, Wales and Scotland, and up to the end of 2002 over five million legal terminations of pregnancy have been carried out for residents of Great Britain. The Abortion Act of 1967 does not apply to Northern Ireland, where only a small number of legal terminations are performed each year on medical grounds under the case law that applied in England and Wales before the Abortion Act 1967. However, some women from Northern Ireland have legal terminations in Great Britain (these abortions are not included in the following

Table 21.4 Legal abortions and abortion rate in Great Britain to women resident in Great Britain; 1988–2002

Triennia	Abortions (*n*)	Abortions per woman*
1988–90	543,217	0.44
1991–93	518,685	0.43
1994–96	513,283	0.44
1997–99	558,479	0.49
2000–02	563,371	0.50

* Calculated by summing age-specific abortion rates to standardise the population age distribution.

analysis). Between 2000 and 2002 4,491 women having an abortion in Great Britain gave their usual address as Northern Ireland.

Table 21.4 shows both the number of legal abortions in Great Britain and the age standardised abortion rate per woman (similar in calculation to a total fertility rate), for last five triennia. Figure 21.1 shows the legal abortion rate for each individual year over the period 1971–2002. The abortion rate shown here is the average number of abortions per woman, if women experienced the abortion rates of a particular year for their entire childbearing years. In 1971, just after the change in law regarding abortions, the abortion rate was 0.28 abortions per woman. Since 1971, the abortion rate has shown an overall upwards trend, although this rise has been interrupted by periods of no growth and sometimes slight decrease in the rate. The abortion rate reached 0.50 abortions per woman aged 15–44 years in 1998 and has subsequently remained at between 0.49 and 0.50.

Following the introduction of legal abortion the number of maternal deaths following illegal abortions fell sharply. In 1970–72 (the first full triennium during which legal abortion was available) there were 37 reported deaths from illegal abortion, falling to one in 1979–80. No maternal deaths from illegal abortion have been reported since, including for this triennium.

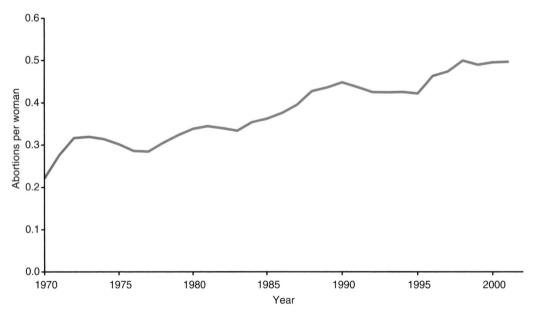

Figure 21.1 Abortion rate for women resident in Great Britain; 1971–2002

Trends in reproductive epidemiology and women's health

Table 21.5 Total number of births (live and still) and total fertility rate; United Kingdom 1976–2002

Triennium	Total births (1000s)	Total fertility rate (per woman)
1976–78	2038.3	1.73
1979–81	2235.2	1.86
1982–84	2182.5	1.77
1985–87	2292.9	1.80
1988–90	2374.0	1.83
1991–93	2343.8	1.80
1994–96	2227.5	1.73
1997–99	2155.3	1.72
2000–02	2027.9	1.64

Note: Total fertility rate is only based on live births and is calculated by summing age-specific fertility rates to standardise for the population age distribution.

Birth rates and fertility trends

Birth rates and fertility trends are important in the context of this Enquiry, as changes in patterns of childbearing may affect the number of maternal deaths. Since the England and Wales Enquiry started in 1952, joined by Scotland and Northern Ireland in 1985, 40.9 million births have been registered in the United Kingdom. The total number of births and the total fertility rate (TFR) for the UK in each triennium since 1976–78 are given in Table 21.5 and Figure 21.2 shows the TFR for the period 1960–2002. The TFR is the average number of children a woman would have if she experienced the fertility rates of a particular year for her entire childbearing years. The TFR standardises for the changing age structure of the population and therefore shows changes in fertility over time more accurately than other period measures of fertility.

Figure 21.2 shows the high fertility of the 1960s 'baby boom', where fertility increased from 1960 peaking in 1964 at 2.95 children per women. During the 1970s there were rapid declines in fertility and the TFR fell to a low of 1.69 in 1977. In the late 1970s,

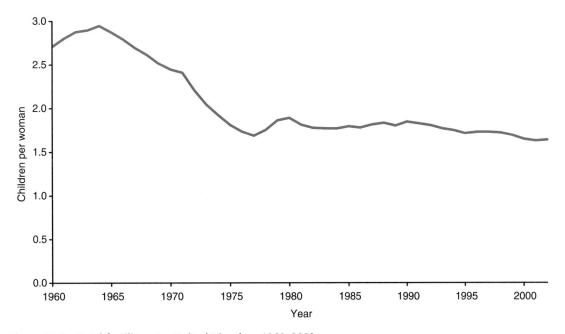

Figure 21.2 Total fertility rate; United Kingdom 1960–2002

the TFR increased briefly before decreasing in the early 1980s to around 1.8 children per woman, remaining around this level throughout the 1980s. Then, throughout the 1990s, the TFR slowly decreased and in 2002 the UK TFR was 1.64 children per woman. Fertility patterns in the four constituent countries of the UK follow the same pattern but the TFR is always higher in Northern Ireland than for the other countries. Data on birth order, from births within marriage,[i] indicate that this is due, at least in part, to women in Northern Ireland having on average more children. In 2000–02, 32% of births within marriage in Northern Ireland were third or higher-order births, compared with 23% of births in England and Wales. In 2000–02 the Northern Irish TFR was 1.78 compared with 1.65 in England and Wales. Scottish fertility has undergone a noticeable decline in the last decade and in 2000–02 the Scottish TFR reached a low of 1.48.

These changes in the TFR since 1977 conceal wider medical and social changes affecting reproductive epidemiology. Reduced perinatal and infant mortality means more babies are surviving into childhood. An increasing proportion of births occur outside marriage and there are changing patterns in the age at which women have children.

Maternities by age

The patterns of fertility by mean age at childbearing and mean age at first birth have changed greatly over the last 50 years. However, some of the change has been due to the changing population distribution. Currently, there are larger numbers of women at older ages, reflecting previous birth generation sizes and this contributes to the trend of increasing mean age at childbearing. In 2002, the mean age at childbearing was 29.3 years. However, if the current age structure of the population is controlled for, then the mean age at childbearing in 2002 was 28.7 years. Figure 21.3 shows the change in the age standardised mean age at childbearing since 1966. The 1960s 'baby boom' was associated with women starting childbearing earlier and therefore mean age at childbearing fell during the late 1960s, reaching a low of 26.4 years in 1974. Since then standardised mean age at childbearing has steadily increased (although at a different rate to the unstandardised age). The rise in standardised mean age at childbearing is a result of fertility rates increasing among women in their thirties and forties and conversely declining for women in their twenties.

Table 21.6 shows the percentage distribution of all live births in England and Wales by age at childbirth and age at first birth for the last five triennia. The data shown in Table 21.6 is only available for England and Wales but the trends shown here are applicable to the UK as a whole. The move towards women having children later in their childbearing years is clearly shown in the table. The percentage of all births that were to women aged 35 years or over more than doubled between 1988–90 and 2000–02, while the percentage of women having a first birth at 35 years or over has nearly trebled since 1988–90. Over the same time, both the percentage of all births and first births occurring to women aged 20–24 years has declined by around ten percentage points. This trend is in part due to changes in the population age structure of women. However, it also reflects other life-course changes, such as increased time spent in education and increasing mean age at marriage.

[i] Birth order data for the different countries of the UK is only available for births within marriage, because the number of previous live births is only recorded at registration for births occurring within marriage. England and Wales produces estimates of birth order for all births, but this data is not published for Northern Ireland or Scotland.

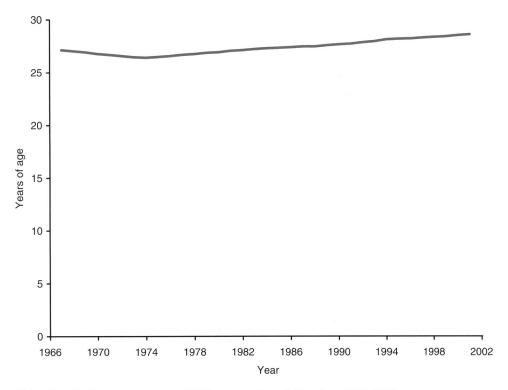

Figure 21.3 Standardised mean age at childbearing; United Kingdom 1966–2002

These changes in timing of childbirth can make an important contribution to maternal mortality because the risk of maternal mortality becomes higher with increasing age at childbirth. Studies have concluded that women aged 35 years or over have a higher frequency of various adverse reproductive events: infertility, spontaneous miscarriage, pregnancy complications (such as caesarean section, high blood pressure, pre-eclampsia), congenital abnormalities, maternal mortality and perinatal mortality, than do younger women.[2]

Table 21.6 Percentage distribution of all live births by age and age at first birth; England & Wales 1988–2002

	1988–90	1991–93	1994–96	1997–99	2000–02
Age (years)					
<20	8	7	7	8	7
20–24	27	24	20	18	18
25–29	35	35	34	30	27
30–34	21	24	28	30	30
35–39	7	8	10	12	15
40+	1	1	2	2	3
Total	100	100	100	100	100
Age (years) at first birth:					
<20	16	14	14	16	15
20–24	33	30	25	23	23
25–29	33	34	34	31	27
30–34	14	17	21	23	24
35+	4	5	6	8	10
Total	100	100	100	100	100

Source: Office for National Statistics.

Table 21.7 Percentage distribution of all live births by parity; England and Wales 1988–2002

Parity	1988–90	1991–93	1994–96	1997–99	2000–02
0	42	41	41	41	42
1	34	34	35	35	35
2	15	15	15	15	15
3	5	6	6	6	5
4	3	3	3	3	3
Total	100	100	100	100	100

Source: Office for National Statistics.

Maternities by parity

Parity is the number of live births a woman has had; that is, a woman who has had one live birth has a parity of one. Patterns of fertility in terms of parity have remained essentially constant over the last five triennia. Table 21.7 shows the distribution of births by mother's parity for the last five triennia. The data shown in Table 21.7 are only available for England and Wales, but the trends shown here are applicable to the UK as a whole. None of the percentages have differed by more than one percentage point over the last five triennia. In 2000–02, the majority of births were to women who had never had a birth before (parity zero) while only 23% of births were to women of a parity of two or higher.

Maternities by marital status

Over the last 50 years there have been large changes in the patterns of maternities by marital status. The number and percentage of all births occurring outside of marriage has greatly increased. This increase has occurred across all four countries of the UK but the patterns of increase and current percentage of births outside marriage differs between the countries, as shown in Figure 21.4. For the past ten years, Wales has had the fastest rate of increase and currently half of all births in Wales occur outside of marriage. Northern Ireland has shown a similar rate of increase, but for the last three decades it has always had the lowest proportion of births occurring outside of marriage of the four countries of the UK (34% in 2002). England and Scotland had a similar rate of increase up until about 1996 but, since then, the percentage of births taking place outside marriage has been increasing faster in Scotland than in England. In 2002, 40% of births occurred outside marriage in England, while this figure was 44% in Scotland.

The increase in births outside marriage has mostly been concentrated in births that are jointly registered, in particular among those where the parents give the same address. In 2002, 59% of births in the UK occurred inside marriage. Of the remaining births that occurred outside marriage, 33% were jointly registered and 7% were registered by the mother alone. The proportion of births occurring outside marriage and registered by one parent has remained at between 6–8% for the last two decades.

Maternities by ethnic origin

Since 1994, ethnic origin has been collected on the Enquiry notification forms. Therefore, to place this data in context, it would be ideal to compare it with the proportion of maternities by the mother's ethnic origin. Unfortunately, however, ethnic origin is not

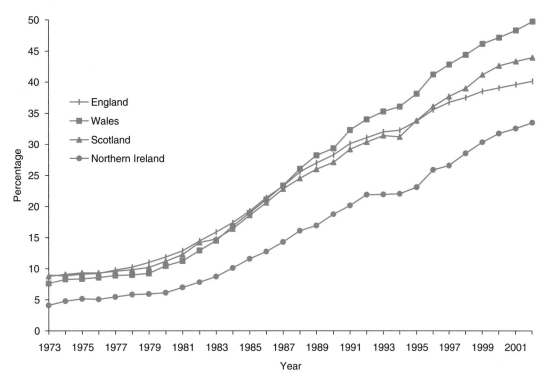

Figure 21.4   Percentage of births outside marriage, countries of the United Kingdom 1973–2002

collected at birth registration. Instead, the parent's countries of birth are recorded. The 2001 Census shows mother's country of birth to be a good indicator of ethnicity. However, increasing proportions of women from different ethnic groups were born in the United Kingdom. Therefore, analysing ethnicity solely using country of birth would miss half of the UK minority ethnic population, as the Census showed 50% of the minority ethnic population were born inside the UK.[3] Ethnic origin is collected by the Hospital Episodes Statistics (HES) but this information is incomplete in many areas, so is not of sufficient quality for analysis. Therefore, to provide a context for with the data recorded by this Enquiry, the population of all women aged 15–44 years in the UK, in 2001 were analysed by their age and ethnic group, as shown in Table 21.8.

In 2001, in total 10.1% of the UK female population aged 15–44 years considered themselves to belong to an ethnic minority. Within these ages, between 8–12% of the population considered themselves to belong to an ethnic minority. Table 21.8 shows that, within the minority ethnic population, there are differing age structures between groups. Black ethnic groups have an older age structure, demonstrated by them making up a larger percentage of the ethnic minority population in older age groups compared with younger age groups. Among 15–19-year-olds only 21% considered themselves to be of Black ethnic origin compared with 32% of 40–44-year-olds. In comparison, Pakistani and Bangladeshi groups have younger age structures.

Maternities by National Statistics socio-economic group

Social and economic deprivation is associated with a higher risk of maternal mortality. The Report for the previous triennium found that women from the most deprived circumstances appeared to have a 20 times greater risk of dying of *Direct* or *Indirect* causes than women from social classes 1 and 2. Therefore, to place the data in this Report in context, ideally an analysis of maternities by maternal social class would be performed.

Table 21.8 Female population of United Kingdom by ethnic group and age; 2001

	Total 15–44 years (1000s)	Total 15–44 years (%)	15–19 years (%)	20–24 years (%)	25–29 years (%)	30–34 years (%)	35–39 years (%)	40–44 years (%)
Black or Black British								
Caribbean	160	13	9	8	9	14	20	18
African	149	12	10	10	12	15	14	12
Other Black	29	2	2	2	2	2	3	2
Asian or Asian British								
Indian	278	22	21	23	23	22	21	25
Pakistani	190	15	19	19	17	14	10	12
Bangladeshi	71	6	7	8	7	5	3	3
Other Asian	58	5	4	4	5	5	5	5
Chinese	75	6	6	7	6	5	6	7
Any mixed background	150	12	17	13	12	11	10	9
Other Ethnic Group	79	6	4	6	8	7	7	7
All ethnic minority groups	1,237	10	11	12	11	10	9	8
White	11,028	90	89	88	89	90	91	92
Total Females (n)	12,266	12,266	1,940	1,697	1,967	2,245	2,321	2,095

Note: the percentages for the individual minority ethnic groups represent the proportional breakdown of 'all ethnic minority groups' total.
Source: Census 2001.

Mother and father's occupations are collected at birth registration and a 10% sample is coded. This information is then used, together with information collected on employment, to derive socio-economic group. However, a large proportion of women at registration state that they are housewives or unemployed. Thus, their socio-economic category may not be representative of their household situation. Therefore, maternities are routinely analysed by the father's socio-economic group rather than the mother's. However, using father's socio-economic group is deficient because it excludes births

Table 21.9 Female population of United Kingdom by NS–SEC and age; 2001

NS–SEC group	16–44 years (1000s)	16–44 years (%)	16–19 years	20–24 years	25–29 years	30–34 years	35–39 years	40–44 years
1. Higher managerial and professional occupations	730	6	0	3	9	8	7	6
2. Lower managerial and professional occupations	2595	22	3	16	28	26	25	25
3. Intermediate occupations	1903	16	7	18	18	17	16	16
4. Small employers and own account workers	388	3	0	1	2	4	5	5
5. Lower supervisory and technical occupations	529	4	2	5	5	5	5	5
6. Semi-routine occupations	1927	16	12	17	15	16	17	18
7. Routine occupations	941	8	6	9	8	8	8	8
8. Never worked and long–term unemployed	664							
L14.1 Never worked	543	5	5	6	5	5	4	4
L14.2 Long-term unemployed	121	1	0	1	1	1	1	1
Not Classified	2237							
L15 Full-time students	1532	13	65	23	4	2	2	1
L17 Not classifiable for other reasons	705	6	0	1	4	7	9	10
Total females	11,915	100	1426	1781	1972	2294	2348	2095

Source: 2001 Census.

that were solely registered by the mother and also in the case of births that were jointly registered by parent's living at separate addresses paternal socio-economic group may not reflect the socio-economic status of the mother and child.

Therefore, to provide a context for the data shown in Chapter 1 of this Report, the UK population of women aged 15–44 years in 2001 was analysed by age and NS-SeC classification, shown in Table 21.9. NS-SeC is the National Statistics Socio-Economic Classification, based on occupation and employment status, introduced by ONS for publication of routine statistics in 2001.[4] Table 21.9 shows from age 25–59 years onwards that socio-economic group distribution is very similar across age groups. The socio-economic group with the largest percentage (25–28%) of the population for 25–29-year-olds and over is the lower managerial and professional group, while for 16–19-year-olds and 20–24-year-olds the largest group is full-time students, who are not classifiable. From age 20–24 years and over, 16–13% of women are classified as belonging to one of the two lowest socio-economic groups.

Maternities by multiplicity

One of the major changes in birth rates in the past two decades has been the increase in multiple births, especially triplet and higher-order births. In the United Kingdom, the number of maternities resulting in twins increased from 7,109 in 1982 to 9,740 in 2002. Triplet and higher-order maternities also increased from 85 in 1982 to 199 in 2002. Multiple births currently make up 1.5% of all live births. Multiple births as a percentage of all live births are now at an all time high. This increase is in part the result of increasing use of *in vitro* fertilisation (IVF) and other assisted conception techniques. IVF births in the UK account for 1% of all births. In the period 1 April 2000 to 31 March 2001, there were 1,579 twin births confirmed following IVF. However, some of this increase in multiple births is associated with increasing age at childbirth, which is, in turn, associated with a higher risk of a multiple birth. Changes in maternities by multiplicity are important due to medical risks associated with multiple births; these include an increased risk of early and late miscarriage, pre-eclampsia, higher rate of caesarean section and an increased chance of hospitalisation before the birth. Also, some parents find it very difficult to cope with twins and especially triplets and this can cause a serious risk of depression following the birth.[5]

Mode of delivery

The proportion of deliveries by caesarean section, whether elective or emergency, has been increasing steadily in England since the 1950s. During the 1950s, around 3% of babies were delivered by caesarean section but this had risen to around 15% by the mid-1990s.[6] The Health Survey for England reported that caesarean sections accounted for 23% of all deliveries in 2002; 9% by planned caesarean and 14% by emergency caesarean. This trend is important in the context of this Enquiry, since complications of a caesarean section may lead to maternal death.

The mode of delivery is highly related to both parity and age (Table 21.10). In 2000–01 5% of deliveries to women aged under 25 years were elective caesareans, a figure that had not changed from 1994–95. The proportion of women opting for a caesarean increases with age. Women aged 35 years and over were three times more likely than women aged less than 25 years to deliver by elective caesarean. Within all age groups,

Table 21.10 Percentage of singleton deliveries by caesarean section by parity and age; England 1994–95, 2000–01

Age (years)	Parity	Method of onset Elective caesareans as percentage of all deliveries (%)		Method of delivery Emergency caesareans as a percentage of all deliveries (except elective caesareans) (%)	
		1994–95	2000–01	1994–95	2000–01
All ages	Total	7	9	9	13
	0	5	6	12	18
	1+	9	11	6	10
Under 25	Total	5	5	7	11
	0	4	4	9	13
	1+	6	7	5	8
25–34	Total	8	9	9	14
	0	5	7	14	21
	1+	9	10	5	10
35 and over	Total	13	15	12	17
	0	11	12	21	29
	1+	13	16	8	13

however, primiparous women were less likely than other women to have an elective caesarean.

The same pattern of increase by age was also seen in the proportion of women whose delivery was by an emergency caesarean. In contrast, however, the proportion of deliveries by emergency caesarean was higher for primiparous women at all ages and in 2000–01 almost one-third of women aged 35 years and over (29%) had their first child delivered by emergency caesarean.

Complications during delivery

Hypertensive disorders and oedema during pregnancy were recorded in about 6% of deliveries in 2002–03. Labour was induced in over half of cases where hypertension was recorded as having complicated pregnancy, compared with one-fifth of all pregnancies.[7]

Twelve percent of deliveries with mention of a complication were recorded as having a long labour; 3% had a prolonged first stage, 8% had a prolonged second stage and the remainder had a delayed delivery due to a multiple birth. Just under two-thirds of women with a prolonged first stage of labour had an emergency caesarean, accounting for 13% of all emergency caesareans. A prolonged second stage of labour most commonly led to an instrumental delivery and these accounted for 40% of instrumental deliveries.

In 2002–03, about 21% of women had an epidural before or during delivery, 2% had a general anaesthetic and 11% a spinal anaesthetic.

There have been some significant changes in anaesthetic use for women having caesareans over the last 15 years. In 1989–90, over 50% of women having a caesarean had a general anaesthetic; by 1997–98 this proportion had fallen to under 20% and fell further to 8% in 2002–03.

Eight percent of women having elective caesareans in 2002–03 had an epidural, a significant drop from 31% in 1989–90. However, to balance these reductions, the use of spinal anaesthetic has risen from 11% in 1989–90 to 64% in 2002–03. Eight percent of women had both a spinal anaesthetic and an epidural.

Other aspects of maternal health:

Obesity

The body mass index (BMI) is the most commonly used measure of obesity. It looks at weight in relation to height, and is defined as weight in kilograms divided by height in square metres. Adults with a BMI of between 25 and 30, inclusive, are deemed to be overweight and those with a BMI over 30 are seen as obese. BMI recordings of between 20 and 25 are seen to represent healthy (or normal) weight.

In 2002, over one-third (34%) of all women were overweight. Almost one-quarter (23%) of all women were classed as being obese, a dramatic rise from the 16% reported in 1993. However, the number has dropped since 2001, when it was at an all time high of 24%. Between 1993 and 2002, the proportion of women classed as obese has risen the most in women aged 25–34 years; a rise of 10% (Figure 21.5).

The percentage of women classed as obese increases with age and reached 43% of women aged 75 years and over in 2002.

Obesity is important to this Enquiry, as women who are very overweight have an increased risk of thromboembolism, hypertension and cardiac problems.

Blood pressure

High blood pressure is a risk factor for both coronary heart disease and stroke. In addition, it is of particular danger to pregnant women and their babies, as it can lead

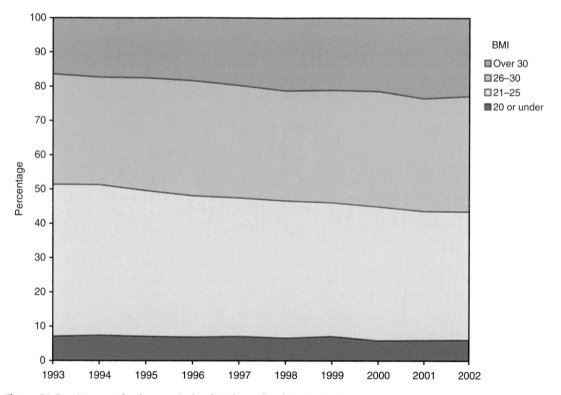

Figure 21.5 Women's body mass index (BMI); England 1993–2002

to eclampsia, a dangerous condition that kills three to five women each year. Blood pressure is considered as hypertensive if the systolic blood pressure is higher than 140 mm/Hg or if the diastolic blood pressure is 90 mm/Hg or over.

In 2002, over one-third (34%) of all women had high blood pressure, a proportion which remained largely unchanged since 1998 (33%). The proportion of women with high blood pressure increased with age, from 4% of 16–24-year-olds to 79% of women aged 75 years and over. From 1998 to 2002, between 58% and 66% of the women classed as having high blood pressure were not taking medication, although the overall proportion of untreated women has decreased slightly since 1998 (from 22% to 20%).

Contraceptive pill usage

In 2002, nearly three-quarters of women aged 16–49 years (72%) used at least one method of contraception. There has been a slight increase in the proportion of women using the contraceptive pill as their primary method of contraception, from 23% in 1986 to around one-quarter (26%) in 2002. This method is particularly common in women between the ages of 18 years and 29 years (53%).[7]

The ONS Omnibus Survey, which carries an annual module on contraception and sexual health, showed that 35% of single women were using a contraceptive pill, compared with 22% of those who were married or cohabiting and 16% of those who were widowed, divorced or separated.

In 2002, 1% of women described their current method of contraception as emergency contraception which includes the morning after pill and emergency intrauterine device. This proportion has remained consistent since the question was first asked in 2000.

Smoking

In 2002, over one-quarter of women (26%) described themselves as current smokers. The proportion of women who smoke has fluctuated between 25% and 27% since 1993. The proportion of current smokers is made up of 8% who described themselves as light smokers (under ten cigarettes a day), 11% describing themselves as medium smokers (10–19 cigarettes a day) and 6% describing themselves as heavy smokers (20 or more per day). The proportion of women who are heavy smokers is the lowest it has been since 1993.[8]

However, evidence suggests that women do reduce their smoking during pregnancy. The Infant Feeding Survey 2000 reported that 35% of women smoked to some degree before pregnancy but this dropped to just 19% throughout pregnancy. This figure has dropped from the 23% reported to have continued smoking during pregnancy in the 1995 Infant Feeding Survey report (Figure 21.6).

Alcohol

The recommended maximum number of alcohol units for women is 14 units per week. However, in 2003, the Department of Health revised their guidelines in an effort to counter the increase in binge drinking and rather than laying down guidelines in terms of a weekly limit, women are now advised not to exceed 2–3 units per day.

The proportion of young women, aged 16–24 years who drink more than the recommended 14 units per week has gone up by half in the last five years to a figure of 32%. However, it is not just young women whose alcohol intake has increased; almost

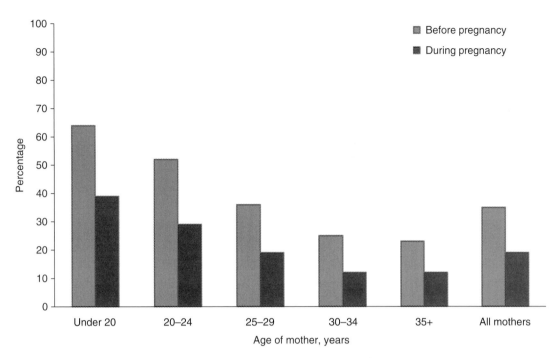

Figure 21.6 Prevalence of smoking before and during pregnancy; England 2000
Source: Infant Feeding Survey 2000

one-third, 31%, of women aged 25–44 years drink more than the recommended amount of units.[7]

For mothers who drank alcohol before pregnancy, 17% consumed less than 1 unit per week, 47% consumed between 1 and 7 units per week, 12% drank 7–14 units per week, and 5% exceeded the recommended safe limit of 14 units per week.

However, 82% of mothers reported reducing their alcohol consumption during pregnancy, over two-thirds of these (67%) within the first month; 97% of mothers consumed no more than 2 units of alcohol per week during their pregnancy and less than 1% consumed more than 7 units.[9]

Postnatal depression and other psychological illness

During the period after childbirth, new mothers experience dramatic physical, social and emotional changes. During this period, mothers are recovering from the physical demands of giving birth as well as adjusting to the new demands of their infant.[2] Information about mothers' health and emotional wellbeing is important to this Enquiry because of the mothers that die due to suicide, either during or after their pregnancy, consequent of postnatal depression and other psychiatric disorders.

The Health Survey for England 2002 looked at women's scores according to the Edinburgh Postnatal Depression Scale (EPNDS).[9] A score of ten or more was seen as a strong indicator of a possible depressive state. The survey found that 24% of all women showed signs of postnatal depression. This proportion varied by family structure with 41% of lone parents having a score of ten or more, compared with 21% of women in two-parent families.

The survey also looked at women's scores according to the General Health Questionnaire (GHQ12) which asks 12 questions with the aim of identifying individuals' psychological wellbeing. A GHQ12 score of four or more is seen as being high, indicating

Table 21.11   Ethnic group by method of onset of delivery and method of delivery; England 2002–03

Method of onset	Method of delivery	Ethnic group			
		Asian	Black	Chinese & other	White
Spontaneous	Spontaneous	60	58	59	53
	Instrumental	7	4	8	8
	Caesarean	7	9	8	7
Induced	Spontaneous	13	12	11	14
	Instrumental	2	1	2	3
	Caesarean	4	5	4	4
Caesarean	Caesarean	8	10	8	10

Source: Hospital Episode Statistics 2002–03.

probable psychiatric illness. Twenty percent of all women had a GHQ12 score of four or more. Women aged 35 years and over were less likely to have a high GHQ12 score; 14% compared with 22% of 16–34-year-olds.

Health of ethnic populations

Information about ethnic group of mother has been collected as a part of Hospital Episode Statistics since 1995 and for 2002–03 this information has been collected for 70% of delivery records. Ethnic group is categorised here as White; Black (aggregate of Black African, Black Caribbean and Black other); Asian (Indian, Pakistani, Bangladeshi); and Chinese and Other (Chinese and Other including mixed ethnic origin).

There were differences between ethnic groups in both onset of labour and type of delivery. White women were less likely than women in the other ethnic groups to have a spontaneous birth without intervention; 53% of White women compared with 58–60% in the other ethnic groups. White women were also less likely than women in any other ethnic group to be induced; 21% compared with 17–19%. Ten percent of White and Black women had planned caesareans compared with 8% of Asian and Chinese and Other women (Table 21.11).

References

1. James WH. The incidence of spontaneous abortion. *Popul Stud* 1970; 24: 241–5.
2. De La Rochebrochard E, Thonneau P. (2002) Paternal age and maternal age are risk factors for miscarriage; results of a multicentre European study. *Hum Reprod* 2002; 17: 1649–56.
3. National Statistics. Census 2001. Focus on people and migration. Overseas-born 1 in 12 in UK were born overseas [www.statistics.gov.uk/cci/nugget.asp?id=767].
4. National Statistics. The National Statistics Socio-economic Classification. 2004 [www.statistics.gov.uk/methods_quality/ns_sec/default.asp].
5. Human Fertilisation and Embryology Authority. Background Papers. Multiple births [www.hfea.gov.uk/PressOffice/Backgroundpapers/MultipleBirths].
6. Department of Health, National Statistics. NHS Maternity Statistics, England: 1989–90 to 1994–95. Department of Health Statistical Bulletin. London: DoH; 1997. [www.publications.doh.gov.uk/public/sb9728.htm].

7. Department of Health, National Statistics. NHS Maternity Statistics, England: 2002–03. Department of Health Statistical Bulletin. London: DoH; 2004 [www.publications.doh.gov.uk/public/sb0410.htm].

8. Office for National Statistics Living in Britain: General Household Survey 2002. London: HMSO; 2004 [www.statistics.gov.uk/StatBase/Product.asp?vlnk=5756].

9. National Statistics. Maternal and Infant Health, Health Survey for England 2002. London: The Stationery Office; 2003 [www.official-documents.co.uk/document/deps/doh/survey02/hse02.htm].

CHAPTER 22

Confidential Enquiries into Maternal Deaths: developments and trends from 1952 onwards

ALISON MACFARLANE

Introduction

It is often stated that confidential enquiries into maternal deaths started in 1952, but what actually happened in that year was a major development in a system which had already been established in 1928 and had its roots in enquiries in the 19th and early 20th centuries (Figure 22.1). Because of concern about the persistently high level of maternal mortality, local enquiries into individual maternal deaths started in Aberdeen in 1917 and led into major national enquiries in Scotland, England and Wales in the 1920s and 1930s.[1-8] These formed part of wider investigations of maternal mortality which looked at the provision of services, maternal morbidity and the social backgrounds of the women who died.

In its final report, published in 1932, the Departmental Committee on Maternal and Morbidity expressed the view that the confidential enquiries into individual deaths were valuable and recommended that they should continue in a modified form. The Ministry of Health responded by sending out a circular in August 1932 to all maternity and child welfare authorities asking them to continue the reporting and enclosing a revised form 97MCW for them to use in compiling confidential reports to be returned directly to the Chief Medical Officer.[9] George Gibberd and Arnold Walker, who had acted as Obstetric Assessors for the Committee's Enquiry agreed to continue their work. Data about maternal deaths from summaries of these enquiries were published in the Annual Report of the Chief Medical Officer and used to inform special enquiries, such as that of the Interdepartmental Committee on Abortion.[10]

Over the same period, the decline in maternal mortality from the late 1930s onwards shown in Figure 22.2 was investigated in analyses of death registration data. In 1939, Richard Titmuss analysed the initial decline by comparing the rate in the years 1935–37 combined with the rate in the years 1929–31 in groups of the more populous counties. He found that the decrease was 31% in the counties of London and Middlesex, 22% in Hertfordshire, Bedfordshire, Essex and Yorkshire, but only 9% in Durham, 6% in Lancashire, and 5% in Warwickshire and Staffordshire, while the rate had risen by 2% in Glamorgan.[11]

A series of analyses in the early 1950s analysed the major downwards trends shown in Figure 22.2.[12-14] They pointed to major therapeutic advances which had played a part, notably prontosil, sulphonamides and penicillin in the case of puerperal deaths from sepsis and blood transfusions in the case of haemorrhage. They also suggested that other factors were likely to have contributed, including social improvements or better access to health care following the 1936 Midwives Act. One of the articles, published in 1951, pointed out that services needed to be organised in a way that would enable women

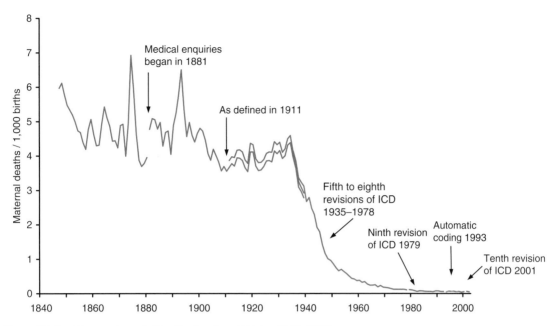

Figure 22.1 Maternal mortality; England and Wales 1847–2002
Source: General Register Office, OPCS and ONS mortality statistics reproduced in *Birth Counts*. Tables A10.1.1–A10.1.4

with complications to access maternity care: "The constant point of view underlying this analysis of maternal deaths is that, despite their infrequency, they should still be regarded as a problem requiring continuous scrutiny and possibly a shift of emphasis in the measures taken to eliminate them".[13]

By the early 1950s, reporting to the Ministry of Health had ceased in some areas and was incomplete in others.[16] This, together with a desire for more detailed information and a

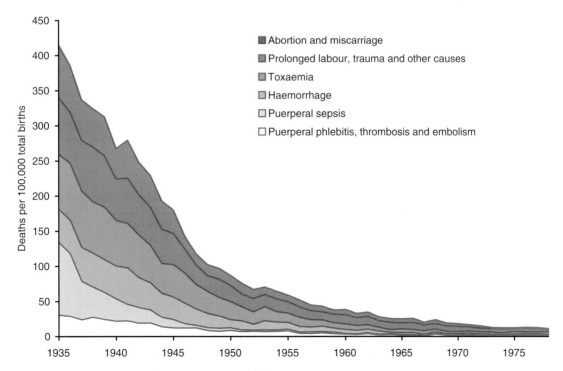

Figure 22.2 Maternal mortality by underlying cause; England and Wales 1935–78
Source: General Register Office and OPCS, Reproduced in *Birth Counts*, Table A10.1.3

review of the clinical care of individual patients led to the establishment of a new system. According to the Ministry, "Its prime purpose was to place the clinical enquiries and assessment of avoidable factors in the hands of practising consultant obstetricians".[15] A *British Medical Journal* editorial, which welcomed the first triennial Report covering the years 1952–54, described the changes made: "In 1951, however, the study, and method of assessment of maternal deaths was broadened and more information obtained. A maternal death is now noted by the medical officer of health of the local health authority and he initiates the inquiry. The local consultant obstetrician obtains all the information possible from those who were in attendance on the patient – midwife, family doctor, hospital or local authority staff".[16]

The new system involved assessment by an experienced obstetrician at regional level in England and at a national level in Wales. The assessors' reports were then sent to the Chief Medical Officer and were finally assessed and classified by the Ministry's consultant advisers on obstetrics. One of these was Arnold Walker, who had been involved with the previous enquiries since 1928. He and another obstetrician, AJ Wrigley, continued as Advisers until they retired in 1966. Similar systems were introduced in Northern Ireland in 1956 and in Scotland in 1965.

A fuller account of developments in Enquiries earlier in the 20th century can be found in Appendix 3 of the 1997–99 Report. This chapter focuses on trends and developments in the triennial enquiries from 1952–54 to 2000–02. In doing so, it follows in the footsteps of the Alec Turnbull's retrospective overview published in the 1982–84 Report, the last for England and Wales on its own. Since 1985–87, reports have covered the United Kingdom as a whole. Because of the small numbers of deaths involved, it was no longer feasible for Scotland and Northern Ireland to continue publishing separate reports. Appendix 3 lists all the Reports published to date.

Scope of the Reports and the agenda for Enquiries from 1952 onwards

A broad picture of the changing agenda of the Enquiry can be gained from the chapter titles in each Report, summarised in Table 22.1. These reflect the way that some causes, such as abortion, ectopic pregnancy and ruptured uterus have become relatively less common and are no longer the subject of whole chapters, while others such as amniotic fluid embolism were not recognised in the 1950s. Other causes of death have increased in relative importance in the context of an overall decline, for a variety of reasons. This includes fuller ascertainment and changes in the agenda to take greater account of the social factors leading to maternal death. The separate chapter on caesarean section was dropped at a time of rising caesarean sections rates because of the incompleteness of data about numbers of deliveries by caesarean section in the United Kingdom.

Another indication of the widening scope of the enquiries is the range of professions represented among the Ministry's consultant advisors and assessors. The two consultant obstetricians were joined by an anaesthetist in 1955–57. In 1980, a pathologist was added to the group. A major expansion occurred in 1985–87 when consultants from each discipline from each of the four countries of the United Kingdom were brought together in a 'clinical subgroup'. The range of disciplines expanded in the 1990s. A physician was added to the Central Assessors in 1991–93 and midwives joined regional

Table 22.1 Chapter headings in the triennial Reports

	1952–54	1955–57	1958–60	1961–63	1964–66	1967–69	1970–72	1973–75	1976–78	1979–81	1982–84	1985–87	1988–90	1991–93	1994–96	1997–99	2000–02
Toxaemia/eclampsia/hypertension	•	•	•	•	•	•	•	•	•	•	•	•	•	•	•	•	•
Haemorrhage	•	•	•	•	•	•	•	•	•	•	•	•	•	•	•	•	•
Pulmonary embolism	•	•	•	•	•	•	•	•	•	•	•	•	•	•	•	•	•
Abortion	•	•	•	•	•	•	•	•	•	•	•						
Ectopic pregnancy					•	•	•	•	•	•	•						
Early pregnancy deaths												•	•	•	•	•	•
Amniotic fluid embolism					•	•	•	•	•	•	•	•	•	•	•	•	•
Sepsis						•	•	•	•	•	•	•	•	•	•	•	•
Sudden death	•																
Ruptured uterus		•	•	•	•	•	•	•	•	•	•						
Genital tract trauma												•	•	•	•	•	•
Miscellaneous causes						•	•	•	•	•	•						
Other direct deaths												•	•	•	•	•	•
Anaesthesia	•	•	•	•	•	•	•	•	•	•	•	•	•	•	•	•	•
Caesarean section	•	•	•	•	•	•	•	•	•	•	•	•					
Cardiac disease	•	•	•	•	•	•	•	•	•	•	•	•					
Asian influenza 1957	•																
Psychiatric causes															•	•	•
Malignancies																•	•
Associated causes						•	•	•	•								
Indirect causes												•	•	•	•	•	•
Fortuitous deaths												•	•	•	•	•	•
'Late' deaths											•	•	•	•	•	•	•
Pathology										•	•	•	•	•	•	•	•
Intensive care														•	•	•	•
Midwifery practice														•	•	•	•
Domestic violence																•	•
Near misses and severe morbidity																•	•
Booking arrangements			•	•	•	•	•	•	•								
Avoidable factors	•	•	•	•													
Substandard care													•				
Factors influencing maternal mortality							•	•	•	•							
Trends in maternal mortality													•	•	•	•	•
Maternal mortality in Europe													•				

panels. A midwife and a psychiatrist were appointed as Central Assessors in 1994–96 and an intensive care specialist in 1997–99.

These professionals have made a major contribution to the enquiries but the crucial role has always been played by the 'women from the Ministry'. Medical staff in the Ministry of Health, subsequently the Department of Health and Social Security and the Department of Health, have been responsible for the day-to-day running of the Enquiries at a national level. Statistical help has been provided successively by the General Register Office, the Office of Population Censuses and Surveys and, since 1996, the Office for National Statistics.

Trends in maternal mortality since 1952

Trends in numbers and rates of maternal death reported to the Enquiries before 1985–87 are shown later and compared with data from civil registration. In trying to interpret trends in mortality over half a century, two major issues arise. The first is changes in definition and the second is completeness of ascertainment.

Table 22.2 Use of revisions of the International Classification of Diseases

Revision of the ICD	Introduced in England and Wales for coding death certificates
Fifth revision	1940
Sixth revision	1950
Seventh revision	1958
Eighth revision	1968
Ninth revision	1979
Tenth revision	2001

Changes in classification

The ways in which maternal and indeed all other deaths are classified changes each time a new revision of the International Classification of Diseases (ICD) is introduced. As well as reflecting changes in perceptions of causality and advances in knowledge, the amount of detail used in coding specific causes may reflect their contribution to overall mortality. Table 22.2 shows the years when each revision was introduced in England and Wales. As the Confidential Enquiry process involves retrospective reviews which can lead to different causes being assigned, this can result in new revisions of the classification being applied to data for years preceding those in which they were used for coding death certificates.

As far as maternal mortality was concerned, the fifth to eighth revisions of the ICD had a fairly consistent structure, making it possible to construct the trends in registered maternal deaths shown in Figure 22.2 and those in deaths reported to the enquiries up to 1978, shown in Table 22.3. A death was either described as a 'true maternal death', with

Table 22.3 Main causes of true maternal deaths reported to confidential enquiries; England and Wales 1952–78

Cause	1952–54	1955–57	1958–60	1961–63	1964–66	1967–69	1970–72	1973–75	1976–78
				Numbers reported					
Abortion	153	141	135	139	133	117	81	29	19**
Pulmonary embolism	138	157	132	129	91	75	61	35	45
Haemorrhage	220*	138	130	92	68	41	27	21	26
Hypertensive diseases of pregnancy	246	171	118	104	67	53	47	39	29
All other causes	369	254	227	228	220	169	139	111	108
All	1,094	861	742	692	579	455	355	235	227
				Rates per million maternities					
Abortion	74.5	66.7	58.8	55.1	51.1	47.6	35.2	15.1	10.9
Pulmonary embolism	67.2	74.3	57.5	51.2	35.0	30.5	26.5	18.2	25.7
Haemorrhage	107.2*	65.3	56.7	36.5	26.2	16.7	11.7	10.9	14.9
Hypertensive diseases of pregnancy	119.8	80.9	51.4	41.3	25.8	21.6	20.5	20.3	16.6
All other causes	179.7	120.2	98.9	90.5	84.6	68.8	60.5	57.8	61.7
All	532.9	407.4	323.4	274.6	222.7	185.2	154.5	122.3	129.8
Deaths known to Registrar General	1,404	1,112	928	816	671	527	387	254	228
Percentage reported to Enquiry	77.9	77.4	80.0	84.8	86.3	86.3	91.7	92.5	99.6*

* Corrected figures
**Including five deaths from anaesthesia associated with operations for abortion for comparison with previous triennia*
Source: Confidential Enquiries into Maternal Deaths in England and Wales and Birth Counts[17] Table 10.4.1

an underlying cause in the chapter used to code conditions of pregnancy, childbirth and the puerperium or as an 'associated death' of a woman known to have been pregnant but having an underlying cause in another chapter of the ICD.[18]

In the ninth revision of the ICD, a major change in structure was introduced, with the introduction of the definitions of 'direct' and 'indirect' maternal deaths set out in Section 1 of this Report.[19] Some of what had been formerly classified as 'associated' deaths were considered 'indirect' and allocated the relevant codes within the chapter of the ICD relating to 'conditions of pregnancy, childbirth and the puerperium' while others were categorised as 'fortuitous'. As Chapter 1 of this Report points out, countries differ in what they include in the 'indirect' category.[20] In particular, suicide and other deaths from psychiatric causes are considered by the compilers of international classifications to be fortuitous rather indirect, but have increasingly been categorised as *Indirect* over the past five triennia in the Confidential Enquiries in the United Kingdom.

The same structure was maintained in the tenth revision of the ICD, used in 2000–02 in this Enquiry.[21] It has also been used from 2000 onwards for coding death certificates in Scotland and from 2001 for coding death certificates in England, Wales and Northern Ireland. Although the term 'late maternal death' did not appear in the ICD until the tenth revision, the concept was used from a much earlier stage, both when reporting data from death registration[17] and in the Confidential Enquiries, as Table 22.1 shows. They have been the subject of a separate chapter since 1979–81, but were discussed in earlier Reports. Although the ICD still uses the term *'Fortuitous'*, the term *'Coincidental'* has been used since 1997–99 to describe these deaths in the Confidential Enquiry Reports.

In the Confidential Enquiries, deaths in earlier triennia were re-categorised retrospectively. Table 22.4, taken from the Report for 1982–84, shows *Direct* maternal deaths in England from 1970–72 to 1976–78 re-categorised in this way and Table 22.5, taken from the same Report, shows how deaths previously classed as associated deaths were categorised subsequently. Tables 22.6 and 22.7 summarise deaths reported to Confidential Enquiries in Scotland and Northern Ireland.

Increasing completeness of ascertainment

Completeness of ascertainment, discussed in Chapter 1 with respect to changes in the methods used to code causes of death on death certificates and linkage studies in England and Wales from the mid-1990s onwards, has always been an issue. In the early years, the major problem was under-reporting compared with death registration. The *British Medical Journal* leader on the 1,094 deaths classified as due to pregnancy and childbirth and 316 deaths classified as due to associated causes in 1952–54 Report commented that "This figure represents only 71% of the total registered maternal deaths. It is to be hoped that in the future all maternal deaths will be included. There is no question of the Ministry searching for a scapegoat and exposing a person or institution to public condemnation: it is only by revealing deficiencies in the maternity services that preventable deaths will be eliminated, administration improved, and maternity made safer".[16]

As Table 22.3 shows, 77.9% of registered true maternal deaths were included in the Enquiries in 1952–54 and this dropped marginally to 77.4% in the next triennium before gradually increasing until 99.6% of true maternal deaths were included in 1976–78. Figure 22.3 compares 'true' maternal mortality rates from death registration and the Enquiry up to 1978, the last year in which the eighth revision of the ICD was used.

Table 22.4 Causes of *Direct* maternal deaths reported to the Confidential Enquiries; England and Wales 1970–84

Causes of *Direct* maternal death	1970–72	1973–75	1976–78	1979–81	1982–84
			Numbers reported		
Pulmonary embolism	51	33	43	23	25
Hypertensive diseases of pregnancy	43	34	29	36	25
Anaesthesia	37	27	27	22	18
Amniotic fluid embolism	14	14	11	18	14
Abortion	73	27	14	14	11
Ectopic pregnancy	34	19	21	20	10
Haemorrhage	30	21	24	14	9
Sepsis, excluding abortion	30	19	15	8	2
Ruptured uterus	11	11	14	4	3
Other direct causes	20	22	19	19	21
All deaths	343	227	217	178	138
			Rates per million pregnancies*		
Pulmonary embolism	17.6	12.8	18.5	9.0	10.0
Hypertensive diseases of pregnancy	14.9	13.2	12.5	14.2	10.0
Anaesthesia	12.8	10.5	11.6	8.7	7.2
Amniotic fluid embolism	4.8	5.4	4.7	7.1	5.6
Abortion	25.3	10.5	6.0	5.5	4.4
Ectopic pregnancy	11.5	7.4	9.0	7.9	4.0
Haemorrhage	10.4	8.1	10.3	5.5	3.6
Sepsis, excluding abortion	10.4	7.4	6.5	3.1	1.0
Ruptured uterus	3.8	4.3	6.0	1.6	1.2
Other direct causes	6.9	8.5	8.2	7.5	8.4
All deaths	118.7	88.0	93.4	70.0	55.0
			Rates per million maternities		
	154.3	122.6	121.8	93.1	72.4
			Thousands		
Estimated number of pregnancies*	2,890.7	2,578.4	2,323.8	2,543.2	2,507.0
Estimated number of maternities	2,222.5	1,851.9	1,781.3	1,910.9	1,905.8

* Pregnancies leading to registrable births, legal abortions or hospital stays for miscarriage or ectopic pregnancy
Source: Confidential Enquiries into Maternal Deaths in England and Wales, 1982–84, Tables 1.7, 18.1 and 18.2 and Birth Counts[17] Table 10.4.2

Table 22.5 Numbers of associated, indirect, and fortuitous deaths, England and Wales, 1952–84

	'Associated'		Indirect	Fortuitous
	All	**Excluding late deaths**		
1952–54	316			
1955–57	339			
1958–60	254			
1961–63	244			
1964–66	176			
1967–69	246	221		
1970–72	251	206		
1973–75	155	111		
1976–78		134	78	56
1979–81		121	90	31
1982–84		105	72	34

Late deaths from 1967–69? onwards are excluded from this table.
Source: *Report on confidential enquiries into maternal deaths in England and Wales, 1982–84*, Table 19.6

Table 22.6 Maternal deaths by diagnostic group; Scotland 1965–85

Diagnostic group	1965–71	1972–75	1976–80	1981–85	1986–90	1965–71	1972–75	1976–80	1981–85	1986–90
	Numbers					Rates per million maternities				
Pulmonary embolism	25	3	7	8	..	38.1	10.3	21.3	24.2	..
Cardiac	18	5	2	8	..	27.5	17.1	6.1	24.2	..
Ectopic	3	5	1	5	..	4.6	17.1	3.0	15.1	..
Amniotic fluid embolism	7	5	6	3	..	10.7	17.1	18.3	9.1	..
Anaesthetic complication	5	7	6	3	..	7.6	24.0	18.3	9.1	..
Pregnancy hypertension	17	3	4	2	..	25.9	10.3	12.2	6	..
Sepsis	18	5	1	1	..	27.5	17.1	3.0	3.0	..
Dystocia	7	0	1	1	..	10.7	–	3.0	3.0	..
Abortion	14	11	5	1	..	21.4	37.7	15.2	3.0	..
Vesicular mole	1	1	0	0	..	1.5	3.4	–	–	..
Haemorrhage	16	9	7	0	..	24.4	30.9	21.3	–	..
Other *Direct* or *Indirect*	35	15	24	12	..	53.4	51.4	73.1	36.3	..
All *Direct* or *Indirect*	166	69	64	44	27	25.3	23.7	19.5	13.3	8.3
Other *Fortuitous*	22	23	19	11	..	3.4	7.9	5.8	3.3	..
All maternal deaths	188	92	83	55	..	28.7	31.5	25.3	16.6	..
Maternities	655,551	291,615	328,304	330,746	325,783					

Source: Scottish Home and Health Department, *Reports on maternal and perinatal deaths in Scotland, 1981–85, 1986–90* and Birth counts[17], Table A10.4.4
The numbers of deaths in 1986–90 were too low for analysis by diagnostic group

Table 22.7 Main causes of true maternal deaths reported to Confidential Enquiries; Northern Ireland 1956–84

Cause	1956–59	1960–63	1964–67	1968–77	1978–84
	Numbers reported				
Abortion	1	2	5	7	1
Ectopic pregnancy	1	1	1	2	2
Haemorrhage	23	9	2	9	3
Hypertensive disease	25	15	9	6	6
Pulmonary embolism	12	6	11	3	0
Sepsis	15	3	2	2	1
Associated with anaesthesia	3	3	2	5	2
Associated with, but not necessarily due to caesarean section	15	10	1	14	*
Rupture of the uterus	3	3	1	2	2
Cardiac disease*	13	13	11	6	3
Miscellaneous	0	0	0	1	3
Total deaths reported to the Enquiry**	116	61	37	54	23
	Rates				
Deaths per 100,000 maternities	–	–	27.2	18.4	12.0
Deaths per 100,000 live births	96.1	47.0	27.4	18.4	12.0
	Numbers reported				
Maternities	–	–	135,819	294,014	191,778
Live births	120,707	129,883	134,878	293,734	192,277

* Not given explicitly for 1978–84
** Numbers and percentages may exceed the total as some deaths were included in more than one category
Source: Confidential Enquiries into Maternal Deaths in Northern Ireland and Birth Counts[17] Table A10.3.5

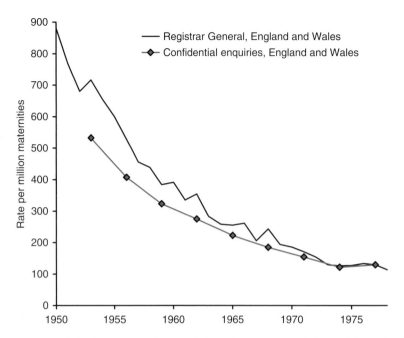

Figure 22.3 'True maternal deaths' reported to Confidential Enquiries and derived from death registration; England and Wales 1950–78
Source: Confidential enquiries and death registration

Crosschecks were made between the two and it was reported that the distribution by very broad cause was similar for death registration and the enquiries. It was difficult to make direct comparisons as the Enquiry Assessors reassigned some of the causes of death on the death certificates in the light of the fuller information assembled for the enquiries. In addition, even in the pre-computer era, the Enquiry brought to light deaths which had not been classified as maternal on death certificates. For example, in 1955–57, there were 361 deaths registered by the Registrar General which had not been reported to the enquiries but an additional 96 deaths which, "due to faulty or incomplete certification of death, were not registered as maternal deaths by the Registrar General".

The situation is now different, as Table 1.1 shows. All the deaths known to the Registrars General are now included in the Enquiries, together with the further deaths which did not originally have maternal underlying causes and those where the pregnancy was not even mentioned. These are ascertained in the ways described in Chapter 1.

Trends up to 2002 in the causes of maternal death which were the leading causes in the early 1950s, are shown in Figure 22.4, drawn on a common scale. For comparative purpose, mortality rates derived from death registration up to 1978 are shown to give a fuller picture of trends in the first 25 years.

The leading cause of death in 1952–54 was those attributed at various periods to toxaemia, hypertension or eclampsia. Rates were already falling in the 1950s, as Figure 22.2 shows, and continued to fall rapidly up the mid 1960s. The decline has been much slower since then and pregnancy-induced hypertension was still one of the leading causes of death in 2000–02.

Mortality attributed to haemorrhage was also high in 1952–54 but already falling, probably because of widening access to blood transfusion. Rates have fluctuated about a similar level since the 1980s and the disappointing upturn in 2000–02 could well be part of this longer-term pattern.

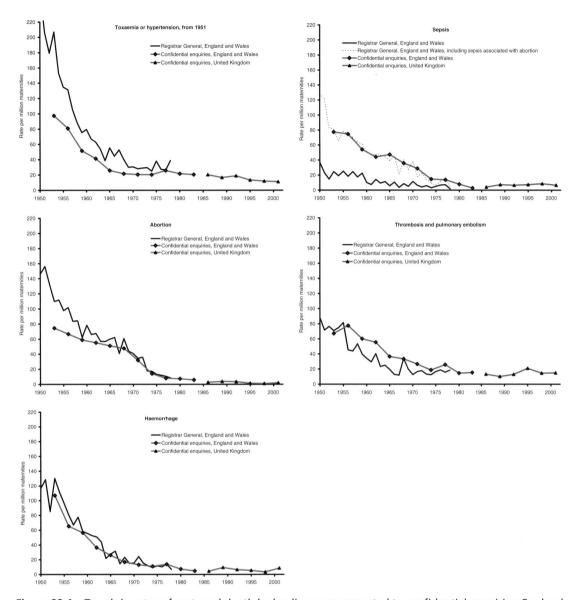

Figure 22.4 Trends in rates of maternal death by leading cause reported to confidential enquiries: England and Wales, 1952–84, United Kingdom 1985–2002 and rates of maternal death registered in England and Wales, 1950–78
Source: Confidential enquiries and death registration

Mortality attributed to thrombosis and pulmonary embolism based on reports to the enquiries was higher than that among registered deaths in seven of the first nine triennia. This, along with the slow nature of the decline, the reported increase in 1994–96 and its persisting position as the leading cause of direct death in 2000–02 may be a consequence of improved ascertainment. Nevertheless the reported rate for 2000–02 remains at nearly a quarter of the rate for 1952–54.

The rate of deaths attributed to abortion and miscarriage declined relatively slowly in the 1950s and 1960s. The role of antibiotics and the changing nature of puerperal sepsis undoubtedly had an impact on death rates from septic abortion.[22] Rates fell quickly, although not instantly, in the aftermath of the implementation of 1967 Abortion Act. Commenting on the first signs of a downturn in 1969, the 1967–69 Report suggested that the availability of contraception under the NHS from 1967 onwards should also have contributed to it. The timing of trends reflects the time it took to establish contraceptive services and safe services for termination of pregnancy and ensure that they were accessible to women who need them.

Deaths from the consequences of miscarriage and abortion had virtually but not completely disappeared from the scene by 2000–02, when the majority of early pregnancy deaths were associated with ectopic pregnancy. Trends in deaths from sepsis overall are difficult to interpret in the early triennia, as deaths from septic abortion were not initially separated from post-abortive sepsis. Overall rates had fallen dramatically since the mid-1930s, as Figure 7.1 (page 110) shows, and the major drop in deaths from abortion contributed substantially to the further decline in the 1970s. After this, the rate levelled off.

Trends in deaths from 'associated causes' are difficult to interpret, because of their subsequent subdivision into *Indirect* and *Fortuitous* and the further subdivision into deaths before 42 days after the end of a pregnancy and *Late* deaths. This is further compounded by changing views about which deaths should be included and increasing levels of ascertainment, notably as a result of changes in the processing of death registration data and the linkage exercise described in Chapter 1. Nevertheless, two aspects stand out from the rest. The first is the decline in numbers of deaths associated with rheumatic heart disease in pregnancy, as the disease itself declined in the 1950s and 1960s. In 1952–54, 38.2% of associated deaths were attributed to cardiac disease as a whole, falling to 16.% in 1973–75. The second is the considerable mortality in 2000–02 from suicide and misadventure in the first year after women gave birth which was revealed by the ONS record linkage exercise.

'Avoidable factors' and 'substandard care'

As the 1952–54 Report commented with respect to the earlier enquiry, "One of the chief features of the investigation initiated by the Departmental Committee was the assessment of what was termed the 'primary avoidable factor' in the circumstances of a maternal death, that is some departure from the (then) accepted standards off satisfactory care, from which ensued the train of events resulting in the death". The same concept was used from 1952–54 onwards, but the procedures and the criteria adopted were made more stringent. Whereas the earlier procedure used a questionnaire "which seldom derived from consultant opinion", from 1952 onwards, a consultant obstetrician was involved in compiling the Report locally, in addition to the obstetricians involved at regional and national levels. It was stated that "practical and generally accepted standards, attainable under average practice conditions, have been applied rather than an ideal". The Report went on to acknowledge that "It is not, of course, suggested that, in all cases in which avoidable factors were considered to be present, death could have been certainly prevented, but the presence of an avoidable factor is regarded as an indication that the risk of death could have been, at least, materially lessened". This was reiterated in subsequent Reports.

The subjective nature of the process was acknowledged on a number of occasions. For example, in the 1967–69 Report, the Assessors commented on this: "For example they have not assessed the use of utus paste to induce abortion as an avoidable factor, even though some consider this to be hazardous; neither has the failure to use anticoagulant drugs in the prevention or treatment of thromboembolic disease been regarded as an avoidable factor". In contrast, an avoidable factor was always considered to be present in illegal abortions.

The Assessors attributed responsibility for avoidable factors to specific categories of staff or to the patient or relatives. The 1952–54 Report stated that "In no case has a patient's refusal to accept termination of pregnancy or to practise contraception been regarded as an avoidable factor". This was reiterated in subsequent Reports and the 1964–66 Report, published in 1969, drew attention to the fact that the National Health Service (Family Planning) Act, which came into force in 1967, had made contraception available under the NHS.

The way in which responsibility was attributed changed over time. The 1958–60 Report commented that. "In order to avoid unjust imputation of blame to persons or to particular professional groups, it was decided in the Report for 1955–57 to ascribe the avoidable factors to the services in which they were made, that is domiciliary or hospital, except where the patient herself contributed to her death. The factors were further subdivided into the period of pregnancy or childbirth in which they occurred. In this Report, it has been decided to ascribe the factor to the person who was responsible for the mistake". This raised questions about the extent to which experienced staff were responsible for actions taken, in their absence, by less experienced staff.

The term 'substandard care' superseded 'avoidable factors' in the 1979–81 Report onwards. "This is because the term was sometimes misinterpreted to mean that avoiding these factors would have prevented the death. The term 'substandard care' has been used to take into account not only failure in clinical care but also some of the underlying factors which may also have produced a low standard of care for the patient. These include shortage of resources for staffing facilities and administrative failure in the maternity services and back-up facilities such as anaesthetic, radiological and pathology services."

Booking arrangements

A recurring feature in the discussion of 'avoidable factors' in the early Reports was booking for delivery, at a time when there were not enough hospital beds for the women who wanted to give birth in hospital. Although the beds should have been allocated on the basis of need for hospital care, this did not necessarily happen in practice. The 1955–57 Report contained may references to the need for better selection of women for hospital care, based on its definition of the 'priority classes', which were categories of women with high maternal mortality rates. It was pointed out in the 1958–60 Report that it was usual to list the indications for hospital care, but the report suggested that it would be simpler to list criteria for delivery at home or in a GP maternity home. These criteria were:

1. As far as can be ascertained, the woman's general physical state is unimpaired.

2. She is pregnant for the second, third or fourth time, the previous pregnancies, labours and puerperia have been normal and she is under 35 years of age.

3. She is a primagravida under 30 years of age.

4. She is rhesus positive or is known to have no antibodies.

5. The home conditions are suitable.

Table 22.8 Numbers of true and associated maternal deaths by initial place of booking, England and Wales; 1961–81

	1961-63	1964–66	1967–69	1970–72	1973–75	1976–78	1979–81
Domiciliary	194	125	68	34	7	6	4
General practioner (all)	96	76	77	60	32	34	24
Separate						10	7
With consultant unit						24	17
Private nursing home		8	1	2	1	1	1
Consultant unit	428	349	352	285	226	224	213
Armed forces hospital		0	0	4	2	2	2
No booking made	218	190	166	148	68	82	46
No information		7	34	16	2	2	9
Total	936	755	698	549	338	351	299

Late deaths are excluded for 1970–72 onwards
Source: Reports on Confidential Enquiries into Maternal Deaths, 1961–63, 1967–69, 1979–81

From 1961–63 to 1976–78, the Reports had a separate chapter on booking arrangements. This was dropped when the structure was organised in 1979–81, on the grounds that "it no longer provided much relevant information". This is not surprising, as, by 1986, when the 1979–81 Report was published, only 0.9% of deliveries in England and Wales took place at home, compared with 28.6% in 1964. Deliveries in isolated GP units had fallen from 12.3% of all deliveries in 1969 to 2.3% in 1986.[17] As Table 22.8 shows, only a handful of deaths in 1979–81 were of women who had booked for home delivery, compared with nearly 200 in 1961–63.

Many of the women for whom no booking had been made died before the 28th week of pregnancy and included a substantial proportion of abortions up to the beginning of the 1970s. The decline in deaths from abortion contributed substantially to the decline of numbers of deaths in this category.

A table of data on deaths by place of booking was included in the 1979–81 Report and has been used in compiling Table 22.8. After 1979–81, the subject of place of delivery was dropped until 1994–96, by which time the percentage of deliveries at home had risen to just over 2% and midwife-led units were replacing the remaining GP maternity units. As Table 22.9 shows, the overwhelming majority of *Direct* and *Indirect* deaths are now of women who give birth in hospital, as that is where over 97 per cent of deliveries took place.

Table 22.9 Numbers of direct and indirect deaths reported to confidential enquiries by place of delivery; United Kingdom 1994–2002

	1994–96	1997–99	2000–02
Consultant unit	152	132	152
Stand-alone GP/midwife-led unit	1	3	1
Accident and emergency	12	11	15
Intensive care unit	2	2	1
Hospital other	0	3	3
Home	2	4	3
Total	169	155	175

Source: Reports on Confidential Enquiries into Maternal Deaths, 1994–96, 1997–99, 2000–02

Social factors

Before the very explicit shift to a greater emphasis on social factors in the 1994–96 Report, the focus of the Reports was predominantly clinical. Nevertheless, the social factors behind maternal death were still apparent to a varying extent. In particular, from the 1950s to the 1970s, the deaths of women who had made no arrangements for delivery included many women who would now be described as 'socially excluded'. Among those repeatedly mentioned were young women, women who had concealed their pregnancies and migrant women. The 1967–69 Report commented that "Of the 166 unbooked women, 37 were of African or West Indian origin, six were Asian and two were non-British European. There is a need for health education among women who because of language barriers or cultural differences may not appreciate the importance of ante-natal care and do not avail themselves of maternity services. The abortion chapter commented that of the 117 deaths from abortion, 40 were to women from the 'New Commonwealth' and 32 of these were due to 'illegal interference'.

Tabulations of maternal deaths by mother's country of birth were included in the Reports for 1970–72 to 1982–84. Each of these showed much higher mortality rates among women born in the 'New Commonwealth' than among those born in the United Kingdom. An analysis of death registration data for the years 1970–78 led to similar conclusions.[23] The 1982–84 Report pointed out that country of birth did not necessarily equate to ethnic origin and the subject was dropped from subsequent Reports until analyses by ethnic origin were attempted in 1994–96. Its absence was noted in a *British Medical Journal* editorial welcoming the Report for 1988–90: "Not quite breaking the surface, but stretching its surface tension, are mentions throughout the Report of 'recent immigrants' or women speaking 'little English'. These may well be numerators in search of a denominator, but the hidden message is clear".[24]

Formal analyses of maternal deaths by social class were included in the Reports for England and Wales for 1970–72 to 1979–81 and the Report for Scotland for 1972–75 also contained a section on social factors. Together with the analyses by country of birth, the analyses for England and Wales probably reflect the influence of Abe Adelstein, head of the Medical Statistics Division of the Office of Population Censuses and Surveys, where work was under way on the Registrar General's Decennial Supplement for 1970–72.[25] The Decennial Supplement and the Confidential Enquiry Reports for 1970–72 and 1979–81 all showed maternal mortality to be highest among women with husbands in manual occupations. After health inequalities disappeared from the national political agenda in the 1980s, these analyses were dropped from the confidential Enquiry Report for 1982–84 on the grounds that "Data on social class are usually based on the occupation of the woman's partner. These data have not been included in this Report because of the increasing difficulty in interpreting social class information on women, many of whom are working and not influenced by their partner's occupation".

No further attempt at analyses by social class was made until 1997–99, when the main finding was not the difference between occupational classes but the differences between the high rates for women who did not have an occupation or a partner with an occupation and the much lower rates for other women.

The inequalities in maternal mortality in the second half of the 20th century contrast with those seen in the 19th century and in the early part of the 20th century. At that time maternal mortality rates were even higher in more affluent districts and among more privileged sections of the population who had access to care which was dangerous than they were among less advantaged women.[26]

International comparisons

From time to time, the Reports have included comparisons with maternal mortality rates for other developed countries. A table of rates was included in the Report for 1967–69, together with a warning that countries vary in their interpretation of international rules for data collection. A further table in the 1970–72 Report showed that England and Wales compared unfavourably with Nordic countries but that rates within England and Wales ranged from 5.9 per 100,000 live births in the Oxford Region to 17.2 per 100,000 live births in the Leeds Region.

The 1988–90 Report included the results of a survey of maternal mortality in countries which were members of the European College of Obstetrics and Gynaecology. The questionnaire asked about the classifications used, the extent to which postmortem examinations were performed and about several aspects of data collection. These included whether the death certificate included a special question on pregnancy and what efforts were made to ensure complete ascertainment of maternal deaths. This survey highlighted considerable discrepancies between countries. The Report warned that caution was needed in comparing data for different countries, especially small countries with few maternal deaths, and called for confidential enquiries to be conducted at a European level. This need for caution was confirmed in a European collaborative study in which international panels of clinicians assessed anonymised data from participating countries, including a subset of UK Enquiry data for 1993, in terms of their classification as *Direct* and *Indirect* and used the results to recalculate direct and indirect mortality rates for the countries concerned.[20]

Severe maternal morbidity

Although maternal morbidity was discussed in the Enquiry Reports published in the 1930s[3,4,6] it did not appear explicitly on the agenda of the current series of Enquiries until 1997–99. A one-off study in the former South East Thames Region,[27] formed part of a European study whose results suggested that, even when working to a common protocol, differences in ascertainment may still affect observed variations between countries.[28] The approach developed in Scotland to routine audit of obstetric haemorrhage, described in Chapter 19 of this Report, is a major step forward and it will be interesting to see what developments follow elsewhere.

Changing maternal mortality

In his preface to the 1967–69 Report, the Chief Medical Officer, Sir George Godber, who had been involved in the implementing the new system in 1952 commented that, "None of us contemplated in 1952 that the number of maternal deaths would be reduced to the extent that it has been. Now we can all see that in the light of this present Report that it may become possible to reduce the number of true maternal deaths below a hundred a year". In a similarly optimistic vein, former Obstetric Assessor, Alec Turnbull, in his overview of the period from 1952–54 to 1982–84 included in the 1982–84 Report, pointed out that maternal mortality had halved in every decade since 1937 from 989 per million maternities in 1951 to 86 in 1984. He predicted that if it continued to decline at the same rate, maternal mortality in England and Wales would reach approximately 44 per million in 1991 and approximately 22 per million in 2001.

Neither of these predictions proved to be true. As the *BMJ* editorial cited earlier pointed out, maternal mortality levelled off from 1985–87 onwards.[24] As this Report makes clear, rising trends at the beginning of the 21st century are not simply a consequence of improvements in ascertainment. Changes in the childbearing population may also play a part. As long ago as 1975, it was suggested that Enquiry data should be standardised for mothers' ages and parity and other relevant factors.[29] Such analyses are needed today to allow for rising age at childbirth, increasing rates of multiple birth and other trends documented in Chapter 21 of this Report. Questions also arise about the use of controls in Confidential Enquiries. So far, the only example use of a comparison group in an enquiry into maternal mortality in the United Kingdom is in the report of the enquiry in Scotland published in 1935.[6]

Like its predecessors, this 50th anniversary Report is intended to stimulate practical action, but, like them, it also raises questions for further debate and investigation.

References

1. Kinloch JP, Smith J, Steven JA. *Maternal Mortality. Report on Maternal Mortality in Aberdeen, 1918–1927, with Special Reference to Puerperal Sepsis*. Edinburgh: Scottish Board of Health; 1928.
2. Scottish Departmental Committee on Puerperal Morbidity. *Report*. Edinburgh: HMSO; 1924.
3. Ministry of Health. *Interim Report of the Departmental Committee on Maternal Mortality and Morbidity*. London: HMSO; 1930.
4. Ministry of Health. *Final Report of the Departmental Committee on Maternal Mortality and Morbidity*. London: HMSO; 1932.
5. Campbell J, Cameron, ID, Jones DM. *High Maternal Mortality in Certain Areas*. Reports on Public Health and Medical Subjects No. 68. London: HMSO; 1932.
6. Douglas, CA, McKinlay PL. *Report on Maternal Morbidity and Mortality in Scotland*. Edinburgh: HMSO; 1935.
7. Ministry of Health. *Report on an Investigation into Maternal Mortality*. Cmd 5422. London: HMSO; 1937.
8. Ministry of Health. *Report of an Investigation into Maternal Mortality in Wales*. Cmd 5423. London: HMSO; 1937.
9. Ministry of Health. *On the State of the Public Health. Annual Report of the Chief Medical Officer for the Year 1932*. London: HMSO; 1933.
10. Ministry of Health, Home Office. *Report of the Interdepartmental Committee on Abortion*. London: HMSO; 1939.
11. Titmuss RM. Puerperal mortality in England and Wales. *Public Health* 1939:LII:353–5.
12. Stocks P. Fifty years of progress as shown by vital statistics. *BMJ* 1950;i:54–7.

13. Webb J, Weston-Edwards P. Recent trends in maternal mortality. *The Medical Officer* 1951;86:201–4.

14. Taylor W, Dauncey M. Changing patterns of mortality in England and Wales. II: maternal mortality. *Br J Prev Soc Med* 1954;8:172–5.

15. Ministry of Health. *Annual Report of the Chief Medical Officer for 1952.* Cmd 9009. London: HMSO; 1953.

16. Maternal mortality. [Editorial]. *BMJ* 1957; August 3:280–1.

17. Macfarlane AJ, Mugford M, Henderson J, Furtado A, Stevens J, Dunn A. *Birth Counts: Statistics of Pregnancy and Childbirth.* Volume 2, Tables. 2nd ed. London: The Stationery Office; 2000.

18. World Health Organization. *International Classification of Diseases. Manual of the International Statistical Classification of Diseases, Injuries and Causes of Death.* Eighth revision. Vol. 1. Geneva: WHO; 1967.

19. World Health Organization. *International Classification of Diseases. Manual of the International Statistical Classification of Diseases, Injuries and Causes of Death.* Ninth revision. Vol. 1. Geneva: WHO; 1977.

20. Salanave B, Bouvier-Colle M-H, Varnoux N, Alexander S, Macfarlane A, The MOMS Group. Classification differences and maternal mortality: a European study. *Int J Epidemiol* 1999;28:64–9.

21. World Health Organization. *International Statistical Classification of Diseases and Related Health Problems.* Tenth revision. Vol. 1. Geneva: WHO; 1992.

22. Loudon I. Puerperal fever, the streptococcus and the sulphonamides. *BMJ* 1987;295:485–90.

23. Marmot MG, Adelstein AM, Bulusu L. *Immigrant Mortality in England and Wales 1970–1978: Causes of Death by Country of Birth.* Studies on Medical and Population Subjects No. 47. London: HMSO; 1984.

24. Keirse M. Maternal mortality: stalemate or stagnant? *BMJ* 1994:308:354–5.

25. Office of Population Censuses and Surveys. *Occupational Mortality: Decennial Supplement 1970–1972 England and Wales.* OPCS Decennial Supplement Series DS No. 1. London: HMSO; 1978.

26. Loudon I. Obstetric care, social class, and maternal mortality. *BMJ* 1986;293:606–8.

27. Waterstone M, Bewley S, Wolfe C. Incidence and predictors of severe obstetric morbidity: case control study. *BMJ* 2001;322:1089–94.

28. Zhang W-H, Alexander S, Bouvier-Colle M-H, Macfarlane A and the MOMS-B Group. Incidence of three conditions of severe maternal morbidity in a European population-based study : the MOMS-B survey. *BJOG.* In press.

29. Newcombe RG. Campbell H, Chalmers I. Maternal deaths. *Lancet* 1975;ii:1099.

Section

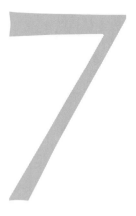

7

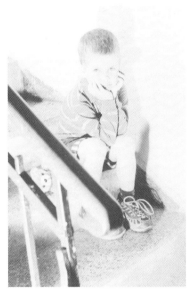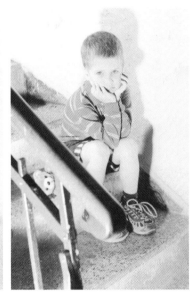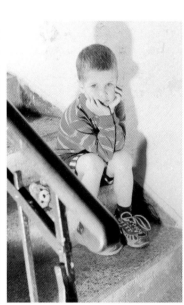

APPENDICES

APPENDIX 1

Method of Enquiry

JOAN NOBLE on behalf of CEMACH

Historical background

This is the sixth Report to cover the whole of the United Kingdom. The English and Welsh reports were published at 3-yearly intervals from 1952 until 1984. The Reports for Scotland were published at different intervals from 1965 to 1985, the last covering both maternal and perinatal deaths. Northern Ireland Reports were started in 1956 and were published 4-yearly until 1967; because of the small number of maternal deaths the next Report covered 10 years from 1968 to 1977 and the last Report covered the 7-year period 1978–1984. The relatively small number of deaths in Scotland and Northern Ireland led to the decision of the four Chief Medical Officers to change to a combined United Kingdom Report after 1984.

From 1984 to 1999 the combined UK Reports were produced by The Confidential Enquiry into Maternal Deaths (CEMD). In April 2003, the CEMD and the Confidential Enquiry into Stillbirths and Infant Deaths (CESDI) merged to form the new Confidential Enquiry into Maternal and Child Health (CEMACH). CEMACH operates with a central office in London and regional offices (nine in England and one each in Wales and Northern Ireland). The central office coordinates the activity of the regional offices, provides the central databases and the direction and leadership for the Enquiry. The management structure of the Enquiry consists of the Board, the Enquiry staff and distinct committees for each area of work. The Board has representation from the Royal College of Obstetricians and Gynaecologists (which hosts the Enquiry), Royal College of Midwifery, Royal College of Pathologists, Faculty of Public Health Medicine, Royal College of Paediatrics and Child Heath and the Royal College of Anaesthetists. This is the first Report of the Maternal Deaths' Enquiry (MDE) to be produced under CEMACH.

CEMACH is commissioned by the National Institute of Clinical Excellence (NICE) to conduct the MDE in England and Wales. Northern Ireland does not come under NICE but contributes funds to cover its participation. In Scotland, the Scottish Programme for Clinical Effectiveness in Reproductive Health acting on behalf of NHS Quality Improvement Scotland (NHSQIS) conducts its own Enquiry programme but sends its cases to be included in the triennial Report and NHSQIS contributes funds towards its participation in the Enquiry.

England and Wales

In the first year of this triennium, the responsibility for initiating an enquiry into a maternal death remained with the Director of Public Health (DPH) of the district in which the woman was usually resident. In the second year before CEMACH was established, this became the responsibility of the CESDI Regional Coordinator and then, once CEMACH was established, it was assumed by the CEMACH Regional Manager (RM).

It is a government requirement that all maternal deaths should be subject to this Confidential Enquiry and all health professionals have a duty to provide the information required. All relevant hospital professionals must participate in the Confidential Enquiries. In participating in the Confidential Enquiry, the professionals concerned are asked for three things:

(i)   to provide a full and accurate account of the circumstances leading up to the woman's death, with supporting records

(ii) to reflect on any clinical or other lessons that have been learned, either personally or as part of the wider institution

(iii) to describe what action may have followed as a result.

Notification of maternal deaths are usually made directly by one or more of the health professionals concerned to the CEMACH RM of the region where the woman was resident. Cases are also reported by coroners, local supervising authority midwifery officers (LSAMO) and others. Ascertainment is checked biannually with the Office of National Statistics for all deaths coded as a maternal death according to the International Classification of Diseases, Injuries and Causes of Death tenth revision (ICD10) and an enquiry is initiated for any case not already reported to CEMACH. Once a case has been notified, a case number is assigned and the enquiry is initiated using a standard form (MDR-UK1) by the CEMACH RM. The enquiry form is sent by the RM to obstetricians, anaesthetists, pathologists, general practitioners, midwives and any other professionals who were concerned with the care of the woman. Copies of case notes are obtained where relevant. Prior to the involvement of CESDI and CEMACH, this information was gathered by the DPH and then circulated by the Regional Obstetrics Assessor to the Regional Assessors. From 2003, under CEMACH, a policy of anonymisation of records has been introduced and once all available information about the death has been collected, all records are anonymised and then circulated by the RM to the Regional Assessors. The Obstetric and Midwifery Assessors review all cases. Anaesthetic Assessors review cases where there was involvement of an anaesthetist or intensive care. Every possible attempt is made to obtain full details of any autopsy and pathological investigations, and these are reviewed by the Pathology Assessor. The Assessors add their comments and opinions regarding the cause or causes of death. The completed form is returned to the CEMACH Central Office by the RM after which it is reviewed by the Director of the MDE and circulated to the Central Assessors. The Central Assessors in obstetrics and gynaecology, midwifery, anaesthetics, pathology, psychiatry and general medicine review, as required, all available recorded facts about each case and assess the factors that may have led to death (Figure A1.1).

Regional assessment

There are 16 sets of Regional Assessors in England and Wales and each set has an obstetrical, anaesthetic, pathology and midwifery assessor. There are between one and three sets of Assessors per region depending on requirements. Assessors are appointed for the term of a triennium (about 4 years, allowing for completion of assessment). Nominations for medical Assessors are sought from presidents of Royal Colleges and nominations for midwives are sought from the Local Supervisory Authority Midwifery Officer. A Regional Assessor must be an active clinical practitioner in the NHS in the

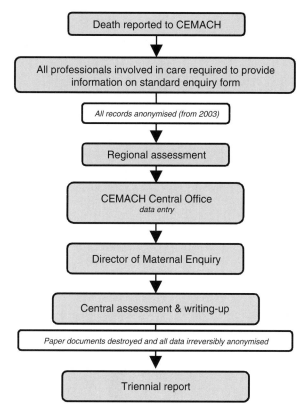

Figure A1.1   Process of enquiry 2000–02

relevant specialty and in good standing with the relevant Royal College or Faculty, consultant level (if medical) or a supervisor of midwives with knowledge and experience of organisation of care. They must be a professional who is well respected by peers, able to realistically commit enough time to assess and return enquiry forms in a timely manner. The position of Regional Assessor is honorary.

The role of Regional Assessor is to review the information reported in the MDE form and any other case documents that have been assembled by the CEMACH RM and make a short report in the relevant section of the enquiry form. This includes a comment on the case, an evaluation of the clinical management and the resources of the organisation responsible for the care. The assessor is also asked to make a judgement as to whether the care was substandard and if so, if this was a contributing factor in the death of the mother.

Since 2003, under CEMACH, all records (including the enquiry form and case notes) are anonymised before regional assessment is undertaken. All information that might identify the mother, the personnel and institutions involved in her care is removed and the case is identified by an assigned number. The anonymised enquiry form and relevant notes are circulated to the Regional Assessors by the CEMACH RM. Once the regional assessment is completed the documents are sent to the CEMACH Central Office for data entry. All cases are then reviewed by the Director of the Maternal Enquiry and circulated to the relevant Central Assessors.

Central assessment

The Central Assessors review each case thoroughly, taking into account the case history, the results of pathological investigations and findings at autopsy given in the enquiry report form before allotting the case to be counted in a specific chapter in the Report. Their assessment occasionally varies with the underlying cause of death as given on the death certificate and classified by the Registrars General using the ICD10. This is because, for example, although the death may have been coded for multiple-organ failure as the terminal event, it could have been precipitated by an obstetric cause, such as septicaemia from an infected caesarean section. Although each maternal death reported to this Enquiry is only counted once and assigned to one chapter, it may also be referred to in other chapters; thus, a death assigned to hypertensive disorder of pregnancy, in which haemorrhage and anaesthesia also played a part, may be discussed in all three chapters.

Authors

Chapters are initially drafted by individual Central Assessors and then discussed in detail by the whole panel before the Report is finalised. Other acknowledged professionals who have a particular and expert interest in specific diseases or areas of practice may be asked to review and comment on the recommendations prior to publication.

Confidentiality

After preparation of the Report and before publication, all maternal death report forms, related documents and files relating to the period of the Report are destroyed and all electronic data is irreversibly anonymised.

Denominator data

Denominator data and other relevant statistical data are supplied by the Office for National Statistics.

Northern Ireland

Maternal deaths are reported to the DPH of the health and social services board in which the woman was resident. The DPH is responsible for organising completion of the maternal death form MDR(UK)1 by those involved in the care and obtaining the autopsy report when one has been conducted. On completion, forms are sent to the Medical Coordinator at the Department of Health, Social Services, and Public Safety. The Medical Coordinator, acting on behalf of the Chief Medical Officer, anonymises the forms and then coordinates the input of the Pathology, Anaesthetic, Midwifery and Obstetric Assessors. A single panel of Assessors deals with all cases, commenting on the case, evaluating the clinical management and the resources of the organisation responsible for the care as well a making a judgement as to whether the care was substandard and if so, if this was a contributing factor in the death of the mother. Assessed case forms are forwarded to the central CEMACH Office and submitted by the MDE Director for central assessment. All papers relating to the cases are destroyed once the reports have been received by the Central CEMACH Office.

Scotland

In Scotland, the system of enquiry is broadly similar except that a single panel of Assessors covers the whole country. A single Assessor representing each of anaesthetics, pathology and midwifery comments on all cases, and each of three Obstetric Assessors comments on cases from a defined geographical area. The panel of assessors meets twice a year (in April and October) to assess and classify each case. The Scottish Programme for Clinical Effectiveness in Reproductive Health (SPCERH) administers the Enquiry on behalf of NHS Quality Improvement Scotland. The Programme office receives copies of the death certificates of all relevant deaths from the General Registrar's Office (Scotland) and then sends an enquiry form to the DPH of the health board of residence of the woman concerned. The enquiry form used is MDR(UK)1. The DPH takes responsibility for organising completion of the form by all professional staff involved in caring for the woman. When this is achieved, it is passed to the appropriate Obstetric Assessor, who determines whether further data are required before the case is submitted for discussion and classification to the full panel of Assessors. In cases where an anaesthetic had been given, an autopsy or pathological investigation undertaken or where there were significant midwifery issues, the Obstetric Assessor passes the form to the Assessors from relevant disciplines for their further comments. The form is then returned to the SPCERH medical coordinator, who retains it from that time until it has been fully considered, classified and used for preparation of the Report. As for the other countries, at all times each form is held under conditions of strict confidentiality and is anonymised before being provided to the UK Central Assessors compiling the Report. Additional information is obtained from statistics collected and analysed by the Information and Statistics Division of NHS Scotland. This is available from routine hospital discharge data collected by general and maternity hospitals. The coverage by Form SMR2, the maternal discharge summary, is now almost universal at 98% of registered births. General practitioners and hospital and community medical and midwifery staff assist in ensuring that deaths occurring at home are included in the MDE.

APPENDIX 2

Assessors for the Maternal Deaths Enquiry and CEMACH Personnel

Director of Enquiry

Dr G Lewis MSc MRCGP FFPH FRCOG

Central Assessors and authors

Obstetrics	Professor J Drife MD FRCOG FRCP (Ed) FRCS (Ed)
	Professor J Neilson MD FRCOG
Anaesthetics	Dr T Thomas Mb ChB FRCA (until 2002)
	Dr G Cooper FRCA FRCOG
	Dr JH McClure FRCA
Intensive Care	Dr S Willatts MD FRCA FRCP (until 2002)
	Dr T Clutton–Brock MRCP FRCA
Pathology	Dr GH Millward–Sadler FRCPath MHSM
Medicine	Professor Michael de Swiet MD FRCP
	Dr C Nelson–Piercy FRCP
Midwifery	Ms Christine Carson RN RM PGDip MSc (until 2002)
	Ms Catherine McCormick RN RM (until 2002)
	Mrs K Sallah RN RM ADM MPH
Psychiatry	Dr M Oates FRCPsych
	Dr M Hepburn FRCOG

CEMACH personnel involved in Enquiry work

Central Office

Chief Executive	Mr R Congdon
Director Development and Analysis (Maternal Enquiry)	Mrs J Noble
Programme Director	Mrs A Miller
Administrative Officer	Mrs M Wilson

CEMACH Regional Managers

East of England	Mrs C Hay
East Midlands	Mrs S Wood
London	Mrs S Roberts

South East	Miss M Gompels
South West	Mrs R Thompson
North East	Mrs M Renwick
Northern Ireland	Dr M Scott
North West	Mrs J Maddocks
Wales	Mrs J Stewart
West Midlands	Mrs P McGeown
Yorkshire and Humber	Mrs L Anson

Regional Assessors

Regional Assessors in Obstetrics

CEMACH Region	Previous CEMD Region	Assessors
East England		Mr B Lim FRCOG
East Midlands		Miss HJ Mellows FRCOG
	East Anglia	Mr PJ Milton MA MD FRCOG (to 2003)
London		Miss G Henson FRCOG
		Mr ME Setchell FRCS FRCOG
		Dr GHW Ward FRCOG
	NW Thames	Mr HG Wagman FRCS (Ed) FRCOG (to 2003)
	SE Thames	Mr JA Elias FRCOG (to 2003)
	SW Thames	Mr PM Coats MRCP FRCS FRCOG DCH (to 2003)
North West		Mr P Donnai MA FRCOG (to 2002)
		Miss P Buck FRCOG
		Mr S Walkinshaw FRCOG
	Mersey	Miss A Garden FRCOG (to 2002)
Northern		Professor JM Davison MSc MD FRCOG
South East		Miss P Hurley FROCG
		Miss C Iffland FRCOG
	Oxford	Miss S Sellers MD FRCOG (to 2002)
	Wessex	Mr CP J Brown FRCOG (to 2003)
South West		Professor PW Soothill FRCOG
		Miss S Sellers MD FRCOG
West Midlands		Professor M Whittle FRCOG (to 2003)
		Mr DHA Redford FRCOG
Yorkshire/Humber		Mr DM Hay FRCOG (to 2003)
		Professor J Walker FRCOG
		Mr SF Spooner FRCOG
East England		Dr A Nicholl FRCA
East Midlands		Dr D Bogod FRCA
London		Dr W Aveling FRCA DRCOG
London		Dr I Findley MBChB DRCOG FRCA
London		Dr S Yentis FRCA
London	NW Thames	Dr AP Rubin FRCA (to 2002)
London	SE Thames	Dr P Groves FRCA (to 2003)
North West		Dr E L Horsman MB ChB FRCA
North West		Dr RG Wilkes MB ChB FRCA
North East	Northern	Dr MR Bryson FRCA (to 2003)

Regional Assessors in Anaesthetics

CEMACH Region	Previous CEMD Region	Assessors
North East		Dr D Hughes FRCA
South East		Dr MB Dobson MRCP FRCA
South East		Dr H Adams FRCA
South East	Wessex	Dr D Brighouse BM MA FRCA (to 2003)
South West		Dr M Wee FRCA
South West		Dr L Shutt FRCA
West Midlands		Dr M Lewis FRCA
Yorkshire/Humber		Dr IF Russell FRCA
Yorkshire/Humber		Dr G Kesseler FFARCS

Regional Assessors in Pathology

CEMACH Region	Previous CEMD Region	Assessors
East England		Dr C Womack FRCPath
East England	East Anglia	Dr PF Roberts FRCP FRCPath (to 2003)
East Midlands	Trent	Dr LJR Brown FRCPath
London		Dr C Corbishley FRCPath
London		Dr M Jarumlowicz FRCPath
London		Dr A Bates MD MRCPath
London	NE Thames	Dr JE McLaughlin BSc BBS FRCPath (to 2003)
London	NW Thames	Dr IA Lampert FRCPath (to 2003)
North West	Mersey	Dr IW McDicken MD FRCPath (to 2003)
North West		Dr R Hale FRCPath
North East		Dr JN Bulmer PhD FRCPath
North West		Dr CH Buckley MD FRCPath (to 2003)
North West		Dr G Wilson FRCPath
South East	Wessex	Dr A Hitchcock FRCPath (to 2002)
South East	SE Thames	Dr N Kirkham MD FRCPath
South East	SW Thames	Dr M Hall FRCPath
South West		Professor PP Anthony FRCPath (to 2003)
South West		Dr C Keen FRCPath
South West		Dr L Hirschowitz FRCPath
South West	Oxford	Dr W Gray FRCPath
West Midlands		Dr DI Rushton FRCPath (to 2002)
West Midlands		Dr T Rollason FRCPath
Yorkshire/Humber		Dr A Andrew FRCPath
Yorkshire/Humber		Dr DR Morgan FRCPath

Regional Assessors in Midwifery

CEMACH Region	Previous CEMD Region	Assessors
East England	East Anglia	Miss E Fern RGN RM MTD (to 2003)
East England		Ms J Fraser MSc DPSM RM RN
East Midlands		Miss JM Savage RN RM

London	*NE Thames*	Ms M McKenna RM RN DPSM (to 2003)
		Ms S Truttero MBA LLB ADM RN RM
		Mrs M Wheeler RN RM ADM BSc (Hons)
North West	*North West*	Miss J Bracken RGN RM MTD (to 2001)
		Ms M Sidebotham RGN RM DPSM/ADM MA
		Ms Angela Pedder RN RM BSc MA
North East	*Northern*	Miss L Robson MA RN RM ADM PGCE (to 2003)
North East		Ms Kath Mannion RM RN ADM BSc MSc
South East	*Wessex*	Mrs M Elliott RN RM (to 2001)
	Wessex	Ms M Newman RN RM (to 2003)
	SE Thames	Mrs I Bryan RN RM DMS (to 2003)
		Ms C Drummond RGN RM
	Oxford	Miss H Pearce RN RM (to 2003)
South West	*Oxford*	Mrs C Osselton RN RM (to 2002)
	South West	Mrs V Beale RN RM Dip Man MSc
		Mrs A Remmers RGN RM MSc
		Ms D Morrall RN RM
West Midlands		Mrs C McCalmont RN RM DPSM
Yorkshire/Humber	*Yorkshire*	Mrs J Duerden MBa RN RM RSCN IHSM (to 2002)
	Yorkshire	Mrs JM Jackson RN RM
		Mrs J Morris BA RN RM ONC DHSM (to 2002)

SCOTLAND

Chairman of Enquiry

Professor MH Hall FRCOG

Medical Coordinator: Scottish Programme for Clinical Effectiveness in Reproductive Health

Dr G Penney FRCOG

CMO's Representative: Scottish Executive Health Department

Dr I Bashford MRCOG

Obstetric Assessors

Professor MH Hall FRCOG
Dr WA Liston FRCOG
Dr CB Lunan FRCOG

Anaesthetic Assessor

Dr JH McClure FRCA

Pathology Assessor

Dr ES Gray FRCPath

Midwifery Assessor

Mrs J Linton RGN RM

NORTHERN IRELAND

Department of Health and Social Services: Northern Ireland

Dr C Willis MB ChB BAO MFPH

Obstetric Assessor

Professor W Thompson BSc MD FRCOG (until 2001)
Miss A Harper FRCOG

Anaesthetic Assessor

Dr IM Bali MD PhD FFARCS

Pathology Assessor

Professor PG Toner DSc FRCPG FRCPath (until 2002)
Dr D O' Hara (until 2003)
Dr G McCusker

Midwifery Assessor

Mrs E Millar RN RM NDNC MHSCert

WALES

Welsh Assembly Government

Dr J Ludlow FFPHM

Obstetric Assessor

Professor RW Shaw MD FRCOG FRCS(Ed) (until 2001)
Mr R Vlies FRCOG

Anaesthetic Assessor

Professor M Harmer MD FRCA (until 2003)
Dr P Clyburn FRCA

Pathology Assessor

Dr R J Kellet FRCPath DMJ (Path) LLM (until 2003)

Dr Lesley Murray FRCPath

Midwifery Assessor

Ms K Isherwood RGN RM ADM (until 2003)
Ms J Keats RN RM

CEMACH Board

Professor M Weindling, Chair
Dr J Chapple, Faculty of Public Health
Mr R Congdon, Chief Executive CEMACH
Dr G Cooper, Royal College of Anaesthetists
Dame Karlene Davis, Royal College of Midwives
Ms S Golightly, Director of Development and Analysis CEMACH (job share)
Dr S Gould, Royal College of Pathologists
Dr M Macintosh, Medical Director CEMACH
Professor N McIntosh, Royal College of Paediatrics and Child Health
Mrs A Miller, Programme Director CEMACH
Mrs J Noble, Director of Development & Analysis CEMACH (job share)
Professor L Parker, Associate Director Confidential Enquiries, National Institute for Clinical Excellence
Professor A Templeton, Royal College of Obstetrics and Gynaecology

APPENDIX 3

Reports of Confidential Enquiries into Maternal Deaths since 1952

England and Wales

Ministry of Health. *Report on Confidential Enquiries into Maternal Deaths in England and Wales,1952–54.* Reports on Public Health and Medical Subjects No. 97. London: HMSO; 1957.

Ministry of Health. *Report on Confidential Enquiries into Maternal Deaths in England and Wales, 1955–57.* Reports on Public Health and Medical Subjects No. 103. London: HMSO; 1960.

Ministry of Health. *Report on Confidential Enquiries into Maternal Deaths in England and Wales, 1958–60.* Reports on Public Health and Medical Subjects No. 108. London: HMSO; 1963.

Ministry of Health. *Report on Confidential Enquiries into Maternal Deaths in England and Wales, 1961–1963.* Reports on Public Health and Medical Subjects No. 115. London: HMSO; 1966.

Ministry of Health. *Report on Confidential Enquiries into Maternal Deaths in England and Wales, 1964–66.* Reports on Public Health and Medical Subjects No. 119. London: HMSO; 1969.

Department of Health and Social Security. *Report on Confidential Enquiries into Maternal Deaths in England and Wales, 1967–69.* Reports on Health and Social Subjects No. 1. London: HMSO; 1972.

Department of Health and Social Security. *Report on Confidential Enquiries into Maternal Deaths in England and Wales, 1970–72.* Reports on Health and Social Subjects No. 11. London: HMSO; 1975.

Department of Health and Social Security. *Report on Confidential Enquiries into Maternal Deaths in England and Wales, 1973–1975.* Reports on Health and Social Subjects No. 14. London: HMSO; 1979.

Department of Health and Social Security. *Report on Confidential Enquiries into Maternal Deaths in England and Wales, 1976–1978.* Reports on Health and Social Subjects No. 26. London: HMSO; 1982.

Department of Health and Social Security. *Report on Confidential Enquiries into Maternal Deaths in England and Wales, 1979–81.* Reports on Health and Social Subjects No. 29. London: HMSO; 1986.

Department of Health and Social Security. *Report on Confidential Enquiries into Maternal Deaths in England and Wales, 1982–84.* Reports on Health and Social Subjects No. 34. London: HMSO; 1989.

Scotland

Scottish Home and Health Department. *A Report on an Enquiry into Maternal Deaths in Scotland, 1965–1971*. Edinburgh: HMSO; 1974.

Scottish Home and Health Department. *A Report on an Enquiry into Maternal Deaths in Scotland, 1972–1975*. Edinburgh: HMSO; 1978.

Scottish Home and Health Department. *A Report on an Enquiry into Maternal Deaths in Scotland, 1976–1980*. Edinburgh: HMSO; 1987.

Scottish Home and Health Department. *Report on maternal and perinatal deaths in Scotland, 1981–1985*. Edinburgh: HMSO; 1989.

Scottish Office Home and Health Department. *Report on maternal and perinatal deaths in Scotland, 1986–1990*. Edinburgh: HMSO; 1994.

Northern Ireland

Government of Northern Ireland, Ministry of Health and Local Government. *A Report on Maternal Deaths in Northern Ireland, 1956–69*. Belfast: HMSO; 1962.

Government of Northern Ireland, Ministry of Health and Social Services. *A Report on an Enquiry into Maternal Deaths in Northern Ireland, 1960–1963*. Belfast: HMSO; 1965.

Government of Northern Ireland, Ministry of Health and Social Services. *A Report on an Enquiry into Maternal Deaths in Northern Ireland, 1964–1967*. Belfast: HMSO; 1968.

Department of Health and Social Services, Northern Ireland. *A Report on an Enquiry into Maternal Deaths in Northern Ireland, 1968–1977*. Belfast: HMSO; 1982.

Department of Health and Social Services Northern Ireland. *A Report on an Enquiry into Maternal Deaths in Northern Ireland, 1978–1984*. Belfast: HMSO; 1988.

United Kingdom

Department of Health, Welsh Office, Scottish Home and Health Department, and Department of Health and Social Services, Northern Ireland. *Report on Confidential Enquiries into Maternal Deaths in the United Kingdom, 1985–87*. London: HMSO; 1991.

Department of Health, Welsh Office, Scottish Home and Health Department, and Department of Health and Social Services, Northern Ireland. *Report on Confidential Enquiries into Maternal Deaths in the United Kingdom 1988–1990*. London: HMSO; 1994.

Department of Health, Welsh Office, Scottish Home and Health Department, and Department of Health and Social Services, Northern Ireland. *Report on Confidential Enquiries into Maternal Deaths in the United Kingdom 1991–1993*. London: HMSO; 1996.

Department of Health, Welsh Office, Scottish Office Department of Health, and Department of Health and Social Services, Northern Ireland. *Why Mothers Die. Report on Confidential Enquiries into Maternal Deaths in the United Kingdom, 1994–1996.* London: The Stationery Office, 1998.

Department of Health, Scottish Executive Health Department, and Department of Health, Social Services and Public Safety, Northern Ireland. *Why Mothers Die. Fifth Report on Confidential Enquiries into Maternal Deaths in the United Kingdom, 1997–1999.* London: RCOG Press; 2001.

INDEX